Disorders of Consciousness

Guest Editor

G. BRYAN YOUNG, MD, FRCP(C)

NEUROLOGIC CLINICS

www.neurologic.theclinics.com

Consulting Editor
RANDOLPH W. EVANS, MD

November 2011 • Volume 29 • Number 4

SAUNDERS an imprint of ELSEVIER, Inc.

W.B. SAUNDERS COMPANY
A Division of Elsevier Inc.

1600 John F. Kennedy Boulevard ● Suite 1800 ● Philadelphia, Pennsylvania 19103-2899

http://www.theclinics.com

NEUROLOGIC CLINICS Volume 29, Number 4
November 2011 ISSN 0733-8619, ISBN-13: 978-1-4557-1031-7

Editor: Donald Mumford

Neurologic Clinics (ISSN 0733-8619) is published quarterly by Elsevier Inc., 360 Park Avenue South, New York, NY 10010–1710. Months of issue are February, May, August, and November. Periodicals postage paid at New York, NY, and additional mailing offices. Subscription prices are $264.00 per year for US individuals, $441.00 per year for US institutions, $130.00 per year for US students, $332.00 per year for Canadian individuals, $530.00 per year for Canadian institutions, $368.00 per year for international individuals, $530.00 per year for international institutions, and $184.00 for Canadian and foreign students/residents. To receive student/resident rate, orders must be accompanied by name of affiliated institution, date of term, and the *signature* of program/residency coordinator on institution letterhead. Orders will be billed at individual rate until proof of status is received. Foreign air speed delivery is included in all *Clinics* subscription prices. All prices are subject to change without notice. **POSTMASTER:** Send address changes to *Neurologic Clinics*, Elsevier Health Sciences Division, Subscription Customer Service, 3251 Riverport Lane, Maryland Heights, MO 63043. **Customer Service: Telephone: 1-800-654-2452 (U.S. and Canada); 314-447-8871 (outside U.S. and Canada). Fax: 314-447-8029. E-mail: journalscustomerservice-usa@elsevier.com (for print support); journalsonlinesupport-usa@elsevier.com (for online support).**

Reprints. For copies of 100 or more of articles in this publication, please contact the Commercial Reprints Department, Elsevier Inc., 360 Park Avenue South, New York, New York, 10010-1710; Tel.: (+1) 212-633-3812; Fax: (+1) 212-462-1935, and E-mail: reprints@elsevier.com.

Neurologic Clinics is also published in Spanish by Nueva Editorial Interamericana S.A., Mexico City, Mexico.

Neurologic Clinics is covered in *Current Contents/Clinical Medicine, MEDLINE/PubMed (Index Medicus), EMBASE/Excerpta Medica, and PsycINFO, and ISI/BIOMED.*

Printed and bound by CPI Group (UK) Ltd, Croydon, CR0 4YY

Transferred to Digital Print 2011

Contributors

CONSULTING EDITOR

RANDOLPH W. EVANS, MD
Clinical Professor, Department of Neurology, Baylor College of Medicine, Houston, Texas

GUEST EDITOR

G. BRYAN YOUNG, MD, FRCP(C)
Professor, Division of Neurology, Department of Clinical Neurological Sciences, University of Western Ontario, London Health Sciences Centre, London, Ontario, Canada

AUTHORS

PAUL ANGARAN, MD, FRCPC
Division of Cardiology, University of Western Ontario, London, Ontario, Canada

MICHAEL J. ANGEL, MD, PhD, FRCP(C)
Lecturer, Division of Neurology, Department of Medicine, University of Toronto, Toronto, Ontario, Canada

JAMES L. BERNAT, MD
Louis and Ruth Frank Professor of Neurocience, Professor of Neurology & Medicine, Dartmouth Medical School, Hanover, New Hampshire; Attending Neurologist, Neurology Department, Dartmouth-Hitchcock Medical Center, Lebanon, New Hampshire

WILLIAM T. BINGHAM, MD, FRCPC
Associate Professor & Pediatric Intensivist, Department of Pediatrics, Royal University Hospital, University of Saskatchewan, Saskatoon, Saskatchewan, Canada

HAL BLUMENFELD, MD, PhD
Departments of Neurology, Neurobiology, Neurosurgery, Yale University School of Medicine, New Haven, Connecticut

MIGUEL BUSSIÈRE, MD, PhD
Assistant Professor, Division of Neurology and Interventional Neuroradiology, Department of Medicine, University of Ottawa, The Ottawa Hospital, Ottawa, Ontario, Canada

SANDRINE DE RIBAUPIERRE, MD
Assistant Professor, Division of Neurosurgery, Department of Clinical Neurological Sciences, University of Western Ontario, London, Ontario, Canada

RAJAT DHAR, MD, FRCPC(C)
Assistant Professor of Neurology, Division of Neurocritical Care, Department of Neurology, Washington University in St. Louis School of Medicine, St Louis, Missouri

JOSEPH T. GIACINO, PhD
Associate Professor, Department of Physical Medicine and Rehabilitation, Harvard Medical School; Director, Rehabilitation Neuropsychology, Spaulding Rehabilitation Hospital; Department of Psychiatry, Massachusetts General Hospital, Boston, Massachusetts

ANDREW M. GOLDFINE, MD
Instructor of Neurology, Department of Neurology and Neuroscience, Weill Cornell Medical College, New York; Burke Medical Research Institute, Weill Cornell Medical College, White Plains, New York

LORNE J. GULA, MD, FRCPC
Division of Cardiology, University of Western Ontario, London, Ontario, Canada

RON HIRSCHBERG, MD
Instructor, Department of Physical Medicine and Rehabilitation, Harvard Medical School; Director, Consultation Physiatry, Massachusetts General Hospital; Staff Physiatrist, Spaulding Rehabilitation Hospital, Boston, Massachusetts

SARA HOCKER, MD
Division of Critical Care Neurology, Mayo Clinic, Rochester, Minnesota

THERESA HUMAN, PharmD, BCPS
Clinical Pharmacist, Neurology/Neurosurgery Intensive Care Unit, Department of Pharmacy, Barnes-Jewish Hospital, St Louis, Missouri

GARY HUNTER, MD, FRCPC
Division of Neurology, University of Saskatchewan, Canada

TREVOR A. HURWITZ, MBChB, MRCP(UK), FRCP(C)
Clinical Professor, Division of Neurology, Department of Psychiatry and Medicine, University of British Columbia; Medical Director, BC Neuropsychiatry Program, British Columbia, Canada

JAMES C. JACKSON, PsyD
Center for Health Services Research; Division of Allergy/Pulmonary/Critical Care Medicine, Department of Psychiatry, Vanderbilt Medical Center; VA Tennessee Valley, Clinical Research Center of Excellence (CRCOE); VA Tennessee Valley Geriatric Research, Education and Clinical Center (GRECC), Nashville, Tennessee

PETER W. KAPLAN, MB, FRCP
Professor of Neurology, Department of Neurology, Johns Hopkins Bayview Medical Center, Baltimore, Maryland

FENELLA J. KIRKHAM, MD, FRCPCH
Professor of Paediatric Neurology, Neurosciences Unit, UCL Institute of Child Health, London; Department of Child Health, Southampton General hospital NHS Trust, Southampton, United Kingdom

GEORGE J. KLEIN, MD, FRCPC
Division of Cardiology, University of Western Ontario, London, Ontario, Canada

ANDREW D. KRAHN, MD, FRCPC
Division of Cardiology, University of Western Ontario, London, Ontario, Canada

PETER LEONG-SIT, MD, FRCPC
Division of Cardiology, University of Western Ontario, London, Ontario, Canada

ALESSANDRO MORANDI, MD, MPH
Center for Health Services Research, Vanderbilt Medical Center, Nashville, Tennessee; Department of Rehabilitation and Aged Care, Ancelle della Carità Hospital, Cremona; Geriatric Research Group, Brescia, Italy

ALEJANDRO A. RABINSTEIN, MD
Division of Critical Care Neurology, Mayo Clinic, Rochester, Minnesota

KAREN L. ROOS, MD
John and Nancy Nelson Professor of Neurology and Professor of Neurological Surgery, Indiana University School of Medicine, Indianapolis, Indiana

EMILY B. RUBIN, JD, MD
Resident, Internal Medicine and Pediatrics, Massachusetts General Hospital, Boston, Massachusetts

VENKATRAMAN SADANAND, PhD, MD, FRCSC, FACS, FAAP
Associate Professor, Department of Neurosurgery, Loma Linda University Medical Center, Loma Linda, California

NICHOLAS D. SCHIFF, MD
Professor of Neurology and Neuroscience, Department of Neurology and Neuroscience, Weill Cornell Medical College, New York, New York

SHASHI S. SESHIA, MD (Bombay), FRCPC&E
Clinical Professor, Division of Pediatric Neurology, Department of Pediatrics, Royal University Hospital, University of Saskatchewan, Saskatoon, Saskatchewan, Canada

SAM D. SHEMIE, MD
Division of Critical Care, Montreal Children's Hospital, McGill University Health Centre; Medical Director, Extracorporeal Life Support Program, Professor of Pediatrics, McGill University, Loeb Chair and Research Consortium in Organ and Tissue Donation, Faculty of Arts, University of Ottawa; Executive Medical Director, Donation, Canadian Blood Services, Montreal, Quebec, Canada

ALLAN C. SKANES, MD, FRCPC
Division of Cardiology, University of Western Ontario, London, Ontario, Canada

JEANNE TEITELBAUM, MD, FRCP
Associate Professor Neurology, McGill University; Clinical Professor of Medicine and Neurology, University of Montreal; Neurologist and Neuro-Intensivist at the Montreal Neurological Institute; Chief of Program for Neurocritical Care, Montreal Neurological Institute, Montreal; Chief of Service for the Stroke Program, Montreal Neurological Institute and Royal Victoria Hospital, Montreal, Quebec, Canada

MICHAEL R. WILSON, MD
Harvard-Partners Neurology Residency, Massachusetts General Hospital, Brigham and Women's Hospital, Boston, Massachusetts

RAYMOND YEE, MD, FRCPC
Division of Cardiology, University of Western Ontario, London, Ontario, Canada

G. BRYAN YOUNG, MD, FRCP(C)
Professor, Division of Neurology, Department of Clinical Neurological Sciences, University of Western Ontario, London Health Sciences Centre, London, Ontario, Canada

Contents

Human consciousness requires brainstem, basal forebrain, and diencephalic areas to support generalized arousal, and functioning thalamocortical networks to respond to environmental and internal stimuli. Disconnection of these interconnected systems, typically from cardiac arrest and traumatic brain injury, can result in disorders of consciousness. Brain injuries can also result in loss of motor output out of proportion to consciousness, resulting in misdiagnoses. The authors review pathology and imaging studies and derive mechanistic models for each of these conditions. Such models may guide the development of target-based treatment algorithms to enhance recovery of consciousness in many of these patients.

This article elucidates a stepwise approach to the patient with an acute alteration in the content or level of consciousness. The article begins with a discussion of the spectrum of diminished responsiveness. It then details which aspects of the history are important in obtaining an evaluation of these patients and reviews the neurologic examination of the comatose patient. A brief overview of the neuroanatomical localization of consciousness is provided. The differential diagnosis of diminished responsiveness is explored, followed by a discussion of the order and importance of laboratory, neuroimaging, and other ancillary tests.

Delirium occurs commonly in both general medical and intensive care unit (ICU) patients, with prevalence rates of up to 80% reported. A common expression of acute brain dysfunction, it is related to wide-ranging untoward outcomes such as prolonged hospitalization, increased costs, higher mortality, and, potentially long-term cognitive impairment. Different risk factors are associated with delirium, including sedation, which has implications for patient management. Multicomponent interventions to prevent delirium, developed in the non-ICU setting, can be adapted to critically ill patients with the purpose of reducing its incidence. Future studies should evaluate target interventions to prevent delirium in the ICU.

This article reviews alterations in consciousness related to intracranial mass lesions. Such lesions can produce impairment of consciousness by their strategic location within components of the ascending reticular activating system or secondarily by compressing or distorting this system, interfering with its synaptic and neurochemical functions. This review concentrates principally on this secondary mechanism.

Severe acquired brain injury has profound impact on alertness, cognition, and behavior. Among those who survive the initial injury, a significant minority fail to fully recover self and environmental awareness, and go on to experience prolonged disorders of consciousness (DOC) that can last a lifetime. Although there are no standards of care to guide clinical management, a growing body of empirical evidence is beginning to accrue to inform clinical decision making. In this article, we review the state of the science as it pertains to diagnosis, prognosis, and treatment of patients with DOC.

Death determined by neurologic criteria or brain death is better understood as brain arrest or the final clinical expression of complete and irreversible neurologic failure. Despite widespread national, international, and legal acceptance of the concept, substantial variation exists in the standards and their application, and there remains a need to clarify and standardize terminology (eg, ancillary and supplementary testing, brain death, or neurologic determination of death). The aim of this article is to review the specific criteria and requirements of brain death, paying special attention to areas of controversy and practice inconsistency.

Recent advances have shown much in common between epilepsy and other disorders of consciousness. Behavior in epileptic seizures often resembles a transient vegetative or minimally conscious state. These disorders all converge on the "consciousness system" —the bilateral medial and lateral fronto-parietal association cortex and subcortical arousal systems. Epileptic unconsciousness has enormous clinical significance leading to accidental injuries, decreased work and school productivity, and social stigmatization. Ongoing research to better understand the mechanisms of impaired consciousness in epilepsy, including neuroimaging studies and fundamental animal models, will hopefully soon enable treatment trails to reduce epileptic unconsciousness and improve patient quality of life.

Coma due to global or focal ischemia or hemorrhage is reviewed. Impaired consciousness due to anoxic-ischemic encephalopathy after cardiac arrest is common but prognostically problematic. Recent guidelines need to be refined for those patients who have received therapeutic hypothermia.

early posttransplant period. Encephalopathy often results from metabolic disturbances and immunosuppressant drug neurotoxicity but can also occur with central pontine myelinolysis and other lesions of the central nervous system (CNS). Seizures are also common and can be related to drug toxicity or herald CNS disorders. A thorough evaluation of any patient who develops seizures or mental status changes after transplantation is warranted to distinguish transient reversible causes from serious CNS disorders.

Treating coma in the mother also means treating the fetus. Pregnant women are subject to causes of coma that may also arise from the effects of pregnancy on organ systems: vascular, cardiac, pulmonary, renal, endocrine, and others. With coma, no investigations are categorically excluded when the mother's health and life are at risk. Pregnancy and hormonal effects on blood volume, blood vessels, and changes in blood pressure explain some special causes of stroke in pregnancy. Others include intracranial hemorrhage and venous occlusive disease, as well as worsening of underlying vessel disease during pregnancy, delivery, and the postpartum period.

Unresponsive patients with or without catatonic motor signs are etiologically heterogeneous, and all require a comprehensive neurodiagnostic assessment to rule out organic causes. Most cases prove to be due to primary psychiatric disorders, mostly mood disorders, especially mania, rather than schizophrenia. These patients respond to lorazepam administered by any route and, failing this, electroconvulsive therapy. Those patients with associated fever and autonomic instability are medical emergencies and need urgent treatment.

The causes of nontraumatic coma (NTC) vary by country, season and period of data collection. Infective diseases are among the major worldwide causes of NTC. Nonaccidental head injury must be in the differential diagnosis. Genetic and ethnic susceptibilities to causes of coma are being recognized. A systematic history and examination are essential for diagnosis, early recognition of herniation syndromes, and management. The management of NTC is discussed, with reference to clinical approach, treatment of seizures, and increased intracranial pressure. Public health measures, education, early diagnosis, and prompt appropriate treatment are the foundations needed to reduce incidence and improve outcome.

Transient global amnesia syndrome was initially described more than a century ago. Although the clinical syndrome is easily recognized and highly consistent in its characteristic features, the underlying pathophysiology has remained elusive. Proposed mechanisms include focal ischemic lesions or local nonischemic energy failures. Diffusion-weighted imaging has been able to demonstrate focal areas of restricted diffusion. Nonetheless, the mechanism of this diffusion restriction is uncertain and does not necessarily indicate ischemia, leaving the exact nature of this seemingly benign disorder in doubt. This review summarizes the pertinent clinical features, proposed pathophysiology, epidemiology, imaging, and future directions in understanding transient global amnesia.

Emily B. Rubin and James L. Bernat

The medical care of patients in disordered states of consciousness, including vegetative and minimally conscious states, raises some of the most intricate ethical questions in medicine. There is inherent ambiguity and uncertainty involved in diagnosing such patients and evaluating their level of awareness and prognosis for recovery. The care of these patients requires the weighing of competing ethical values, including respect for personal autonomy, protection of vulnerable patients, nonmaleficence, and the just use of limited medical resources. We highlight some of the major ethical issues in caring for patients with severe brain injury.

FORTHCOMING ISSUES

RECENT ISSUES

RELATED INTEREST

Psychiatric Clinics December 2010
Traumatic Brain Injury: Defining Best Practice
Silvana Riggio, MD, and Andy Jagoda, MD, *Guest Editors*

THE CLINICS ARE NOW AVAILABLE ONLINE!

Access your subscription at:
www.theclinics.com

Preface

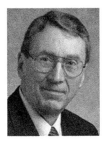

G. Bryan Young, MD, FRCP(C)
Guest Editor

Neurologists and neurosurgeons are practical people. We don't often gaze at our navels and wonder if consciousness is "real or an illusion."[1] We accept that "being conscious" includes an essential alertness and an awareness of ourselves and the world, however imperfectly we do this, and that such awareness arises as a function of brain activity. Admittedly, we do not fully understand how awareness and awareness that we are aware happen, but presumably such functions are the net result of neuronal processing and integration of activity of numerous modules and centers. The "whole is more than the sum of its parts" is probably a fair statement.

Our ability to determine whether consciousness is present or not was revolutionized by the work of Adrian Owen and colleagues, who showed that a patient who was declared "vegetative" was able to generate different brain responses, detected by functional magnetic resonance imaging (fMRI), to imagine she was playing tennis or walking through rooms of her house.[2] Although not able to show any motor response, upon which we have traditionally depended, she was able to show evidence of language comprehension and processing with a sophisticated level of imagining. Indeed, such patients, who amount to about 10% of those previously declared "vegetative," are able to generate accurate binary responses to various questions using the above imagining technique.[3]

This should serve as a wake-up call for us to do better, to more accurately determine whether there is the innate capacity or potential for consciousness, ie, the ultimate prognosis for patients. We should be able to do this without relying on fMRI for each unresponsive patient.[4]

This monograph is devoted to disorders of consciousness, both reversible and irreversible. The neurological basis of consciousness is reviewed by Drs Goldfine and Schiff. A clinical approach is given by Drs Hocker and Rabinstein. The impairment of consciousness by mass lesions, anoxic-ischemic encephalopathy, stroke, seizures, central nervous system infections and inflammatory diseases, general metabolic disorders, intoxications (to appear in a forthcoming issue), trauma, and syncope are dealt with in excellent articles by experts in their respective fields. In addition, causes of impaired consciousness in childhood diseases, pregnancy, and transplantation are discussed. Various states of impaired consciousness, including psychogenic

Neurol Clin 29 (2011) xiii–xiv
doi:10.1016/j.ncl.2011.08.005

unresponsiveness, delirium, transient global amnesia, stupor, coma, and brain death, are addressed by experts in individual articles. Finally, the all important ethical issues involving end-of-life decision-making fall to Drs Rubin and Bernat. Ethical discussions take us back to the philosophy of what consciousness is and how important it is in human existence. However, ethical considerations go beyond consciousness to quality-of-life issues. Perhaps "being conscious" is not enough when all other aspects of life are denied. Also, the processing of information to command, which we can to some extent assess with technology, is not equivalent to the generation of spontaneous thought. Can we ever truly assess the higher aspects of "thinking" in the absence of a motor action?

We hope you enjoy this volume and that it will update your knowledge and stimulate you to think about consciousness in a more comprehensive and meaningful way.

G. Bryan Young, MD, FRCP(C)
Division of Neurology
Department of Clinical Neurological Sciences
University of Western Ontario
London Health Sciences Centre, 339 Windermere Road
London, ON N6A 5A5, Canada

E-mail address:
bryan.young@lhsc.on.ca

REFERENCES

1. Blackmore S. Consciousness: A Brief Insight. New York: Sterling; 2010.
2. Owen AM, Coleman MR, Boly M, et al. Detecting awareness in the vegetative state. Science 2006;313(5792):1402.
3. Monti MM, Vanhaudenhuyse A, Coleman MR, et al. Willful modulation of brain activity in disorders of consciousness. N Engl J Med 2010;362:579–89.
4. Ropper AH. Cogito ergo sum by MRI. N Engl J Med 2010;362:348–9.

Consciousness: Its Neurobiology and the Major Classes of Impairment

Andrew M. Goldfine, MD[a,b],*, Nicholas D. Schiff, MD[a]

KEYWORDS

- Consciousness • Vegetative state • Minimally conscious state
- Traumatic brain injury • Arousal

Disorders of consciousness encompass a wide range of syndromes whereby patients demonstrate a globally impaired ability to interact with the environment. We briefly review the subset of disorders of consciousness that result from permanent brain injury, such as ischemic stroke, global ischemia, and traumatic brain injury (TBI). Disorders of consciousness may also arise as functional (rather than structural) disturbances of consciousness, including generalized and complex partial seizures as well as metabolic and toxic delirium. These functional disturbances are not discussed here but have been reviewed by Posner and colleagues.[1]

In this review, we first review brain structures that support the normal conscious state to develop a framework to demonstrate how their dysfunction can lead to disorders of consciousness. We then present the nosology of the different disorders of consciousness, including coma, vegetative state (VS), the minimally conscious state, and akinetic mutism. The pathology and brain imaging data that give insight into the pathophysiology associated with each diagnostic category are reviewed. Knowledge of the underlying mechanisms of the disorders can enhance the ability to prognosticate and promote recovery from these devastating conditions.

This work was supported by NIH-NICHD 51912, the James S McDonnell Foundation. AMG is supported by grant KL2RR024997 of the Clinical & Translational Science Center at Weill Cornell Medical College.

[a] Department of Neurology and Neuroscience, Weill Cornell Medical College, LC 803, 1300 York Avenue, New York, NY 10065, USA

[b] Burke Medical Research Institute, Weill Cornell Medical College, 785 Mamaroneck Avenue, White Plains, NY 10605, USA

* Corresponding author. Burke Medical Research Institute, Weill Cornell Medical College, 785 Mamaroneck Avenue, White Plains, NY 10605.

E-mail address: andygoldfine@gmail.com

Neurol Clin 29 (2011) 723–737

doi:10.1016/j.ncl.2011.08.001

0733-8619/11/$ – see front matter © 2011 Elsevier Inc. All rights reserved.

BIOLOGIC BASIS OF CONSCIOUSNESS: MECHANISMS OF AROUSAL AND CEREBRAL INTEGRATIVE FUNCTION
A Clinically Relevant Definition of Consciousness

Normal human consciousness is defined as the presence of a wakeful arousal state and the awareness and motivation to respond to self or environmental events. In the intact brain, arousal is the overall level of responsiveness to environmental stimuli. Arousal has a physiologic range from stage 3 non–rapid eye movement (REM) sleep during which strong stimuli are required to elicit a response, to states of high vigilance, during which subtle stimuli can be detected and acted upon.[2] Whereas arousal is the global state of responsiveness, awareness is the brain's ability to perceive specific environmental stimuli in different domains, including visual, somatosensory, auditory, and interoceptive (eg, visceral and body position). The focal loss of awareness, such as language awareness in aphasia or spatial awareness in left-sided neglect, does not significantly impair awareness in other modalities. Motivation is the drive to act on internal or external stimuli that have entered conscious awareness. In the next section, we describe the brain regions that support these three aspects of consciousness and show that they are not independent, but rather interact extensively with each other.

Underlying Substrates of Arousal and Conscious Awareness

The initial discovery that specific brain areas could drive overall cerebral activity appeared in the work of Moruzzi and Magoun.[3] These investigators proposed the existence of an ascending reticular activating system (ARAS) in the upper brainstem tegmentum (reticular formation) and central thalamus that promoted widespread cortical activation.[4] Subsequent work has revealed that the ARAS is not a monolithic activating system, but a collection of interdependent subcortical and brainstem areas that have specific roles in arousal and awareness.[5] The core areas for maintaining an awake state seem to be the glutamatergic and cholinergic neurons in the dorsal tegmentum of the midbrain and pons.[6] These areas activate the central thalamus (primarily intralaminar nuclei) and basal forebrain. The central thalamus and basal forebrain subsequently activate the cortex through glutamatergic and cholinergic projections, respectively. In addition to supporting arousal, the basal forebrain is active during REM sleep and the central thalamus plays a role in conscious awareness (below).

Other brain regions are also involved in arousal but have a more modulatory role, including the nuclei in the upper brainstem that use norepinephrine, dopamine, serotonin, and other neurotransmitters. These nuclei act on the basal forebrain, thalamus, striatum, and cortex.[2,5] The hypothalamus is also involved in the sleep-wake transition[7] and its histaminergic outputs help maintain the awake state. Overall, the large number of regions involved in arousal provide redundancy, so that selective damage to one region, even if bilateral, only rarely results in permanent unconsciousness.

Whereas the level of arousal reflects the overall state of activity in the brain, conscious awareness is a more dynamic and complex process involving various cerebral networks at any one time. There are several competing theories on how we become aware of environmental and internal stimuli, although it is widely believed to depend on interactions between the cortex and specific and nonspecific (eg, intralaminar) thalamic nuclei.[8–10]

Conscious awareness and arousal states also interact. Without arousal, there is no awareness, and in states of high arousal, awareness can be focused on one modality at the expense of others.[11] For example, animal models have been used to demonstrate that in addition to a core generalized arousal, there are also more specific forms of arousal, such as hunger, sexual behavior, and fear, which enhance responses to specific stimuli.[12,13] Conversely, awareness also influences arousal, such as the abrupt increase in arousal when an alarm goes off.

Stimuli are not acted on as reflexes, but typically require motivation to enter conscious awareness through a process called intention or goal-directed behavior.[14,15] Lesion and functional brain imaging studies demonstrate that goal-directed behavior is primarily driven by the medial frontal and anterior cingulate cortices.[16–18] These cortical regions are supported in producing goal-directed behavior by striatopallidal-thalamic loops as well as the ventral tegmental area and the periaqueductal gray of the brainstem (**Fig. 1**).[19] The arousal systems discussed previously also act directly on the goal-directed behavior network, primarily through innervation of the striatum and frontal cortex.[18,20]

In summary, studies indicate that the normal conscious state includes volition, processing of sensory information, and a generalized level of arousal. As discussed later, brain injury can produce disorders of consciousness from injury at any of these levels.

NOSOLOGY AND PATHOPHYSIOLOGY OF DISORDERS OF CONSCIOUSNESS

The disorders of consciousness discussed in this article are syndromes that are behaviorally defined, and each is thought to reflect a specific pathophysiologic model (**Table 1**). However, the models are imprecise and do not apply in every case. As such, we will begin with an overview of the behavioral assessment of levels of consciousness, followed by more detailed descriptions for each syndrome. Pathology and imaging data are used to support mechanistic models underlying each behavioral syndrome.

General Concepts in the Assessment of Consciousness

The determination of level of consciousness at the bedside is primarily a judgment of responsiveness across multiple sensory modalities (eg, vision, somatosensation, and

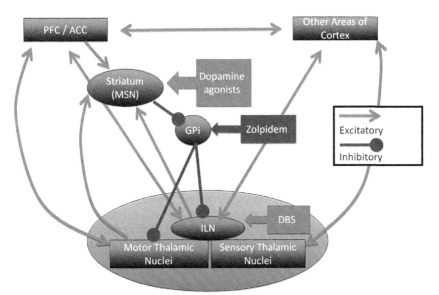

Fig. 1. A network that drives goal-directed behavior together with targets for specific interventions. ACC, anterior cingulate cortex; GPi, globus pallidus pars interna; ILN, intralaminar nuclei of the thalamus; MSN, medium spiny neurons; PFC, prefrontal cortex. Blue arrows represent glutamatergic synapses and red represents GABAergic synapses unless otherwise noted.

Table 1
Summary of behavioral features and pathophysiologies of disorders of consciousness syndromes from permanent brain injury

Syndrome	Behavioral Description	Pathophysiology
Coma	Eyes closed, immobile, or reflex movements	Global dysfunction of corticothalamic loops from diffuse cellular dysfunction, disconnection, or loss of upper brainstem arousal tone. If the entire brain or brainstem is permanently nonfunctional, then diagnosis is brain death rather than coma
Vegetative state	Alternating eyes-closed/ eyes-open states, reflex movements	Same as coma, except that it implies some functioning of the upper brainstem
Minimally conscious state	Low-level and typically intermittent interaction with the environment. Emergence from MCS is defined as recovery of functional object use or consistent communication	Diverse but typically diffuse injury to white matter and/or thalamus. Varying degrees of cortical injury
Akinetic mutism	Severe form has eye tracking only (fits within MCS), whereas milder forms have decreased initiation of goal-directed behavior with relatively retained response to commands	Dysfunction of prefrontal cortex or its subcortical connections (striatum, globus pallidus, or central thalamus) or of white matter connecting these areas
Locked-in state[a]	Complete or almost complete loss of motor output resulting in the appearance of a disorder of consciousness	Classically the loss of corticospinal tract in ventral pons, but can also be from diffuse white matter injury in the setting of trauma

[a] Not a disorder of consciousness.

auditory) and cognitive domains (eg, language and learned movements). The lowest level of behavior to be documented is whether eye opening is spontaneous or requires stimulation (eg, loud sounds or noxious touch). Higher-level behaviors include responses that are contingent on sensory stimuli. These range from eyes tracking a mirror and withdrawal from painful touch, to accurately following commands and the use of objects (eg, a comb or toothbrush).[21] The level of effort required to alert the patient and the speed of their response should also be noted, because these observations guide subjective and objective assessments of arousal. Inaccuracy in specific cognitive domains (eg, aphasia and apraxia) reflects focal impairments in awareness, rather than global disorders of consciousness.

One caveat to behavioral testing of arousal is that all of the patient responses require a capacity for motor output and adequate arousal. Patients with functional or structural interruption of motor systems at any level may not be able to follow the commands, despite full comprehension and intention. Patients with a minimal residual ability to communicate (eg, eye blinks) but who have generally intact consciousness, are deemed to be in the locked-in state (LIS).[1] There are also patients with both impaired motor output and arousal from diffuse brain injury, which contribute to a high misdiagnosis rate in disorders of consciousness.[22,23] To ensure accurate diagnosis in patients with diffuse brain injury, it is essential to examine patients at maximal levels of arousal using techniques such as deep tendon massage or postural repositioning.[24] Patients should also be examined at multiple time points or videotaped by family to capture periods of high alertness.

Coma and VS Represent Loss of Corticothalamic Function

The most common disorder of consciousness that immediately follows severe brain injury is coma. Coma is a state that is characterized by eyes-closed unresponsiveness: comatose patients fail to respond to even the most vigorous stimulation.[1] When given noxious stimulation, patients may not move at all or may display stereotyped/reflexive movements only. The pathophysiology of coma is generally the same as VS (discussed below), except that some patients have loss of some or all brainstem function. For patients with loss of all brainstem and cerebral function, the diagnosis is brain death. Coma prognosis is complex and depends on the causes and the severity of injury as well as the multiple medical factors that led to the initial injury.[1] Brain death does not have a prognosis because it is simply equivalent to death.

If patients survive coma, they either recover consciousness within days or transition to VS within 30 days after injury. VS is a behaviorally-defined state, similar to coma, whereby patients show no evidence of self or environmental awareness.[25] It is also similar to coma because patients can have spontaneous or stimulus-induced, stereotyped movements, and may retain brainstem regulation of visceral autonomic function that would suggest that the lower brainstem is intact. The only behaviorally salient difference from coma is that VS patients cycle daily through eyes-open and eyes-closed periods. This does not imply that VS patients have normal sleep-wake cycles; rather, their electroencephalograms (EEGs) display a monotonous slow pattern regardless of whether the eyes are open or closed, or they only have fragmented components of normal electrographic sleep-wake phenomenology.[26,27] The periods of eye opening reflect only a crude arousal pattern that involves upper brainstem nuclei.

VS may represent a transitional state on the way to recovery of consciousness or could be a chronic condition in cases of more severe brain injuries. Persistent vegetative state (PVS)[25] is a term used for patients who have remained in VS for an arbitrarily defined duration of 30 days.[28] Another commonly used term is permanent vegetative state, which is applied to patients in VS after global ischemia for 3 months or TBI for 1 year.[28] Permanent VS is more of a prognosis than a diagnosis, as these time durations reflect only a reduced probability of recovery. We prefer to define patients in persistent VS simply by the etiology and duration, avoiding the use of absolute terms, such as permanent.

There are three main pathologic findings in patients with prolonged VS from structural injury. The most common is diffuse cortical and thalamic cell loss, which occurs in the setting of global ischemia caused by cardiac arrest.[29] The second is widespread damage to long axons, known as diffuse axonal injury (DAI), which occurs from TBI.[30] DAI has been shown in animal models to occur as a result of rapid acceleration-deceleration injury of the axons, sometimes in conjunction with delayed axonal disconnections.[31] The third and least common pattern of injury is extensive damage to the upper brainstem and thalamus, which usually occurs as a result of basilar artery stroke.[32,33] The common link between these three injury types and VS is the loss of corticothalamic function, either from cell death, disconnection, or loss of brainstem drive.

In vivo imaging studies further support the model of VS that represents diffuse cortico-thalamic dysfunction. Fluorodeoxyglucose (FDG)-positron emission tomography (PET) is a measure of energy consumption, and in the brain it primarily represents the neuronal firing rate at the synapse.[34] Patients in PVS have been shown to have global metabolic rates reduced by 50% or more compared to healthy controls.[35] In general, metabolic rates exhibit less reduction in the brainstem and more reduction in the cortex and subcortical nuclei, with the most consistent reduction occurring in the medial parietal and frontal areas.[36] Comparable reductions in cerebral metabolic rate have been identified during generalized anesthesia[37,38] and slow-wave sleep in healthy controls.[39,40]

To examine corticothalamic functioning more directly, investigators have used $H_2^{15}O$-PET, functional magnetic resonance imaging (fMRI), and event-related potential analysis to measure brain responses to sensory inputs.[41] Studies using simple and complex auditory stimuli[42–44] and noxious stimuli[45] have demonstrated a pattern of activation of brainstem and primary sensory cortical regions in some patients with VS without the activation of higher-order sensory or association areas. These results suggest that patients with VS may have some residual thalamocortical activity, but do not possess enough to produce the global integrative function that is required for conscious awareness.

These imaging tools have also been used to provide insight into an ambiguous area between VS and consciousness. Schiff and colleagues[46] described 3 patients who demonstrated complex motor behaviors but were still considered to be in VS. All were found to have an overall low resting metabolism (20–50% of normal by FDG-PET), yet had residual islands of cortical and subcortical higher metabolism in areas consistent with their behaviors. In all patients, these brain structures showed marked abnormalities at the level of response to simple sensory stimuli as measured by magnetoencephalography, which demonstrated a loss of the integrity of even early cortical processing. These patients, similar to those studied by Laureys and colleagues,[44,47] revealed that some preservation of basic corticothalamic processing may coexist with behavioral unconsciousness and this does not contravene a clinical diagnosis of VS.

The Minimally Conscious State Represents a Low Level of Residual Corticothalamic Integrity or an Inability to Maintain Cerebral Integrative Function

The next level of recovery on the continuum from VS to full consciousness is the minimally conscious state (MCS). The Aspen Neurobehavioral Workgroup defined MCS in 2002 as "a condition of severely altered consciousness in which minimal but definite behavioral evidence of self or environmental awareness is demonstrated."[48] This condition has been operationally defined by a set of behavioral tests known as the JFK Coma Recovery Scale Revised (CRS-R),[21] and is discussed by Hirschberg and Giacino elsewhere in this issue. MCS includes a more heterogeneous group of patients than VS, because the operational definition allows for a wide range of behaviors, whereas VS only includes reflexive movements. In MCS, low-end behaviors include visual tracking to a mirror, localization of noxious touch, and inaccurate verbalization, whereas high-end behaviors include consistent movement to command and choosing correctly between 2 objects. Patients with only low-end behaviors can be difficult to differentiate from VS, because these behaviors may be subtle and infrequent.[22,49,50] This differentiation is essential because patients in MCS have significantly better prognoses for recovery than those in VS.[51,52]

Pathology and anatomic imaging literature have revealed that MCS is typically associated with similar injury patterns as VS, but with sufficient surviving neurons and connectivity between cortex, thalamus, and brainstem arousal centers to support some level of behavioral responsiveness.[53,54] In the setting of TBI, one study found that across the continuum of VS to MCS to full consciousness, patients were less likely to have severe DAI and more likely to have focal brain injuries, such as hematomas and contusions.[53] Notably, these investigators reported overlap in pathologic findings across all levels of consciousness, which demonstrated that current anatomic methods cannot completely account for the variances in behavior.

Functional imaging (fMRI and $H_2{}^{15}O$-PET) and neurophysiologic methods have proved to be more sensitive than anatomic methods in distinguishing patients in VS from those in MCS, because they measure corticothalamic function. For example, when presented with sensory stimuli, MCS patients activate higher-order association cortices, similar to healthy controls, whereas VS patients, at best, activate primary sensory cortices.[55,56] However, compared to healthy controls, MCS patients require a higher level of arousal (ie, more alerting stimuli) to produce similar patterns of activation.[42] This requirement for a higher level of arousal is consistent with behavioral data, which show that these patients fluctuate in their level of responsiveness[57] and suggest an underlying inability to maintain cerebral integrative functioning.

Akinetic Mutism and Related Syndromes are Disorders of Goal-Directed Behavior

Akinetic mutism, in its originally described form, fits in the category of MCS,[58] although milder variants, including abulia,[59,60] are categorized as fully conscious states.[61] Patients with these conditions have intact arousal and often the appearance of vigilance, but have severe poverty of movement despite lack of damage to motor systems. Severe cases can only be distinguished from VS by the preservation of visual tracking through smooth pursuit eye movements. The underlying cause in most cases is injury to the bilateral medial frontal lobes and anterior cingulate cortex from a mass lesion or anterior cerebral artery infarct. These syndromes can also arise from bilateral injury to the basal ganglia,[62,63] dorsal and central thalamus, or midbrain,[64] as these areas are tightly integrated with the frontal lobes in the generation of goal-directed behavior. As discussed below, the circuits involving these areas play a significant role in recovery of consciousness from a wide range of injuries.

Patients with Severely Damaged Motor System may be Widely Miscategorized

Functional brain imaging studies have led to a new but currently undefined category of disordered consciousness: patients who are behaviorally in VS or MCS, yet demonstrate imaging evidence of high-level cognitive processes, including command following and, in 2 instances, communication.[65–67] These studies used fMRI (although EEG may also be used[68]) to reveal changes in cortical activity when patients are asked to imagine a motor performance or spatial navigation task (**Fig. 2** shows example results). The most striking example of covert conscious function came from a patient who initially fulfilled the behavioral criteria for VS, but was able to answer 5 out of 6 autobiographical questions correctly using the mental imagery of playing tennis as a 'yes' response and walking around his house as a 'no' response.[66] Only a few such patients have been identified, because there are no obvious historical or anatomic imaging markers to predict covert consciousness. Furthermore, the assessments currently used require levels of memory and attention not present even in some fully conscious subjects.[67] The clinical implications of these findings are also not clear, because it is not yet possible to turn these fMRI or EEG paradigms into a bedside communication device. Moreover, it is not known if the ability to follow commands identified through fMRI predicts an emergence to full consciousness. However, once these measurements are obtained, it is clear that the patients have interacted with their environment, thereby placing them in a vague category between high-level MCS and LIS.

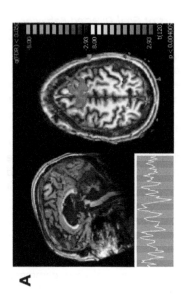

A

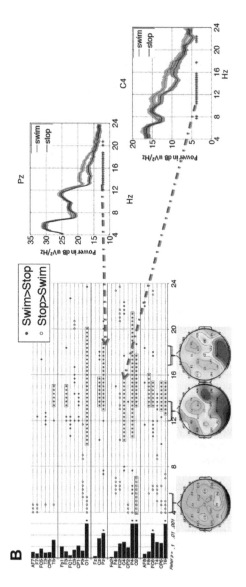

B

MECHANISTIC CONSIDERATIONS IN THE PROGNOSIS AND TREATMENT OF PATIENTS WITH DISORDERS OF CONSCIOUSNESS
Prognosis from Disorders of Consciousness

The pathophysiologies described earlier help to explain the mechanisms by which some patients recover and why others do not, and give an interpretive framework for the successes of specific interventions in improving arousal. In brief, the three types of pathophysiologies linked to disorders of consciousness from permanent brain injury discussed earlier are: (1) loss of cortical and thalamic neurons from global ischemia, (2) DAI in the setting of rapid acceleration/deceleration that leads to the disconnection of corticothalamic loops, and (3) damage to the upper brainstem and central thalamic neurons leading to loss of arousal tone for corticothalamic loops. In addition, dysfunction of medial frontal systems from any of these three mechanisms, as well as others, may result in MCS and globally impaired levels of function near the operational criteria for MCS (ie, akinetic mutism).

Global ischemia generally has the worst prognosis of the injury types discussed because of the marked sensitivity of cortical and thalamic neurons to hypoxia and ischemia.[29] In this setting, the key issue is typically the prediction of recovery to avoid futile attempts at sustaining life in patients who are often otherwise quite ill.[69] Previously, this declaration could be made purely on clinical grounds within 3 days after an injury,[70] but with the addition of therapeutic hypothermia,[71,72] these criteria no longer apply.[73] Prognosis after hypothermia is difficult, most likely because the neurons spared by hypothermia remain functionally impaired for long time periods, leading to a later demonstration of recovery. As a result, new prognostic algorithms need to be developed, which will likely require more time after injury as well as new imaging and electrophysiological techniques. If patients survive and transition to MCS, treatment strategies are similar to those discussed below.

Patients with DAI presenting with coma have a wide range of outcomes, from prolonged VS to independent functioning.[28,69] The time course of recovery is also variable, ranging from days to years. Interestingly, one patient regained full consciousness and language after 19 years in MCS.[74] There are no reliable predictors of recovery in this population, although rough guidelines suggest that patients in MCS have a higher likelihood of recovery than those in VS, especially if MCS occurs within the first year.[51,52] This is a better prognosis than for patients with global ischemia, for whom recovery to independence is exceedingly rare if the patient remains in VS for 3 months. The mechanism by which the brain recovers from DAI is still not clear.[75] Possible contributors to recovery include the regrowth of corticothalamic axons[74–77] and the remapping of intracortical connections to maximize spared pathways.[78]

Fig. 2. Noninvasive imaging evidence of command following in a patient with severe brain injury who was behaviorally locked in. (*A*) fMRI demonstrating increased activity (*orange*) in supplementary motor and other cortical areas when the patient was asked to imagine swimming versus a resting baseline. (*B*) Spectral analysis of EEG in the same patient performing the imagination of the swimming task at a different time. Example power spectra for 2 channels are on the right; the image on the left summarizes significant spectral changes across all channels and frequencies tested. Head maps below summarize amplitude of power change across all channels at the frequencies listed directly above. (*Adapted from* Bardin JC, Fins JJ, Katz DI, et al. Dissociations between behavioural and functional magnetic resonance imaging-based evaluations of cognitive function after brain injury. Brain 2011;134(Pt 3):769–82; Goldfine AM, Victor JD, Conte MM, et al. Determination of awareness in patients with severe brain injury using EEG power spectral analysis. Clin Neurophysiol 2011. Available at: http://www.ncbi.nlm.nih.gov/pubmed/21514214. Accessed July 17, 2011; with permission.)

In cases of upper brainstem and central thalamic injury, recovery of function depends on the ability of the remaining arousal centers to restore patterned cortico-thalamic activity. If return of consciousness occurs, patients may be left with severe cognitive deficits, depending on the degree of thalamic injury.[79] Similar to DAI, there are a wide range of reported outcomes, but anatomic and functional imaging techniques do not allow prediction of the potential for recovery in most cases.

TREATMENT STRATEGIES FOR PATIENTS WITH DISORDERS OF CONSCIOUSNESS

Akinetic mutism offers a model for approaches that improve the level of consciousness (see **Fig. 1**). In akinetic mutism, the injury to the cortico-striatopallidal-thalamocortical circuit involving the medial frontal lobe can produce dysfunction as severe as in patients with much more widespread injury.[58,61] Increasing the function of this circuit through medication or brain electrical stimulation can drive activity widely through the cerebrum.[80] For example, dopaminergic agents (eg, amantadine, levo-dopa, bromocriptine, or apomorphine) that enhance striatal background activity, have been shown to raise the level of consciousness and improve recovery rates in patients with various severe brain injuries (reviewed by Hirschberg and Giacino elsewhere in this issue). Zolpidem, an agonist of a subset of γ-aminobutyric acid(A) (GABA$_A$) receptors, has also been demonstrated to dramatically improve consciousness in patients with diffuse brain injury.[81,82] The mechanism of action of zolpidem is thought to occur through cortical activation, both directly[83] and indirectly, by inhibiting the globus pallidus interna from inhibiting thalamocortical firing.[84] Another successful approach through the same network, although only reported in a single patient, is direct activation central thalamic outflow via deep brain stimulation (DBS).[85,86]

There are no clear guidelines for medical management to attempt to speed recovery of consciousness, as almost all data are from case series. Accordingly, we offer some approaches that have been proved to be successful in our experience. For a medically stable patient with a disorder of consciousness, the first goal is to rule out potential inhibitors of recovery. This includes undiagnosed seizure disorders, particularly because they can be difficult to detect behaviorally in patients with impaired motor output. Medications can also be culprits in worsening arousal, especially those with anticholinergic, antihistaminergic, barbiturate, and benzodiazepine properties as well as some antiepileptic and antispasticity agents.[87]

To promote recovery of consciousness, we recommend amantadine 200–400 mg, split between early morning and early afternoon doses. Amantadine has a relatively benign safety profile and is the only medication tested to date in patients in VS and MCS in a well-powered, randomized, double-blind, clinical trial,[88] although the results have not yet been published. A selective serotonin reuptake inhibitor may also be added, based on animal model[89] and clinical trial[90] evidence for enhancing plasticity, although there is no strong evidence in patients with disorders of consciousness. Zolpidem can be given as 5 or 10 mg doses with a response expected within 1 hour, though only rarely.[91] Zolpidem is apparently safe, though there are no long-term data and the potential for habituation exists. Medications should be trialed individually, with a gradual titration of doses. Patients should have well-documented formal examinations using the CRS-R before and after initiation and dose changes, and any side effects should be noted. In addition, physical, occupational, and speech therapy should be used when appropriate, including daily joint stretching to avoid contractures, which can severely limit movement when the motor system recovers.

SUMMARY

Fins[92] has argued against a nihilistic approach to patients with chronic disorders of consciousness, as if the loss of function is invariably permanent and there is nothing more to be gained from diagnostic testing and treatment. We agree that these patients deserve a more systematic approach to assessment, prognosis, and treatment. The evidence described in this review shows that these conditions include a wide range of pathologies, causes, prognoses, and proven treatments. Diagnostic testing can be used to determine the degree of injury and suggest residual capacity for cognitive function. Future work will allow the use of imaging modalities to predict recovery and development of tools to communicate with those who have lost all motor function.

REFERENCES

1. Posner JB, Saper CB, Schiff ND, et al. Plum and Posner's diagnosis of stupor and coma. 4th edition. New York: Oxford University Press; 2007.
2. Steriade MM, McCarley RW. Brain control of wakefulness and sleep. 2nd edition. New York (NY): Kluwer Academic/Plenum Publishers; 2005.
3. Moruzzi G, Magoun HW. Brain stem reticular formation and activation of the EEG. Electroencephalogr Clin Neurophysiol 1949;1(4):455–73.
4. Magoun HW. The waking brain. Springfield (IL): Charles C Thomas; 1958.
5. Parvizi J, Damasio A. Consciousness and the brainstem. Cognition 2001;79(1–2): 135–60.
6. Steriade M, Glenn LL. Neocortical and caudate projections of intralaminar thalamic neurons and their synaptic excitation from midbrain reticular core. J Neurophysiol 1982;48(2):352–71.
7. Mignot E, Taheri S, Nishino S. Sleeping with the hypothalamus: emerging therapeutic targets for sleep disorders. Nat Neurosci 2002;5(Suppl):1071–5.
8. Llinás R, Ribary U, Contreras D, et al. The neuronal basis for consciousness. Philos Trans R Soc Lond B Biol Sci 1998;353(1377):1841–9.
9. Jones EG. Thalamic circuitry and thalamocortical synchrony. Philos Trans R Soc Lond B Biol Sci 2002;357(1428):1659–73.
10. Tononi G, Edelman GM. Consciousness and complexity. Science 1998;282 (5395):1846–51.
11. Broadbent DE. Perception and communication. London (UK): Pergamon Press; 1958.
12. Garey J, Goodwillie A, Frohlich J, et al. Genetic contributions to generalized arousal of brain and behavior. Proc Natl Acad Sci U S A 2003;100(19):11019–22.
13. Pfaff D. Brain arousal and information theory: neural and genetic mechanisms. 1st edition. Cambridge (MA): Harvard University Press; 2005.
14. Searle JR. Intentionality, an essay in the philosophy of mind. Cambridge (UK): Cambridge University Press; 1983.
15. Brentano F. Psychology from an empirical standpoint. 2nd edition. New York (NY): Routledge; 1995.
16. Frith CD, Friston K, Liddle PF, et al. Willed action and the prefrontal cortex in man: a study with PET. Proc Biol Sci 1991;244(1311):241–6.
17. Paus T, Koski L, Caramanos Z, et al. Regional differences in the effects of task difficulty and motor output on blood flow response in the human anterior cingulate cortex: a review of 107 PET activation studies. Neuroreport 1998;9(9):R37–47.
18. Paus T, Zatorre RJ, Hofle N, et al. Time-related changes in neural systems underlying attention and arousal during the performance of an auditory vigilance task. J Cogn Neurosci 1997;9(3):392–408.

19. Panksepp J. Affective neuroscience: the foundations of human and animal emotions. 1st edition. New York: Oxford University Press; 2004.
20. Kinomura S, Larsson J, Gulyás B, et al. Activation by attention of the human reticular formation and thalamic intralaminar nuclei. Science 1996;271(5248): 512–5.
21. Giacino JT, Kalmar K, Whyte J. The JFK coma recovery scale-revised: measurement characteristics and diagnostic utility. Arch Phys Med Rehabil 2004;85(12): 2020–9.
22. Schnakers C, Vanhaudenhuyse A, Giacino J, et al. Diagnostic accuracy of the vegetative and minimally conscious state: clinical consensus versus standardized neurobehavioral assessment. BMC Neurol 2009;9(1):35.
23. Smart CM, Giacino JT, Cullen T, et al. A case of locked-in syndrome complicated by central deafness. Nat Clin Pract Neurol 2008;4(8):448–53.
24. Elliott L, Coleman M, Shiel A, et al. Effect of posture on levels of arousal and awareness in vegetative and minimally conscious state patients: a preliminary investigation. J Neurol Neurosurg Psychiatry 2005;76(2):298–9.
25. Jennett B, Plum F. Persistent vegetative state after brain damage. A syndrome in search of a name. Lancet 1972;1(7753):734–7.
26. Bekinschtein T, Cologan V, Dahmen B, et al. You are only coming through in waves: wakefulness variability and assessment in patients with impaired consciousness. Prog Brain Res 2009;177:171–89.
27. Kobylarz EJ, Schiff ND. Neurophysiological correlates of persistent vegetative and minimally conscious states. Neuropsychol Rehabil 2005;15(3–4):323–32.
28. The Multi-Society Task Force on PVS. Medical aspects of the persistent vegetative state. N Engl J Med 1994;330(21):1499–508.
29. Adams JH, Graham DI, Jennett B. The neuropathology of the vegetative state after an acute brain insult. Brain 2000;123(7):1327–38.
30. Adams JH, Graham DI, Murray LS, et al. Diffuse axonal injury due to non-missile head injury in humans: an analysis of 45 cases. Ann Neurol 1982;12(6): 557–63.
31. Gennarelli TA, Thibault LE, Adams JH, et al. Diffuse axonal injury and traumatic coma in the primate. Ann Neurol 1982;12(6):564–74.
32. Ingvar DH, Sourander P. Destruction of the reticular core of the brain stem. A patho-anatomical follow-up of a case of coma of three years' duration. Arch Neurol 1970;23(1):1–8.
33. Castaigne P, Lhermitte F, Buge A, et al. Paramedian thalamic and midbrain infarct: clinical and neuropathological study. Ann Neurol 1981;10(2):127–48.
34. Eidelberg D, Moeller JR, Kazumata K, et al. Metabolic correlates of pallidal neuronal activity in Parkinson's disease. Brain 1997;120(8):1315–24.
35. Levy DE, Sidtis JJ, Rottenberg DA, et al. Differences in cerebral blood flow and glucose utilization in vegetative versus locked-in patients. Ann Neurol 1987;22(6): 673–82.
36. Laureys S, Goldman S, Phillips C, et al. Impaired effective cortical connectivity in vegetative state: preliminary investigation using PET. Neuroimage 1999;9(4): 377–82.
37. Blacklock JB, Oldfield EH, Di Chiro G, et al. Effect of barbiturate coma on glucose utilization in normal brain versus gliomas. Positron emission tomography studies. J Neurosurg 1987;67(1):71–5.
38. Alkire MT, Haier RJ, Barker SJ, et al. Cerebral metabolism during propofol anesthesia in humans studied with positron emission tomography. Anesthesiology 1995;82(2):393–403 [discussion: 27A].

39. Maquet P, Dive D, Salmon E, et al. Cerebral glucose utilization during sleep-wake cycle in man determined by positron emission tomography and [18F]2-fluoro-2-deoxy-D-glucose method. Brain Res 1990;513(1):136–43.
40. Maquet P, Degueldre C, Delfiore G, et al. Functional neuroanatomy of human slow wave sleep. J Neurosci 1997;17(8):2807–12.
41. Cruse D, Owen AM. Consciousness revealed: new insights into the vegetative and minimally conscious states. Curr Opin Neurol 2010;23(6):656–60.
42. Schiff ND, Rodriguez-Moreno D, Kamal A, et al. fMRI reveals large-scale network activation in minimally conscious patients. Neurology 2005;64(3):514–23.
43. Bekinschtein TA, Dehaene S, Rohaut B, et al. Neural signature of the conscious processing of auditory regularities. Proc Natl Acad Sci U S A 2009;106(5):1672–7.
44. Laureys S, Faymonville M-E, Degueldre C, et al. Auditory processing in the vegetative state. Brain 2000;123(8):1589–601.
45. Laureys S, Faymonville ME, Peigneux P, et al. Cortical processing of noxious somatosensory stimuli in the persistent vegetative state. Neuroimage 2002;17(2):732–41.
46. Schiff ND, Ribary U, Moreno DR, et al. Residual cerebral activity and behavioral fragments can remain in the persistently vegetative brain. Brain 2002;125(6):1210–34.
47. Laureys S, Lemaire C, Maquet P, et al. Cerebral metabolism during vegetative state and after recovery to consciousness. J Neurol Neurosurg Psychiatry 1999;67(1):121–2.
48. Giacino JT, Ashwal S, Childs N, et al. The minimally conscious state: definition and diagnostic criteria. Neurology 2002;58(3):349–53.
49. Andrews K, Murphy L, Munday R, et al. Misdiagnosis of the vegetative state: retrospective study in a rehabilitation unit. BMJ 1996;313(7048):13–6.
50. Vanhaudenhuyse A, Schnakers C, Brédart S, et al. Assessment of visual pursuit in post-comatose states: use a mirror. J Neurol Neurosurg Psychiatry 2008;79(2):223.
51. Estraneo A, Moretta P, Loreto V, et al. Late recovery after traumatic, anoxic, or hemorrhagic long-lasting vegetative state. Neurology 2010;75(3):239–45.
52. Luauté J, Maucort-Boulch D, Tell L, et al. Long-term outcomes of chronic minimally conscious and vegetative states. Neurology 2010;75(3):246–52.
53. Jennett B, Adams JH, Murray LS, et al. Neuropathology in vegetative and severely disabled patients after head injury. Neurology 2001;56(4):486–90.
54. Kampfl A, Schmutzhard E, Franz G, et al. Prediction of recovery from posttraumatic vegetative state with cerebral magnetic-resonance imaging. Lancet 1998;351(9118):1763–7.
55. Boly M, Faymonville ME, Peigneux P, et al. Auditory processing in severely brain injured patients: differences between the minimally conscious state and the persistent vegetative state. Arch Neurol 2004;61(2):233–8.
56. Bekinschtein T, Niklison J, Sigman L, et al. Emotion processing in the minimally conscious state. J Neurol Neurosurg Psychiatry 2004;75(5):788.
57. Hart T, Whyte J, Millis S, et al. Dimensions of disordered attention in traumatic brain injury: further validation of the moss attention rating scale. Arch Phys Med Rehabil 2006;87(5):647–55.
58. Cairns H, Oldfield RC, Pennybacker JB, et al. Akinetic mutism with an epidermoid cyst of the 3rd ventricle. Brain 1941;64(4):273–90.
59. Fisher CM. Honored guest presentation: abulia minor vs. agitated behavior. Clin Neurosurg 1983;31:9–31.

60. Stuss DT, Alexander MP. Is there a dysexecutive syndrome? Philos Trans R Soc Lond B Biol Sci 2007;362(1481):901–15.

61. Schiff ND, Plum F. The role of arousal and "gating" systems in the neurology of impaired consciousness. J Clin Neurophysiol 2000;17(5):438–52.

62. Bhatia KP, Marsden CD. The behavioural and motor consequences of focal lesions of the basal ganglia in man. Brain 1994;117(4):859–76.

63. Mega MS, Cohenour RC. Akinetic mutism: disconnection of frontal-subcortical circuits. Neuropsychiatry Neuropsychol Behav Neurol 1997;10(4):254–9.

64. Segarra JM. Cerebral vascular disease and behavior: the syndrome of the mesencephalic artery (basilar artery bifurcation). Arch Neurol 1970;22(5):408–18.

65. Owen AM, Coleman MR, Boly M, et al. Detecting awareness in the vegetative state. Science 2006;313(5792):1402.

66. Monti MM, Vanhaudenhuyse A, Coleman MR, et al. Willful modulation of brain activity in disorders of consciousness. N Engl J Med 2010;362(7):579–89.

67. Bardin JC, Fins JJ, Katz DI, et al. Dissociations between behavioural and functional magnetic resonance imaging-based evaluations of cognitive function after brain injury. Brain 2011;134(Pt 3):769–82.

68. Goldfine AM, Victor JD, Conte MM, et al. Determination of awareness in patients with severe brain injury using EEG power spectral analysis. Clin Neurophysiol 2011. Available at: http://www.ncbi.nlm.nih.gov/pubmed/21514214. Accessed July 17, 2011.

69. Jennett B. The vegetative state: medical facts, ethical and legal dilemmas. Cambridge (UK): Cambridge University Press; 2002.

70. Levy DE, Caronna JJ, Singer BH, et al. Predicting outcome from hypoxic-ischemic coma. JAMA 1985;253(10):1420–6.

71. Bernard SA, Gray TW, Buist MD, et al. Treatment of comatose survivors of out-of-hospital cardiac arrest with induced hypothermia. N Engl J Med 2002;346(8):557–63.

72. The Hypothermia after Cardiac Arrest Study Group. Mild therapeutic hypothermia to improve the neurologic outcome after cardiac arrest. N Engl J Med 2002;346(8):549–56.

73. Rossetti AO, Oddo M, Logroscino G, et al. Prognostication after cardiac arrest and hypothermia: a prospective study. Ann Neurol 2010;67(3):301–7.

74. Voss HU, Uluç AM, Dyke JP, et al. Possible axonal regrowth in late recovery from the minimally conscious state. J Clin Invest 2006;116(7):2005–11.

75. Povlishock JT, Katz DI. Update of neuropathology and neurological recovery after traumatic brain injury. J Head Trauma Rehabil 2005;20(1):76–94.

76. Bendlin BB, Ries ML, Lazar M, et al. Longitudinal changes in patients with traumatic brain injury assessed with diffusion-tensor and volumetric imaging. Neuroimage 2008;42(2):503–14.

77. Sidaros A, Engberg AW, Sidaros K, et al. Diffusion tensor imaging during recovery from severe traumatic brain injury and relation to clinical outcome: a longitudinal study. Brain 2008;131(2):559–72.

78. Dancause N, Barbay S, Frost SB, et al. Extensive cortical rewiring after brain injury. J Neurosci 2005;25(44):10167–79.

79. Katz DI, Alexander MP, Mandell AM. Dementia following strokes in the mesencephalon and diencephalon. Arch Neurol 1987;44(11):1127–33.

80. Schiff ND. Recovery of consciousness after brain injury: a mesocircuit hypothesis. Trends Neurosci 2010;33(1):1–9.

81. Clauss RP, van der Merwe CE, Nel HW. Arousal from a semi-comatose state on zolpidem. S Afr Med J 2001;91(10):788–9.
82. Brefel-Courbon C, Payoux P, Ory F, et al. Clinical and imaging evidence of zolpidem effect in hypoxic encephalopathy. Ann Neurol 2007;62(1):102–5.
83. McCarthy MM, Brown EN, Kopell N. Potential network mechanisms mediating electroencephalographic beta rhythm changes during propofol-induced paradoxical excitation. J Neurosci 2008;28(50):13488–504.
84. Schiff ND, Posner JB. Another "Awakenings." Ann Neurol 2007;62(1):5–7.
85. Schiff ND, Giacino JT, Kalmar K, et al. Behavioural improvements with thalamic stimulation after severe traumatic brain injury. Nature 2007;448(7153):600–3.
86. Schiff ND. Central thalamic deep-brain stimulation in the severely injured brain: rationale and proposed mechanisms of action. Ann N Y Acad Sci 2009;1157: 101–16.
87. Goldstein LB. Common drugs may influence motor recovery after stroke. The Sygen In Acute Stroke Study Investigators. Neurology 1995;45(5):865–71.
88. Meythaler JM, Brunner RC, Johnson A, et al. Amantadine to improve neurorecovery in traumatic brain injury-associated diffuse axonal injury: a pilot double-blind randomized trial. J Head Trauma Rehabil 2002;17(4):300–13.
89. Vetencourt JFM, Sale A, Viegi A, et al. The antidepressant fluoxetine restores plasticity in the adult visual cortex. Science 2008;320(5874):385–8.
90. Chollet F, Tardy J, Albucher J-F, et al. Fluoxetine for motor recovery after acute ischaemic stroke (FLAME): a randomised placebo-controlled trial. Lancet Neurol 2011;10(2):123–30.
91. Whyte J, Myers R. Incidence of clinically significant responses to zolpidem among patients with disorders of consciousness: a preliminary placebo controlled trial. Am J Phys Med Rehabil 2009;88(5):410–8.
92. Fins JJ. Constructing an ethical stereotaxy for severe brain injury: balancing risks, benefits and access. Nat Rev Neurosci 2003;4(4):323–7.

A Clinical and Investigative Approach to the Patient with Diminished Responsiveness

Sara Hocker, MD[a],*, Alejandro A. Rabinstein, MD[b]

KEYWORDS

• Coma • Encephalopathy • Diagnosis • Evaluation

Neurologists are frequently faced with the task of determining the etiology of "altered mental status." While the term "altered mental status" in itself is problematic, the incidence with which we are asked this question points to a great need for neurologists to have a practical approach to these patients so that, as with the neurologic examination, when it is done the same way every time important findings are not missed. Consciousness has been described by physicians for centuries as a continuum of states of being. Alterations can range from the alert patient with a disturbance in the content of consciousness caused by a failure of multiple cortical areas leading to difficulty in integration of what is perceived, to the patient with a disturbance of arousal in which there is dysfunction of the reticular formation in the brainstem and thalamus, leading to decreased alertness. These components can occur in isolation or in association with one another, and both can present with varying degrees of magnitude.

In this article the authors first attempt to provide the clinician with a focused approach to the patient with diminished responsiveness using the neurologic examination and what is known about the physiology of consciousness to aid in the formulation of a differential diagnosis. Only acute alterations in consciousness are discussed. Second, the rational use of laboratory, neuroimaging, and other ancillary studies used to confirm a diagnosis are discussed.

The authors have nothing to disclose.
[a] Division of Critical Care Neurology, Mayo Clinic, 200 First Street SW, Rochester, MN 55905, USA
[b] Mayo Clinic, 200 First Street SW, Rochester, MN 55905, USA
* Corresponding author.
E-mail address: Hocker.Sara@mayo.edu

doi:10.1016/j.ncl.2011.07.003
0733-8619/11/$ – see front matter © 2011 Elsevier Inc. All rights reserved.
neurologic.theclinics.com

FOCUSED HISTORY

Clues obtained in the history may decrease the time it takes to find the cause of coma and initiate its treatment, which may in some instances become the difference between severe impairment and return to normal function. Most information will be obtained from family members, paramedics, police, or other witnesses to the onset of diminished responsiveness or preceding events. It is always important to determine the acuity of the change. The differential diagnosis of a sudden change in consciousness or content of thought is very different from that which occurs over a period of days to weeks or even that which is fluctuating. If there were no witnesses to the onset of events, information should be sought about when the patient was last seen to be normal. If there was an insidious or fluctuating decline, it is important to gather a description of the patient's recent behavior at work or home with particular attention to changes in personality, automatic-appearing behaviors, or changes in level of alertness. The knowledge that a similar or the same event has happened before can be particularly helpful. Details on medical and social history, as well as prescription or recreational drug use and exposure to toxic substances or travel should be investigated.

LOCALIZATION AND PHYSIOLOGY OF DIMINISHED RESPONSIVENESS

When a neurologist is called to evaluate the patient with diminished responsiveness, a multitude of terms may be used to describe the patient. Patients may be described as confused, agitated, delirious, stuporous, unresponsive, unconscious, or comatose. Perhaps most frequently they are described as having altered mental status. In general, for the neurologist it is simplest to think in terms of alertness and awareness.

Maintaining alertness is primarily a function of the ascending reticular activating system (ARAS), which projects from the brainstem tegmentum through synaptic relays in the rostral intralaminar and thalamic nuclei to the cerebral cortex. Awareness is primarily a function of the cortex, with contributions from the precuneus and anterior cingulate gyrus. Encephalopathy is a broad term used to denominate a syndrome of diffuse cerebral dysfunction, which may be caused by various factors that reduce energy metabolism through decreases in the synthesis of acetylcholine, glutamate, or γ-aminobutyric acid (GABA).[1,2] These factors may include, for example, acute derangements of metabolic or endocrine systems, generalized tonic-clonic, complex partial, or nonconvulsive status epilepticus, and drug toxicity. The term encephalopathy does not imply complete lack of awareness or response. Coma is a state in which the patient is unconscious, unaware, and unresponsive to external stimuli, and results from structural damage to the ARAS, anterior cingulate cortex, and association cortex (precuneus and cuneus), or from profound diffuse cerebral dysfunction. A patient in coma may have eye opening to pain with no eye tracking or fixation, reflexive motor responses to noxious stimuli, and preservation or absence of brainstem reflexes.

Important mimickers of coma include the locked-in syndrome, extreme abulia, and psychogenic coma. The locked-in syndrome can be easily missed if the patient is not asked to blink or perform vertical eye movements. The syndrome is caused by a lesion of the ventral pons resulting in de-efferentation of the motor tracts with sparing of the ARAS. Thus, locked-in patients have preservation of consciousness, can blink and move their eyes vertically to commands, and can see, hear, and feel pain. This condition typically occurs with acute basilar artery occlusion or pontine hemorrhages; however, it can rarely be seen with neuromuscular conditions such as botulism, acute inflammatory demyelinating polyradiculoneuropathy (Guillain-Barré syndrome),[3] or paralysis from neuromuscular blocking agents with inadequate sedation during surgical procedures under general anesthesia. Abulia, or akinetic mutism, is a state in which the patient does not initiate speech or movement but may have preserved awareness.[4] This presentation results from lesions of the anterior cingulate gyrus. Psychogenic unresponsiveness typically lasts only 1 to 2 days, often with unexpected "sudden awakening" and complete amnesia for the episode and events preceding the episode. **Fig. 1** summarizes the localization of diminished responsiveness.

Prolonged states of unconsciousness including the persistent vegetative state and the minimally conscious state are not discussed in this article.

EXAMINATION

The neurologic examination of the patient with diminished responsiveness begins with inspection of the patient in the absence of any stimulation, with particular attention to the pattern of respirations in spontaneously breathing patients, and the posture and movements of the patient, if any. Cluster breathing and central neurogenic hyperventilation indicate bilateral cortical or pontine lesions, whereas ataxic breathing indicates a lesion in the pontine tegmentum. A Cheyne-Stokes breathing pattern is the least localizing. Multifocal myoclonus of the face and extremities can indicate diffuse brain dysfunction due to metabolic derangements or nonconvulsive status epilepticus. The level of alertness may help differentiate between the two conditions. Spontaneous generalized myoclonus may indicate anoxic-ischemic brain injury or, less commonly, lithium, cyclosporine, or pesticide toxicity. Stimulus-induced myoclonus may be seen in encephalopathic patients with Creutzfeldt-Jakob disease.

Next, the level of alertness and awareness should be determined. The patient may be alert but inattentive, sleepy but easily arousable, or unable to follow any but the simplest of commands and have an expression of bewilderment. This semiology is consistent with encephalopathy, or diffuse cerebral dysfunction. In a comatose patient, the level of alertness should be described in terms of eye opening. The patient may open the eyes to loud voice or gentle tactile or noxious stimulation, or may have no eye opening at all, indicating various levels of impaired alertness. The examiner should note whether the patient fixates and tracks.

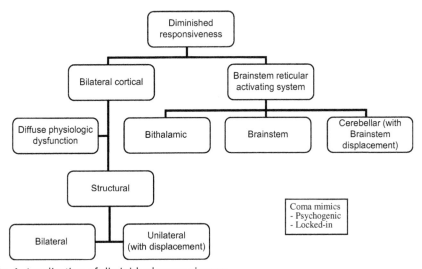

Fig. 1. Localization of diminished responsiveness.

Fundoscopy may provide diagnostic clues. For instance, retinal hemorrhages can be seen with aneurysmal subarachnoid hemorrhage, and acute papilledema may indicate increased intracranial pressure. The size, reactivity, symmetry, and position of the pupils, position of the eyes in primary gaze, presence of corneal, oculocephalic, and oculovestibular reflexes, as well as the presence and symmetry of grimace to pressure of the supraorbital nerve or temporomandibular joint capsule[5] should be examined to evaluate for possible structural brain injury or herniation, and to determine brainstem function.

The motor response can range from following commands in each extremity to localizing pain, to abnormal flexion, or extension responses. As important as the type of motor response is whether there is symmetry of the motor response.

A coma scale such as the FOUR score[6] (**Table 1**) may be used to ensure that the minimum requirements of a coma examination are obtained. The Glasgow Coma Scale should not be used as a surrogate for the neurologic examination, as it gives very little information about the functioning of the brainstem and cannot diagnose the locked-in syndrome.

There are no completely reliable tests for psychogenic unresponsiveness, although there are many techniques that may be helpful. These methods include closed eyes

Table 1
The FOUR score

Activity/Response	Score
Eye Response	
Eyelids open or opened, tracking or blinking to command	4
Eyelids open but not tracking	3
Eyelids closed but open to loud voice	2
Eyelids closed but open to pain	1
Eyelids remain closed with pain	0
Motor Response	
Thumbs-up, fist or peace sign	4
Localizing to pain	3
Flexion response to pain	2
Extension response to pain	1
No response to pain, or generalized myoclonus status	0
Brainstem Reflexes	
Pupil and corneal reflexes present	4
One pupil wide and fixed	3
Pupil or corneal reflexes absent	2
Pupil and corneal reflexes absent	1
Absent pupil, corneal, and cough reflex	0
Respiration	
Not intubated, regular breathing pattern	4
Not intubated, Cheyne-Stokes breathing pattern	3
Not intubated, irregular breathing	2
Breathes above ventilator rate	1
Breathes at ventilator rate or apnea	0

that open by tickling the inside of the nares, abnormal nonphysiologic movements, and the hand-drop test in which one arm is lifted and held over the face and when "dropped" by the examiner slides to the side of the patient rather than on to the body.

All patients with diminished responsiveness should be examined for signs of meningeal inflammation. The general examination should focus on external signs of trauma, vital signs, inspection of the skin, and attention to the breath odor, which may provide clues to toxic or systemic etiology.

DIFFERENTIAL DIAGNOSIS

On completion of the general and neurologic examination the clinician should be able to categorize the patient as having either structural intracranial disease or diffuse cerebral dysfunction (**Table 2**). The patient with structural intracranial disease will typically have focal or lateralizing signs on examination; however, the absence of focal deficits does not necessarily exclude structural damage. For example, patients with anoxic-ischemic encephalopathy, acute hydrocephalus, meningitis, or encephalitis may have acute changes in responsiveness without focal deficits. Therefore, the initial test in a patient with an acute decrease in responsiveness and stable airway, breathing, and circulation, after measuring serum glucose, must be a form of brain imaging, most often a noncontrast computed tomography (CT) scan of the head. By contrast, patients with focal neurologic deficits in association with an acute decrease in the level of consciousness do not always have a structural cause, as exemplified by patients with severe hypoglycemia or seizures with postictal deficits. **Fig. 2** shows the typical neuroimaging findings seen with anoxic-ischemic encephalopathy.

In is important to keep in mind that hypertensive encephalopathy is almost never the sole reason for unexplained coma, but rather may be a physiologic response to increased intracranial pressure resulting in decreased cerebral perfusion.

ANCILLARY TESTS

Having used the history and examination to formulate a differential diagnosis, selected neuroimaging and specific laboratory tests may be obtained to narrow the differential and, in most instances, find the explanation for acute changes in responsiveness.

All patients with acute changes in consciousness that are severe enough to prompt neurologic consultation deserve the following initial studies after or during stabilization of the airway, breathing, and circulation: serum chemistry including blood urea nitrogen, creatinine, glucose and electrolytes, serum osmolality, arterial blood gas, liver function tests including an ammonia level, complete blood count, prothrombin time, activated prothrombin time urine toxicology screen, serum alcohol level, and electrocardiogram. The reason for the serum osmolality measurement is to look for the presence of a gap between measured and calculated osmolality, which will be a clue that an atypical alcohol is present. In selected cases thyroid function tests, serum levels of specific drugs, urine ketoacids, blood cultures, and cortisol levels may be indicated.

After considering the available information obtained from these initial studies or while awaiting the results, a CT scan of the head should be obtained. It is a common dictum that an immediate CT scan of the brain is required in the comatose patient. This scan may reveal when the cause of coma is a structural lesion, and it is particularly useful for documenting a new mass, diffuse or multiple hemispheric lesions, edema, hemorrhage, hydrocephalus, or brain tissue shifts. Contrast is rarely performed or indicated in the acute setting.

Table 2
Differential diagnosis of diminished responsiveness

Structural Intracranial Disease	Diffuse Cerebral Dysfunction

Bilateral
  Anoxic-ischemic encephalopathy
  Subarachnoid hemorrhage
  Multiple traumatic brain contusions
  Traumatic brain injury
  Multiple cerebral infarcts
  CNS infection (meningitis, encephalitis, or PML)
  Gliomatosis
  Lymphoma
  Multiple brain metastases
  Acute disseminated encephalomyelitis
  Cerebral edema
  Acute hydrocephalus
  Acute leukoencephalopathy
  Posterior reversible encephalopathy syndrome
  Air or fat embolism
	Seizures (nonconvulsive status epilepticus or postictal state)
	
	Acute metabolic-endocrine derangement
	  Acute electrolyte shifts (hypoglycemia, hyperglycemia, hyponatremia, hypernatremia, hypercalcemia)
	  Addison disease
	  Acute hypothyroidism (myxedema)
	  Acute panhypopituitarism
	  Acute uremia
	  Hypercapnia
	  Profound acid-base disturbance
	  Sepsis
	  Acute liver failure
	  Thiamine deficiency (Wernicke encephalopathy)

Unilateral (with displacement of the contralateral hemisphere)
  Intraparenchymal hematoma
  Subdural or epidural hematoma
  Hemorrhagic contusion
  Large vessel ischemic stroke
  Cerebral venous thrombosis
  Cerebral abscess
  Brain tumor
	Toxic Cause
	  Carbon monoxide
	  Cyanide poisoning
	  Ethanol or atypical alcohols
	  Anticholinergic drug poisoning
	  Cholinergic agents (organophosphates, nerve gases)
	  Opioids
	  Sedative-hypnotic drugs (benzodiazepines, barbiturates)
	  Neuroleptics (butyrophenones, phenothiazines)

Bithalamic
  Bilateral thalamic infarcts (sequential unilateral infarcts, venous infarcts in deep cerebral venous thrombosis or occlusion of the artery of Percheron)
	Antidepressants (tricyclics, MAO inhibitors)
	  Sympathomimetics (amphetamines, cocaine, theophylline)
	  Extreme hypothermia
	  Gas inhalation
	  Acute (lethal) catatonia
	  Neuroleptic malignant syndrome
	  Serotonin syndrome

Brainstem
  Pontine hemorrhage
  Basilar artery occlusion and brainstem infarct
  Central pontine myelinolysis (after rapid correction of hyponatremia)
  Brainstem hemorrhagic contusion	

Cerebellum (with displacement of brainstem)
  Cerebellar infarction
  Cerebellar hemorrhage
  Cerebellar abscess
  Cerebellar tumor (typically metastasis or glioma in adults)	

Abbreviations: CNS, central nervous system; MAO, monoamine oxidase; PML, progressive multifocal leukoencephalopathy.

Adapted by Wijdicks EF. The comatose patient. New York: Oxford University Press; 2008; with permission from BMJ Publishing Group Limited.

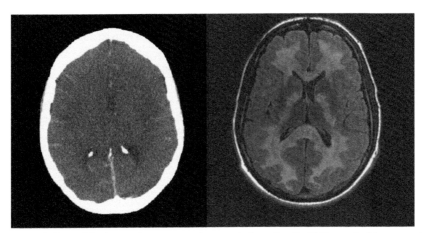

Fig. 2. Radiological findings of severe anoxic encephalopathy. (*Left*) Computed tomography scan of the head showing lack of gray-white matter differentiation, absence of sulci, and pseudosubarachnoid hemorrhage. (*Right*) Magnetic resonance imaging scan of the brain demonstrating diffuse fluid-attenuated inversion recovery signal change within the white matter of both cerebral hemispheres and cortical spinal tracts. (*Adapted by* Wijdicks EF. The comatose patient. New York: Oxford University Press; 2008; with permission from BMJ Publishing Group Limited.)

In patients presenting with signs or symptoms suggestive of central nervous system infection as well as patients presenting with thunderclap headache or meningeal irritation who have a normal CT of the head and normal coagulation indices, a lumbar puncture should be performed urgently and the cerebrospinal fluid (CSF) should be sent for analysis of cell count, glucose, protein, Gram stain, and cultures, as well as polymerase chain reaction for viruses when these are suspected. If subarachnoid hemorrhage is suspected the CSF should be centrifuged to assess for xanthochromia. Additional CSF should be saved for potential future testing if possible. Because a delay in diagnosis of bacterial meningitis may result in severe neurologic morbidity or mortality, the CT scan of the head should be obtained first to minimize the risk of precipitating or exacerbating a pressure gradient that may result in brain herniation.[7]

In patients with a normal CT scan, a magnetic resonance imaging (MRI) scan is more sensitive for the diagnosis of certain conditions, and has markedly reduced the number of patients with uncertain etiology early in the course of coma (**Table 3**).

Magnetic resonance angiography (MRA) can be used to confirm suspected basilar artery occlusion, and magnetic resonance venography (MRV) may be indicated to confirm the patency of the cerebral veins and sinuses. Both MRA and MRV are potentially useful in selected cases, and the decision to obtain these additional tests depends on the initial findings on MRI. Cerebral angiography is indicated only in cases of suspected cerebral vasculitis, ruptured aneurysm, arterial venous malformation, or possible basilar artery occlusion that are being considered for intervention.

Any comatose patient who has had witnessed seizure-like activity at some point in the course of events needs an electroencephalogram (EEG) to evaluate for the presence of nonconvulsive status epilepticus. However, in the absence of a witnessed seizure, the clinical manifestations of status may be very subtle or even absent. EEG should be ordered urgently in any patient with previous history of seizure disorder and unexplained coma, regardless of whether convulsive movements have been observed, as well as in comatose patients without a history of seizure disorder who

Table 3
Examples of the value of MRI scanning in disorders manifested with alteration of consciousness

Neurologic Disease	MRI Findings[a]
Prolonged status epilepticus	Cortical or hippocampal hyperintensities
Anoxic-ischemic encephalopathy[11,12]	Symmetric white matter hyperintensities
Brainstem ischemia	Hyperintensities in the thalamus, occipital lobes, and brainstem
Acute toxic leukoencephalopathies[13]: Chemotherapy drugs, antimicrobial agents (amphotericin B), immunosuppressive drugs (cyclosporine, tacrolimus, methotrexate), drugs of abuse (toluene, cocaine, heroin, ecstasy, psilocybin, methadone, oxycodone), environmental toxins (carbon monoxide, arsenic, carbon tetrachloride)	Diffuse confluent hyperintense lesions in white matter, basal ganglia
Acute demyelination syndromes: Acute disseminated encephalomyelitis (ADEM) Osmotic demyelination[14]	Patchy, multifocal, poorly marginated hyperintense lesions in white matter, basal ganglia Thalamic, striatal, pontine, and cerebellar lesions
Wernicke encephalopathy[15–17]	Hyperintensity of the mammillary bodies and periaqueductal gray matter
Traumatic brain injury	Lesions in corpus callosum, white matter
Herpes simplex encephalitis	Temporal, frontal lobe hyperintensities

[a] All changes described as seen on fluid-attenuated inversion recovery sequence.

have normal brain imaging and no major metabolic abnormalities or toxic exposures.[16] EEG has little specificity apart from the diagnosis of seizures. Diffuse slowing and even triphasic waves, which were once thought to be synonymous with metabolic causes of encephalopathy, can be seen with a structural cause of coma. That said, the presence of triphasic waves should indicate the need for further evaluation focused on metabolic disorders.[8] Similarly, periodic lateralized epileptiform discharges are nonspecific and only suggest a focus of irritable cortex, as seen with herpes simplex encephalitis or mass lesions. EEG should also be considered in patients with a known structural cause of diminished responsiveness when there is a discrepancy between the depth of the depression of consciousness and the severity of the primary diagnosis.[9,10]

The most challenging and uncomfortable scenario for the clinician is the patient in coma with a normal CT and MRI and no obvious metabolic or toxic cause. At this point, it is important to review the history, and neurologic and constitutional signs at presentation, then repeat the examination. A fluctuating examination may provide diagnostic clues. Diagnoses to consider in these patients include lupus cerebritis, immune-mediated encephalitis, which typically presents over weeks and occurs most often in young patients, and limbic encephalitis due to paraneoplastic, voltage-gated potassium channel encephalopathy or nonparaneoplastic anti–N-methyl-D-aspartate (NMDA) receptor antibody encephalitis. When limbic encephalitis is considered, the patient should undergo full-body positron emission tomography (PET) scanning and a pelvic examination or pelvic CT, as PET scanning will not detect an ovarian teratoma that has been associated with anti-NMDA receptor encephalitis.

When other alternative explanations are not available, an unidentified toxin should be considered and a specialist in toxicology should be consulted if available.[16]

SUMMARY

Considering the vast number of causes of diminished responsiveness, the best approach is to methodically work through a comprehensive evaluation beginning with a focused history and general and neurologic examinations followed by localization of the lesion, formulation of a differential diagnosis, and the rational use of laboratory, neuroimaging, and other ancillary tests to confirm diagnosis. Despite the improvement in technology that has helped enhance our understanding of the many causes of changes in consciousness, the diagnosis remains a clinical task in many instances.

REFERENCES

1. Sharshar T, Polito A, Checinski A, et al. Septic-associated encephalopathy—everything starts at a microlevel. Crit Care 2010;14(5):199.
2. Bismuth M, Funakoshi N, Cadranel JF, et al. Hepatic encephalopathy: from pathophysiology to therapeutic management. Eur J Gastroenterol Hepatol 2011; 23(1):8–22.
3. Rigamonti A, Basso F, Stanzani L, et al. Guillain-Barré syndrome mimicking brain death. J Peripher Nerv Syst 2009;14(4):316–9.
4. Shetty AC, Morris J, O'Mahony P. Akinetic mutism—not coma. Age Ageing 2009; 38(3):350–1.
5. Wijdicks EF. Temporomandibular joint compression in coma. Neurology 1996;46: 1774.
6. Wijdicks EF, Bamlet W, Maramattom B, et al. Validation of a new coma scale—the FOUR score. Am Neurol 2005;58:585–93.
7. Van Crevel H, Hijdra A, de Gans J. Lumbar puncture and the risk of herniation: when should we first perform CT? J Neurol 2001;249:129–37.
8. Brenner RP. The interpretation of the EEG in stupor and coma. Neurologist 2005; 11:271–84.
9. Vespa PM, Nuwer MR, Nenov V, et al. Increased incidence and impact of nonconvulsive and convulsive seizures after traumatic brain injury as detected by continuous electroencephalographic monitoring. J Neurosurg 1999;91:750–60.
10. Dennis LJ, Claassen J, Hirsch LJ, et al. Nonconvulsive status epilepticus after subarachnoid hemorrhage. Neurosurgery 2002;51:1136–43.
11. Torbey MT, Bhardwaj A. MR imaging in comatose survivors of cardiac resuscitation. AJNR Am J Neuroradiol 2002;23:738.
12. Arbelaez A, Castillo M, Mukherji SK. Diffusion weighted MR imaging of global cerebral anoxia. AJNR Am J Neuroradiol 1999;20:999–1007.
13. Filley CM, Kleinschmidt-DeMasters BK. Toxic leukoencephalopathy. N Engl J Med 2001;345(6):425–32.
14. Chua GC, Sitoh YY, Lim CC, et al. MRI findings in osmotic myelinolysis. Clin Radiol 2002;57:800–6.
15. Suzuki S, Ichijo M, Fujii H, et al. Acute Wernicke's encephalopathy: comparison of magnetic resonance images and autopsy findings. Intern Med 1996;35:831–4.
16. Rabinstein AA, Wijdicks EF. Coma: raised intracranial pressure and hydrocephalus. In: Warlow C, editor. The Lancet handbook of treatment in neurology. London: Elsevier Ltd; 2006. p. 179–200.
17. Wijdicks EF. The comatose patient. New York: Oxford University Press; 2008.

Delirium in the Intensive Care Unit: A Review

Alessandro Morandi, MD, MPH[a,b,c,*], James C. Jackson, PsyD[a,d,e,f,g]

KEYWORDS

- Delirium • Intensive care unit • Risk factors • Sedation
- Prevention • Multicomponent treatment
- Pharmacologic treatment • Antipsychotics

This article provides an overview of the literature currently available concerning the epidemiology, definition, diagnosis, pathophysiology, and the management of delirium, with a specific focus on delirium in the intensive care unit (ICU), though the literature and principles described herein generally apply to non-ICU settings and will be relevant to clinicians and researchers working in medical settings outside of critical care. Delirium is a complex and multifaceted syndrome, and though it has a long history in the annals of medicine, key questions pertaining to delirium remain unanswered. Answers to these questions, however, are increasingly being pursued, as reflected in a sharp spike in the number of articles published on delirium in the last decade.

EPIDEMIOLOGY OF DELIRIUM

Delirium is highly prevalent in medical populations, with rates of up to 80% reported in the highest risk groups (eg, medical ICU cohorts). As with most conditions, rates vary depending on illness severity and diagnostic methods including, and notably, the tools that are used.[1–3] Delirium is associated with adverse outcomes generally, but in ICU

Drs Morandi and Jackson have no conflicts of interest to report.
^a Center for Health Services Research, Vanderbilt Medical Center, 1215 21st Avenue South MCE Suite 6100, Nashville, TN 37232-1269, USA
^b Department of Rehabilitation and Aged Care, Ancelle della Carità hospital, Cremona, Italy
^c Geriatric Research Group, Brescia, Italy
^d Division of Allergy/Pulmonary/Critical Care Medicine, Vanderbilt Medical Center, Nashville, TN, USA
^e Department of Psychiatry, Vanderbilt Medical Center, Nashville, TN, USA
^f VA Tennessee Valley, Clinical Research Center of Excellence (CRCOE), TN, USA
^g VA Tennessee Valley Geriatric Research, Education and Clinical Center (GRECC), TN, USA
* Corresponding author. Center for Health Services Research, Vanderbilt Medical Center, 1215 21st Avenue South MCE Suite 6100, Nashville, TN 37232-1269.
E-mail address: morandi.alessandro@gmail.com

settings it is particularly concerning due in part to the breadth of untoward consequences to which it is linked. These factors include, but are not limited to, self-extubation and removal of catheters,[4] greater duration of hospitalization,[5–7] increased cost,[8] higher 6-month mortality,[9–11] and long-term cognitive impairment.[12,13] Many of these outcomes appear to be associated with delirium duration as opposed to simply the presence versus absence of delirium, suggesting a possible "dose-response" relationship. For reasons that remain unclear, delirium continues to be significantly unrecognized.

DEFINITION OF DELIRIUM

The definitive reference for delirium is the *Diagnostic and Statistical Manual of Mental Disorders* (Fourth Edition, Text Revised) (DSM-IV-TR).[14] According to the DSM-IV-TR, delirium is a condition characterized by: (1) a disturbance of consciousness with inattention, accompanied by (2) acute change in cognition (ie, memory deficits, disorientation, language disturbances, and perceptual disturbances) not accounted for by preexisting, established, or evolving dementia (though cognitive changes can take various forms in delirium, changes in attention are most typically observed); (3) development over a short period of time (hours to days) with fluctuation over time; (4) evidence that the disturbance is caused by the direct physiologic consequences of a general medical condition. Although a consensus about the technical definition of delirium exists, it is described variously and often with imprecision (eg, acute confusional state, ICU psychosis, acute brain dysfunction, encephalopathy, and so forth). Delirium symptoms are frequently similar to and often strongly mimic symptoms of other neuropsychiatric or frankly neurologic disorders. As such, the ability to make a proper diagnosis of delirium is often predicated on information about the baseline cognitive status from the family, caregivers, or other informants. In some cases depression and delirium can be difficult to differentiate, particularly among those with a hypoactive presentation. Farrell and Ganzini[15] showed that 42% of the patients referred to a psychiatric service for evaluation or treatment of a depressive disorder were found to be delirious. In some cases, acute psychosis in schizophrenia and delirium tremens can also be misidentified as delirium. In the case of schizophrenia, individuals are generally not disoriented and do not characteristically have the classic attentional derailments displayed in delirium, while often demonstrating paranoia—a condition rare among hospitalized delirious patients. Delirium tremens (due to alcohol withdrawal) (1) usually presents 48 to 96 hours after cessation of drinking; (2) can last up to 2 weeks; (3) can be worse overnight; (4) level of consciousness and disorientation are impaired and fluctuating; (5) reduced attention and global amnesia are present; (6) cognition and speech are impaired; and (7) hallucinations (usually tactile, visual) and delusions (persecutory) can be present.

DELIRIUM SUBTYPES

Delirium can be expressed in the context of distinct subtypes, typically referred to as hypoactive, hyperactive, and mixed.[16–18] Hypoactive delirium, often unrecognized, is characterized by symptoms of lethargy and minimal psychomotor activity. Hyperactive delirium, by contrast, is marked by significant agitation. Individuals with mixed expressions fluctuate between the hypoactive and hyperactive expressions. For example, Peterson and colleagues[19] reported that in a cohort of elderly medical ICU patients 43.5% were hypoactive, 54.9% were hyperactive, and fewer than 2% were mixed.

Subsyndromal Delirium

Questions persist about a condition existing between the boundaries of "normal" and "delirious." Popularly referred to as subsyndromal delirium (SSD),[20-23] this phenomenon is one in which symptoms never progress to meet the DSM-IV-TR requirements. Though relatively little studied, a recent investigation[24] showed that individuals with syndromal symptoms have worse outcomes than their "normal" counterparts. This finding suggests a continuum of severity[20,23] across a spectrum from "normal" to "frank" delirium.

ISSUES IN THE DIAGNOSIS OF DELIRIUM

Diagnosis of delirium is done in various ways, with diagnoses often made in the context of clinical interviews (eg, psychiatric or geriatric consultations). Less commonly, formal neuropsychological tests are used. Debate exists regarding the appropriateness of this approach, because attention—widely thought to be the key feature of delirium—influences other domains of cognition (eg, memory, executive functioning, processing speed) so powerfully. In some contexts, notably the ICU, several brief screening tools are used, such as the Intensive Care Delirium Screening Check List (ICDSC)[2] and the confusion assessment method for the ICU (CAM-ICU).[1,3] These tools can be used by nonspecialists and can be used to quickly identify delirium in ICU patients. Descriptions of the CAM-ICU and ICDSC can be found at www.icudelirium.org.

The ICDSC was originally validated in medical and surgical ICU patients against a consulting psychiatrist who served as the standard reference rater.[2] The ICDSC is a highly sensitive tool, with a specificity of 64%. It has a total score ranging from 0 to 8, with delirium defined as a score of 4 or more.

The CAM-ICU, a variant of the Confusion Assessment Method (CAM),[25] from which it was adapted, was designed to be used with intubated patients and validated against content experts who based their delirium diagnoses on the DSM-IV. Psychometric properties are strong,[1,3] with high sensitivity (93%–100%), specificity (89%–100%), and interrater reliability (κ = 0.96, 95% confidence interval [CI] 0.92–0.99). The CAM-ICU is used via a 2-step approach (**Fig. 1**), with level of consciousness typically assessed via the Richmond Agitation Sedation Scale (RASS),[26,27] a 10-point scale ranging from −5 (no response to voice or physical evaluation) to +4 (overtly combative, violent, immediate danger for staff). Scores of 0 reflect normal mental status. Patients with RASS scores of −4 or −5 cannot be assessed as, by definition, they are comatose. The CAM-ICU consists of 4 features, each of which parallel DSM-related criteria, with an acute change or fluctuation in mental status (Feature 1), accompanied by inattention (Feature 2), and either disorganized thinking (Feature 3) or altered level of consciousness (Feature 4).

PATHOPHYSIOLOGY

The pathophysiology of delirium remains a subject of much debate, with many theories and perspectives having been proposed.[28-33]

Studies of pathophysiology to date have involved brain modifications via neuroimaging, inflammation and sepsis, genetics, and the role of biomarkers and neurotransmitters.

Neuroimaging

Little work has been done on the neuroimaging of delirium, though early evidence suggests that delirium may be caused by diffused brain dysfunction rather than

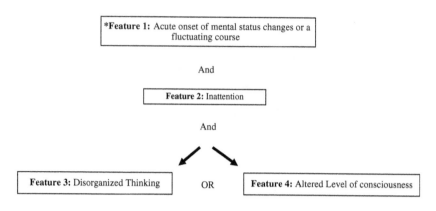

Fig. 1. The Confusion Assessment Method for the ICU (CAM-ICU). The diagnosis of delirium requires the presence of acute onset of changes or fluctuations in the course of mental status (Feature 1) and inattention (Feature 2), plus either disorganized thinking (Feature 3) or an altered level of consciousness. * The level of consciousness (arousal) is first evaluated with the Richmond Agitation Sedation Scale (RASS). The RASS is a 10-point scale ranging from −5 (no response to voice or physical evaluation) to +4 (overtly combative, violent, immediate danger for staff), with RASS score of 0 denoting a calm and alert patient. The patient comatose (RASS −5 or −4) cannot be assessed for delirium. The patient with a RASS score of −3 or greater (−2 to +4) can be assessed by the CAM-ICU. (*Adapted with permission from* Dr. E. Wesley Ely, http://www.icudelirium.org/).

localized disruption.[34,35] Two studies have demonstrated decreased cerebral blood flow in multiple areas of the brain in studies of delirious patients.[36,37] Other investigations have reported structural abnormalities in those experiencing delirium (eg, cerebral ventricles, gross white and gray matter atrophy, cortical and subcortical lesions, or ventricular enlargement).[36–40]

Inflammation and Sepsis

Sepsis-related inflammation likely contributes to the development of delirium in the ICU. Numerous mechanisms underlying this contribution have been proposed, with one prominent suggestion being that the inflammatory cascade occurring in sepsis may decrease essential oxygen delivery and nutrient to cells by impairing capillary flow.[41–43] Inflammatory mediators (ie, tumor necrosis factor α, interleukin-1, and other cytokines and chemokines) can result in disseminated intravascular coagulation, with leukocyte-vascular endothelium adhesion and induced endothelial damage. Sepsis-induced encephalopathy has been thought to be attributable to the degradation of the blood-brain barrier,[44] and the prolonged exposure to the lipopolysaccharide[45] may impair the synaptic transmission and neuronal excitability in the hippocampus. While these investigations suggest a link between delirium and sepsis, clearly more studies are needed to better evaluate the role of the inflammatory process and the coagulopathy related to sepsis and delirium.

Biomarkers, Neurotransmitters, Sedatives, and Analgesic Medications

The correlation between delirium, biomarkers, and different neurotransmitters is very poorly understood although data exist regarding potential interactions of delirium with acetylcholine, amino acids, and neurotransmitters such as monoamines and γ-amino-butyric acid (GABA). A comprehensive discussion of these interactions is beyond the scope of this review, although the authors offer several brief observations in the context of an overview. With regard to acetylcholine, it has been suggested that greater anticholinergic activity due to overuse of anticholinergic medications is associated with a subsequent increase in delirium symptom severity,[46] though the specific nature of this association needs to be further investigated. Similarly, limited evidence supports a possible association between amino acid precursors, and some investigators have proposed that the alteration of the availability of large neutral amino acids (LNAA) may be involved in the development of delirium.[47–49] Multiple neurotransmitters are also thought to be involved in delirium, including monoamines (eg, serotonin, dopamine, norepinephrine), imbalances in acetylcholine, glutamate, and GABA, with monoamines, in particular, modulating neurotransmission and thereby affecting behavior, cognitive functioning, and mood.[50] With regard to GABA, the primary inhibitory neurotransmitter in the central nervous system (CNS), its release has been hypothesized to be linked with delirium. As several agents widely used in the ICU (eg, benzodiazepines and propofol) have high affinity for GABAergic receptors, their relationship with delirium in the ICU is of significant interest. Recently, Pandharipande and colleagues[51] evaluated the relationship between administration of sedatives and analgesics and delirium in an ICU cohort, demonstrating that lorazepam is an independent risk factor for daily transition to delirium (odds ratio = 1.2, 95% CI 1.2–1.4). While sedative agents such as benzodiazepines and propofol act on the GABA receptor and are implicated in the genesis of delirium, novel GABA receptor-sparing agents (ie, dexmedetomidine) may be an alternative for sedation of ICU patients. Pandharipande and colleagues[52] reported that medical and surgical ICU patients sedated with dexmedetomidine have 4 more days alive without delirium or coma (median days, 7 vs 3.0; $P = .01$) than patients sedated with lorazepam. With regard to opiates data remain unclear, as findings to date have been inconsistent.[53,54]

The role of gene predisposition has also been investigated in the pathogenesis of delirium. Indeed the gene encoding for apolipoprotein E (APO-E) is a gene that has been evaluated for a possible relationship with ICU delirium. APO-E is known to be implicated with a higher susceptibility of Alzheimer disease as well as poorer cognitive outcomes after cardiac surgery, though results in this regard are somewhat equivocal.[55] Ely and colleagues[56] evaluated the relationship between APO-E genotypes and delirium in medical ICU patients, showing that the APO-E4 carriers were delirious for 2 more days than those without APO-E polymorphisms (median [interquartile range]: 4 [3–4.5] days versus 2 [1–4 days]; $P = .05$). Alternatively, one recent investigation found that among elderly medical patients, APO-E4 carriers were not found to have a higher risk of delirium.[57]

MANAGEMENT OF DELIRIUM: PREVENTION AND TREATMENT

Most studies conducted in the last several years evaluating preventative and treatment protocols for delirium have included non-ICU patients. ICU patients present a higher incidence of delirium, and a multifactorial approach should be considered to identify the presence of risk factors. The authors first describe the risk factors for delirium and available preventive and treatment protocols.

Risk Factors

Risk factors are typically considered to be in one of two categories: predisposing and precipitating. Though studied extensively in general medical populations, risk factors for delirium have been relatively little investigated in critically ill medical, surgical, and trauma patients.[4,6,56,58] As such, ICU clinicians and researchers should rely on evidence from the broader risk-factor literature, as appropriate. In a study by Dubois and colleagues[4] hypertension and history of smoking emerged as strong predictors of delirium in medical and surgical ICU cohorts. Elsewhere, Ouimet and colleagues[6] demonstrated that percentage of days with abnormal bilirubin level, exposure to morphine, and the epidural route of analgesia were also associated with delirium. Aldemir and colleagues[58] have reported a link between delirium and laboratory abnormalities such as hypocalcemia (<8 mg/mL), hyponatremia (<130 mmol/L), elevated levels of serum urea nitrogen (>100 mg/dL), hyperbilirubinemia (>10 mg/dL total bilirubin), and anemia (hematocrit <25%) in surgical ICU patients. Multiple other risk factors have been reported including age (>65 years), the presence of dementia at baseline, severity of illness, fever (38°C), infections, respiratory diseases, hypotension (symptomatic, or systolic blood pressure <80 mm Hg), and metabolic acidosis.[51,58,59]

Other risk factors have been elucidated in non-ICU cohorts but have not yet been shown to be associated with ICU delirium. These factors include use of physical restraints, use of bladder catheter, malnutrition (serum albumin level <30 g/L), impairment of vision (visual acuity <20/70), more than 3 medications added (during the 24–48-hour period before delirium onset), fracture on admission, and any iatrogenic event (eg, any diagnostic procedure or therapeutic intervention or any harmful occurrence that was not a natural consequence of the patient's illness).[60–62]

Analgesics and sedatives

ICU patients often receive analgesics and sedatives for the treatment of pain, the provision of comfort, and for anxiety reduction (particularly in the context of mechanical ventilation).[63] Some of these medications can have a detrimental effect and are risk factors for delirium. In particular, a strong association has been demonstrated between delirium and exposure to certain medications such as lorazepam, midazolam, and meperidine.[4,6,51,53,54] These studies highlight the importance of evaluating and treating pain, and suggest there could be potential advantages to the use of alternative sedatives such as α2-agonists for patients in the ICU.[52]

Sleep

Adequate sleep is critically important to ICU patients, though it is well known that sleep deprivation is common. Some evidence suggests that ICU patients "sleep" only 2 hours per day.[64] Although the link between sleep and delirium is unclear, evidence indicates that mechanical ventilation and sedative and analgesic exposure likely contribute to sleep-cycle alteration.[65] As sedatives common in the ICU such as lorazepam and midazolam are delirium risk factors and may act via sleep disruption, greater attention should be given to this association as a site of future intervention.

Impact of risk factors

Both predisposing and precipitating factors may interact to increase the risk of the development of delirium in individual patients. This notion has been articulated by Inouye and Charpentier,[60] who have posited that delirium develops in the context of the interplay between "vulnerability" and the severity of a given "insult." Put simply, individuals are admitted to the hospital with a set of predisposing factors that may make them particularly susceptible to developing delirium. In such patients, typically those who are both elderly and suffering from mild or moderate cognitive impairment, a single insult (eg, use of restraint) could be the factor contributing to delirium. Alternatively, patients resistant to the development of delirium could still experience this syndrome because of precipitating factors such as severity of illness, administration of sedatives, and immobilization, which could be seen as the precipitating cause of delirium. Clinicians could count also on the acronym ICUDELIRIUM(S) (**Table 1**) to easily remember the main risk factors and conditions linked to delirium and then create a risk stratification, as indicated by Inouye,[66] in which one point is given to each risk factor present at admission and a patient is classified as being at low (no risk factors), intermediate (1 or 2 risk factors), and high risk (3 or 4 risk factors) of developing delirium.

Prevention Protocols: Multicomponent and Pharmacologic Interventions

Multicomponent prevention protocols

Delirium is usually a multifactorial syndrome, often driven by various risk factors. Therefore, a multicomponent intervention approach designed to address primary risk factors may be the most effective. To date, no interventions have been conducted for this specific purpose in an ICU setting, but information may be gleaned from studies of general hospital and surgical patients (**Table 2**).

The Hospital Elder Life Program (HELP)[67] is a well-known study conducted with a focus on assessing the efficacy of a multicomponent approach to delirium treatment

---

Table 1
Mnemonic for risk factors and causes of ICUDELIRIUM(S)

Iatrogenic exposure	• Consider any diagnostic procedure or therapeutic intervention or any harmful occurrence that was not a natural consequence of the patient's illness
Cognitive impairment	• Preexisting dementia, or MCI or depression
Use of restraints and catheters	• Reevaluate the use of restraints and bladder catheters daily
Drugs	• Evaluate the use of sedatives (eg, benzodiazepines or opiates) and medications with anticholinergic activity • Consider the abrupt cessation of smoking or alcohol • Consider withdrawal from chronically used sedatives
Elderly	• Evaluate patients older than 65 years with greater attention
Laboratory abnormalities	• Especially hyponatremia, azotemia, hyperbilirubinemia, hypocalcemia, and metabolic acidosis
Infection	• Sepsis and severe sepsis • Especially urinary, respiratory tract infections
Respiratory	• Consider respiratory failure (Pco_2 >45 mm Hg or Po_2 <55 mm Hg or oxygen saturation <88%) • Consider causes such as COPD, ARDS, PE
Intracranial perfusion	• Consider presence of hypertension or hypotension • Consider hemorrhage, stroke, tumor
Urinary/fecal retention	• Consider urinary retention or fecal impaction, especially in elderly and postoperative patients
Myocardial	• Consider myocardial causes: myocardial infarction, acute heart failure, arrhythmia
Sleep and sensory deprivation	• Consider the alterations of the sleep cycle and sleep deprivation • Consider the nonavailability of glasses (poor vision) • Consider the nonavailability of hearing devices (poor hearing)

Abbreviations: ARDS, acute respiratory distress syndrome; COPD, chronic obstructive pulmonary disease; MCI, mild cognitive impairment; PE, pulmonary embolism.

Table 2
Delirium management in the ICU[a]

	Interventions	Setting and Study Design
Step 1: Prevention		
1. Evaluation of risk factors		
2. Multicomponent protocols		
Multicomponent strategy[67]	Targeted intervention on cognitive impairment, sleep deprivation, immobilization, psychoactive medications, vision impairment, hearing impairment, dehydration	Non-ICU clinical trial
Proactive geriatric consultation[68]	Daily visits with geriatrics for entire hospital duration, with target recommendations used	Non-ICU clinical trial
Nursing-led model[95]	(1) Nursing detection of delirium with validated tools. (2) Nursing evaluation of potential causes of delirium when delirium is diagnosed. (3) Proactive plan for preventing and managing the common risk factors involving nurses and physicians. (4) Create an environment that enhances reintegration and help the patient to reduce confusion and agitation	Non-ICU clinical trial
3. Pharmacologic protocols		
Haloperidol[71]	Haloperidol 0.5 mg 3 times a day, started at admission and continued until 3 days after surgery	Non-ICU (hip surgery patients) randomized, placebo-controlled trial
Risperidone[72]	Risperidone 1 mg after surgery	Non-ICU (postcardiac surgery) double-blind, placebo-controlled randomized trial
Sedation with dexmedetomidine[52]	Dexmedetomidine to a maximum dose of 1.5 μg/kg per hour	ICU randomized trial
Step 2: Treatment		
Pharmacologic treatment		
Haloperidol[63]	Haloperidol 2–5 mg (0.5–2 mg in the elderly) intravenously, followed by double repeated doses every 15–20 min if agitation persists up to a maximum of 20 mg/d	SCCM Guidelines[63]
Olanzapine[86]	Olanzapine, starting dose 5 mg (2.5 mg over 65 years) and titrated on clinical judgment	ICU randomized trial, no placebo group
Risperidone[87]	Risperidone, starting dose 0.5 mg twice a day, up to a maximum of 2.5 mg/d	ICU and non-ICU, blind clinical trial. No placebo group

Abbreviation: SCCM, Society of Critical Care Medicine.
[a] The data included in this table are obtained combining ICU and non-ICU studies.

and management. The study consisted of an intervention aimed at 6 delirium risk factors (ie, cognitive impairment, sleep deprivation, immobilization, psychoactive medications, vision impairment, hearing impairment, and dehydration). Delirium incidence was reduced in the intervention group in comparison with the usual care group (9.9% vs 15%). No differences were noted between groups with regard to delirium severity of recurrence rates, however. In a similar vein, Marcantonio and colleagues[68] studied the effects of randomizing hip surgery patients to proactive geriatric consultation versus usual care, finding that those receiving geriatric consultation (a very comprehensive array of assessments and/or interventions) experienced a 36% relative risk reduction in incident delirium but no benefits with regard to abbreviated delirium duration or delirium severity. Other studies[69,70] have demonstrated that multifactorial interventions are effective in reducing the duration, but not the incidence, of delirium.

Pharmacologic prevention protocols

To date two studies[71,72] have evaluated the efficacy of antipsychotics for delirium prevention. Data are unclear regarding the use of anticholinergic drugs (ie, rivastigmine and donepezil) for delirium prevention and treatment.[73,74]

Kaslivaart and colleagues[71] conducted a randomized, double-blind, placebo-controlled trial in hip surgery patients and showed that that low-dose prophylactic haloperidol (0.5 mg 3 times a day, started at admission and continued until 3 days after surgery) was ineffective compared with placebo in reducing the incidence of postoperative delirium, though it reduced delirium severity (as measured by the DRS-R-98, with a mean difference of 4.0; 95% CI 2.0–5.8; P = .001).

Prakanrattana and Prapaitrakool[72] concluded, in a double-blind, placebo-controlled randomized trial, that a single dose (1 mg) of risperidone following coronary artery bypass surgery reduced postoperative delirium incidence (11.1% vs 31.7%, respectively; P = .009, relative risk = 0.35, 95% CI 0.16–0.77).

The chronic use of rivastigmine in patients affected by dementia may help prevent delirium in high-risk elderly patients admitted to a medical ward.[74] Donepezil was shown to be ineffective in delirium prevention and treatment in a randomized controlled trial including a cohort of an older population without dementia undergoing elective total joint replacement surgery.[73]

Of interest is that benzodiazepines are frequently used as sedatives in the ICU although they themselves have been shown to be deliriogenic.[6,51,53,54] Pandharipande and colleagues[52] piloted an approach using a new sedation protocol with dexmedetomidine, a highly selective α2-agonist, versus lorazepam in medical and surgical ICU patients. Individuals treated with dexmedetomidine spent fewer days in coma and more time neurologically "normal" (defined as without coma or delirium) than their counterparts sedated via lorazepam. This preliminary work suggests a need for larger trials aiming to prove α2-receptor agonists (eg, dexmedetomidine, clonidine) to be alternative sedative agents less likely to cause delirium than the benzodiazepines.

Pharmacologic Treatment

The use of medications in the treatment of delirium is common, and should be considered following a thorough assessment of relevant predisposing and precipitating risk factors. At present, haloperidol is the drug of choice for the treatment of delirium as indicated by the Guidelines of the Society of Critical Care Medicine[63] and of the American Psychiatry Association (APA),[75] though its efficacy has not been tested in a placebo-controlled trial. Several open trials[76–85] have evaluated the efficacy of typical and atypical antipsychotic delirium treatment, but only two have included a cohort of ICU patients.[86,87]

Skrobik and colleagues[86] studied the safety and clinical utility of olanzapine (starting dose 5 mg daily) versus haloperidol (starting dose 2.5–5 mg every 8 hours) for the treatment of ICU delirium. Olanzapine and haloperidol were associated with reduction in delirium symptoms over time. However, recommendation for it and other atypical antipsychotics as a treatment for delirium in the critical care setting is limited by the current trial and absence of placebo-controlled data. Han and Kim[87] evaluated, in a double-blind trial, the efficacy of risperidone (starting dose 0.5 mg twice a day) versus haloperidol (starting dose 0.75 mg twice a day) for treatment of delirium in 24 medical, oncology, and ICU patients, concluding that no significant differences existed between groups on outcome measures including delirium severity scores. More recently two randomized clinical trials including placebo in their design, have investigated the role of typical and atypical antipsychotics for the treatment of delirium in critically ill patients.[88,89]

Devlin and colleagues[88] compared the efficacy of the addition of a regimen of as needed haloperidol plus quetiapine (50 mg every 12 hours and titrated on a daily basis by increments of 50 mg every 12 hours to a maximum dose of 200 mg every 12 hours) vs as needed haloperidol plus placebo in the treatment of 36 ICU delirious patients. Medications were titrated to effect, such that if a patient required open-label haloperidol for agitation in the last 24-hours the dose of the study drug was increased. Patients treated with quetiapine had faster resolution of delirium compared to the placebo (Median [IQR] 1.0 [0.5–3.0] days for quetiapine vs 4.5 [2.0–7.0] days for placebo, $P = .001$).

In a second trial Girard and colleagues[89] conducted the Modifying the Incidence of Delirium (MIND) Trial, which randomized 103 medical and surgical mechanically ventilated ICU patients to treatment with haloperidol (5 mg), ziprasidone (40 mg) or placebo. Duration of delirium was similar between groups (haloperidol: 14.0 vs ziprasidone 15.0 vs placebo 12.5, $P = .66$). This trial was conducted as a pilot, feasibility, study and therefore was not powered to answer to determine the efficacy of antipsychotics in the treatment of delirium. A larger scale trial is now being performed (NCT01211522).

From the data currently available, atypical (eg, olanzapine, risperidone, quetiapine, ziprasidone) and typical antipsychotics (eg, haloperidol) may or may not be helpful in the treatment of delirium. Typical and atypical antipsychotics, especially in elderly patients with dementia, have been associated with increased mortality[90–93] and confer potential side effects more generally. To date the studies that have evaluated the short-term used of antipsychotics for the treatment of delirium have not shown an increased risk of death. However, these studies did not focus on the side effects of these drugs in geriatric ICU patients with dementia. As such, future studies of antipsychotics should include this particular aspect as an outcome measure.

SUMMARY

Delirium is recognized as a common form of acute brain dysfunction in medically ill patients in general and critically ill patients in particular, leading researchers to view it as the "sixth vital sign."[94] Mechanisms implicated in the pathophysiology of delirium are still elusive. Intriguing data are available with respect to the interaction between sepsis, acetylcholine levels, the interaction between drugs that altering GABA levels, and delirium. Several risk factors are thought to be associated with delirium, including specific medications for sedation or pain management, widely used in an ICU setting; their use should therefore be carefully evaluated. Current multicomponent protocols and pharmacologic interventions designed for the non-ICU setting can potentially be adapted for a critical-care setting. Future studies in the ICU setting should build on current work, to (1) assess the efficacy of multicomponent protocols to prevent delirium and (2) assess the safety and efficacy of antipsychotics versus placebo in the prevention and treatment of delirium, while carefully evaluating the outcomes in elderly patients with dementia.

Key Points

1. Medically ill patients, particularly populations at high risk (eg, ICU patients) should receive a complete evaluation of predisposing and precipitating risk factors, giving particular attention to the exposure to pain medications and sedatives

2. It is mandatory to assess and diagnose delirium in the ICU with the use of available tools such as the ICDSC and the CAM-ICU

REFERENCES

1. Ely EW, Inouye SK, Bernard GR, et al. Delirium in mechanically ventilated patients: validity and reliability of the confusion assessment method for the intensive care unit (CAM-ICU). JAMA 2001;286(21):2703–10.
2. Bergeron N, Dubois MJ, Dumont M, et al. Intensive Care Delirium Screening Checklist: evaluation of a new screening tool. Intensive Care Med 2001;27(5): 859–64.
3. Ely EW, Margolin R, Francis J, et al. Evaluation of delirium in critically ill patients: validation of the Confusion Assessment Method for the Intensive Care Unit (CAM-ICU). Crit Care Med 2001;29(7):1370–9.
4. Dubois MJ, Bergeron N, Dumont M, et al. Delirium in an intensive care unit: a study of risk factors. Intensive Care Med 2001;27(8):1297–304.
5. Ely EW, Gautam S, Margolin R, et al. The impact of delirium in the intensive care unit on hospital length of stay. Intensive Care Med 2001;27(12):1892–900.
6. Ouimet S, Kavanagh BP, Gottfried SB, et al. Incidence, risk factors and consequences of ICU delirium. Intensive Care Med 2007;33(1):66–73.
7. Thomason JW, Shintani A, Peterson JF, et al. Intensive care unit delirium is an independent predictor of longer hospital stay: a prospective analysis of 261 non-ventilated patients. Crit Care 2005;9(4):R375–81.
8. Milbrandt EB, Deppen S, Harrison PL, et al. Costs associated with delirium in mechanically ventilated patients. Crit Care Med 2004;32(4):955–62.
9. Ely EW, Shintani A, Truman B, et al. Delirium as a predictor of mortality in mechanically ventilated patients in the intensive care unit. JAMA 2004;291(14): 1753–62.
10. Lin SM, Liu CY, Wang CH, et al. The impact of delirium on the survival of mechanically ventilated patients. Crit Care Med 2004;32(11):2254–9.
11. McNicoll L, Pisani MA, Inouye SK. One-year outcomes following delirium in older ICU patients. J Am Geriatr Soc 2004;52:S2.
12. Jackson JC, Gordon SM, Hart RP, et al. The association between delirium and cognitive decline: a review of the empirical literature. Neuropsychol Rev 2004; 14(2):87–98.
13. Jackson JC, Gordon SM, Girard TD, et al. Delirium as a risk factor for long term cognitive impairment in mechanically ventilated ICU survivors. Am J Respir Crit Care Med 2007;175:A22.

14. American Psychiatric Association. Diagnostic and statistical manual of mental disorders, text revision. 4th edition. Washington, DC: American Psychiatric Association; 2000.
15. Farrell KR, Ganzini L. Misdiagnosing delirium as depression in medically ill elderly patients. Arch Intern Med 1995;155(22):2459–64.
16. Lipowski ZJ. Delirium in the elderly patient. N Engl J Med 1989;320(9):578–82.
17. Lipowski ZJ. Delirium: acute confusional states. Rev. ed. New York: Oxford University Press; 1990.
18. Meagher DJ, Trzepacz PT. Motoric subtypes of delirium. Semin Clin Neuropsychiatry 2000;5(2):75–85.
19. Peterson JF, Pun BT, Dittus RS, et al. Delirium and its motoric subtypes: a study of 614 critically ill patients. J Am Geriatr Soc 2006;54(3):479–84.
20. Cole M, McCusker J, Dendukuri N, et al. The prognostic significance of subsyndromal delirium in elderly medical inpatients. J Am Geriatr Soc 2003;51(6): 754–60.
21. Levkoff SE, Liptzin B, Cleary PD, et al. Subsyndromal delirium. Am J Geriatr Psychiatry 1996;4:320–9.
22. Levkoff SE, Yang FM, Liptzin B. Delirium: the importance of subsyndromal states. Prim Psychiatr 2004;11:40–4.
23. Marcantonio ER, Ta T, Duthrie E, et al. Delirium severity and psychomotor types: their relationship with outcomes after hip fracture repair. J Am Geriatr Soc 2002; 50:850–7.
24. Ouimet S, Riker R, Bergeon N, et al. Subsyndromal delirium in the ICU: evidence for a disease spectrum. Intensive Care Med 2007;33(6):1007–13.
25. Inouye SK, van Dyck CH, Alessi CA, et al. Clarifying confusion: the confusion assessment method. A new method for detection of delirium. Ann Intern Med 1990;113(12):941–8.
26. Ely EW, Truman B, Shintani A, et al. Monitoring sedation status over time in ICU patients: reliability and validity of the Richmond Agitation-Sedation Scale (RASS). JAMA 2003;289(22):2983–91.
27. Sessler CN, Gosnell MS, Grap MJ, et al. The Richmond Agitation-Sedation Scale: validity and reliability in adult intensive care unit patients. Am J Respir Crit Care Med 2002;166(10):1338–44.
28. Flacker JM, Lipsitz LA. Serum anticholinergic activity changes with acute illness in elderly medical patients. J Gerontol A Biol Sci Med Sci 1999;54(1):M12–6.
29. Gunther ML, Morandi A, Ely EW. Pathophysiology of delirium in the intensive care unit. Crit Care Clin 2008;24(1):45–65, viii.
30. Inouye SK, Ferrucci L. Elucidating the pathophysiology of delirium and the interrelationship of delirium and dementia. J Gerontol A Biol Sci Med Sci 2006;61(12): 1277–80.
31. Van Der Mast RC. Pathophysiology of delirium. J Geriatr Psychiatry Neurol 1998; 11:138–45.
32. Trzepacz PT. Delirium. Advances in diagnosis, pathophysiology, and treatment. Psychiatr Clin North Am 1996;19(3):429–48.
33. Trzepacz PT. Is there a final common neural pathway in delirium? Focus on acetylcholine and dopamine. Semin Clin Neuropsychiatry 2000;5:132–48.
34. Gunther ML, Jackson JC, Wesley EE. Loss of IQ in the ICU brain injury without the insult. Med Hypotheses 2007;69(6):1179–82.
35. Robertsson B, Olsson L, Wallin A. Occurrence of delirium in different regional brain syndromes. Dement Geriatr Cogn Disord 1999;10(4):278–83.

36. Fong TG, Bogardus ST Jr, Daftary A, et al. Cerebral perfusion changes in older delirious patients using 99mTc HMPAO SPECT. J Gerontol A Biol Sci Med Sci 2006;61(12):1294–9.
37. Yokota H, Ogawa S, Kurokawa A, et al. Regional cerebral blood flow in delirium patients. Psychiatry Clin Neurosci 2003;57(3):337–9.
38. Alsop DC, Fearing MA, Johnson K, et al. The role of neuroimaging in elucidating delirium pathophysiology. J Gerontol A Biol Sci Med Sci 2006;61(12): 1287–93.
39. Hopkins RO, Gale SD, Weaver LK. Brain atrophy and cognitive impairment in survivors of acute respiratory distress syndrome. Brain Inj 2006;20(3):263–71.
40. Koponen H, Hurri L, Stenback U, et al. Computed tomography findings in delirium. J Nerv Ment Dis 1989;177(4):226–31.
41. Goyette RE, Key NS, Ely EW. Hematologic changes in sepsis and their therapeutic implications. Semin Respir Crit Care Med 2004;25:645–59.
42. Opal SM, Esmon CT. Bench-to-bedside review: functional relationships between coagulation and the innate immune response and their respective roles in the pathogenesis of sepsis. Crit Care 2003;7(1):23–38.
43. Terborg C, Schummer W, Albrecht M, et al. Dysfunction of vasomotor reactivity in severe sepsis and septic shock. Intensive Care Med 2001;27(7):1231–4.
44. Sharshar T, Carlier R, Bernard F, et al. Brain lesions in septic shock: a magnetic resonance imaging study. Intensive Care Med 2007;33(5):798–806.
45. Hellstrom IC, Danik M, Luheshi GN, et al. Chronic LPS exposure produces changes in intrinsic membrane properties and a sustained IL-beta-dependent increase in GABAergic inhibition in hippocampal CA1 pyramidal neurons. Hippocampus 2005;15(5):656–64.
46. Han L, McCusker J, Cole M, et al. Use of medications with anticholinergic effect predicts clinical severity of delirium symptoms in older medical inpatients. Arch Intern Med 2001;161(8):1099–105.
47. Balan S, Leibovitz A, Zila SO, et al. The relation between the clinical subtypes of delirium and the urinary level of 6-SMT. J Neuropsychiatry Clin Neurosci 2003;15: 363–6.
48. Flacker JM, Lipsitz LA. Large neutral amino acid changes and delirium in febrile elderly medical patients. J Gerontol A Biol Sci Med Sci 2000;55:B249–52.
49. Van Der Mast RC, van den Broek WW, Fekkes D, et al. Incidence of and preoperative predictors for delirium after cardiac surgery. J Psychosom Res 1999;46: 479–83.
50. Bloom FE, Kupfer DJ, Bunney BS, et al. Amines. Psychopharmacology: the fourth generation of progress. New York: Raven Press; 1995. p. 1287–359.
51. Pandharipande P, Shintani A, Peterson J, et al. Lorazepam is an independent risk factor for transitioning to delirium in intensive care unit patients. Anesthesiology 2006;104(1):21–6.
52. Pandharipande PP, Pun BT, Herr DL, et al. Effect of sedation with dexmedetomidine vs lorazepam on acute brain dysfunction in mechanically ventilated patients: the MENDS randomized controlled trial. JAMA 2007; 298(22):2644–53.
53. Marcantonio ER, Juarez G, Goldman L, et al. The relationship of postoperative delirium with psychoactive medications. JAMA 1994;272(19):1518–22.
54. Pandharipande P, Cotton BA, Shintani A, et al. Prevalence and risk factors for development of delirium in surgical and trauma intensive care unit patients. J Trauma 2008;65(1):34–41.

55. Corder EH, Saunders AM, Strittmatter WJ, et al. Gene dose of apolipoprotein E type 4 allele and the risk of Alzheimer's disease in late onset families. Science 1993;261(5123):921–3.
56. Ely EW, Girard TD, Shintani AK, et al. Apolipoprotein E4 polymorphism as a genetic predisposition to delirium in critically ill patients. Crit Care Med 2007; 35(1):112–7.
57. van Munster BC, Korevaar JC, de Rooij SE, et al. The association between delirium and the apolipoprotein E ε4 allele in the elderly. Psychiatr Genet 2007; 17(5):261–6.
58. Aldemir M, Ozen S, Kara IH, et al. Predisposing factors for delirium in the surgical intensive care unit. Crit Care 2001;5(5):265–70.
59. McNicoll L, Pisani MA, Zhang Y, et al. Delirium in the intensive care unit: occurrence and clinical course in older patients. J Am Geriatr Soc 2003;51(5):591–8.
60. Inouye SK, Charpentier PA. Precipitating factors for delirium in hospitalized elderly persons. Predictive model and interrelationship with baseline vulnerability. JAMA 1996;275(11):852–7.
61. Inouye SK. Predisposing and precipitating factors for delirium in hospitalized older patients. Dement Geriatr Cogn Disord 1999;10(5):393–400.
62. Schor JD, Levkoff SE, Lipsitz LA, et al. Risk factors for delirium in hospitalized elderly. JAMA 1992;267(6):827–31.
63. Jacobi J, Fraser GL, Coursin DB, et al. Clinical practice guidelines for the sustained use of sedatives and analgesics in the critically ill adult. Crit Care Med 2002;30(1):119–41.
64. Aurell J, Elmqvist D. Sleep in the surgical intensive care unit: continuous polygraphic recording of sleep in nine patients receiving postoperative care. Br Med J (Clin Res Ed) 1985;290(6474):1029–32.
65. Gabor JY, Cooper AB, Crombach SA, et al. Contribution of the intensive care unit environment to sleep disruption in mechanically ventilated patients and healthy subjects. Am J Respir Crit Care Med 2003;167(5):708–15.
66. Inouye SK. Prevention of delirium in hospitalized older patients: risk factors and targeted intervention strategies. Ann Med 2000;32(4):257–63.
67. Inouye SK, Bogardus ST Jr, Charpentier PA, et al. A multicomponent intervention to prevent delirium in hospitalized older patients. N Engl J Med 1999;340(9):669–76.
68. Marcantonio ER, Flacker JM, Wright RJ, et al. Reducing delirium after hip fracture: a randomized trial. J Am Geriatr Soc 2001;49(5):516–22.
69. Lundstrom M, Edlund A, Karlsson S, et al. A multifactorial intervention program reduces the duration of delirium, length of hospitalization, and mortality in delirious patients. J Am Geriatr Soc 2005;53(4):622–8.
70. Milisen K, Foreman MD, Abraham IL, et al. A nurse-led interdisciplinary intervention program for delirium in elderly hip-fracture patients. J Am Geriatr Soc 2001; 49:523–32.
71. Kalisvaart KJ, de Jonghe JF, Bogaards MJ, et al. Haloperidol prophylaxis for elderly hip-surgery patients at risk for delirium: a randomized placebo-controlled study. J Am Geriatr Soc 2005;53(10):1658–66.
72. Prakanrattana U, Prapaitrakool S. Efficacy of risperidone for prevention of postoperative delirium in cardiac surgery. Anaesth Intensive Care 2007;35(5):714–9.
73. Liptzin B, Laki A, Garb JL, et al. Donepezil in the prevention and treatment of post-surgical delirium. Am J Geriatr Psychiatry 2005;13(12):1100–6.
74. Dautzenberg PL, Mulder LJ, Olde Rikkert MG, et al. Delirium in elderly hospitalised patients: protective effects of chronic rivastigmine usage. Int J Geriatr Psychiatry 2004;19(7):641–4.

75. American Psychiatric Association. Practice guideline for the treatment of patients with delirium. Am J Psychiatry 1999;156(Suppl 5):1–20.

76. Breitbart W, Tremblay A, Gibson C. An open trial of olanzapine for the treatment of delirium in hospitalized cancer patients [abstract]. Psychosomatics 2002;43: 175–82.

77. Horikawa N, Yamazaki T, Miyamoto K, et al. Treatment for delirium with risperidone: results of a prospective open trial with 10 patients. Gen Hosp Psychiatry 2003;25(4):289–92.

78. Kim KS, Pae CU, Chae JH, et al. An open pilot trial of olanzapine for delirium in the Korean population. Psychiatry Clin Neurosci 2001;55(5):515–9.

79. Kim KY, Bader GM, Kotlyar V, et al. Treatment of delirium in older adults with quetiapine. J Geriatr Psychiatry Neurol 2003;16(1):29–31.

80. Lee KU, Won WY, Lee HK, et al. Amisulpride versus quetiapine for the treatment of delirium: a randomized, open prospective study. Int Clin Psychopharmacol 2005;20(6):311–4.

81. Mittal D, Jimerson NA, Neely EP, et al. Risperidone in the treatment of delirium: results from a prospective open-label trial. J Clin Psychiatry 2004;65(5):662–7.

82. Pae CU, Lee SJ, Lee CU, et al. A pilot trial of quetiapine for the treatment of patients with delirium. Hum Psychopharmacol 2004;19(2):125–7.

83. Parellada E, Baeza I, de Pablo J, et al. Risperidone in the treatment of patients with delirium. J Clin Psychiatry 2004;65:348–53.

84. Sasaki Y, Matsuyama T, Inoue S, et al. A prospective, open-label, flexible-dose study of quetiapine in the treatment of delirium. J Clin Psychiatry 2003;64(11): 1316–21.

85. Sipahimalani A, Masand PS. Olanzapine in the treatment of delirium. Psychosomatics 1998;39:422–30.

86. Skrobik YK, Bergeron N, Dumont M, et al. Olanzapine vs haloperidol: treating delirium in a critical care setting. Intensive Care Med 2004;30(3):444–9.

87. Han CS, Kim YK. A double-blind trial of risperidone and haloperidol for the treatment of delirium. Psychosomatics 2004;45(4):297–301.

88. Devlin JW, Roberts RJ, Fong JJ, et al. Efficacy and safety of quetiapine in critically ill patients with delirium: a prospective, multicenter, randomized, double-blind, placebo-controlled pilot study. Crit Care Med 2010;38(2):419–27.

89. Girard TD, Pandharipande PP, Carson SS, et al. Feasibility, efficacy, and safety of antipsychotics for intensive care unit delirium: the MIND randomized, placebo-controlled trial. Crit Care Med 2010;38(2):428–37.

90. Gill SS, Bronskill SE, Normand SL, et al. Antipsychotic drug use and mortality in older adults with dementia. Ann Intern Med 2007;146(11):775–86.

91. Rochon PA, Normand SL, Gomes T, et al. Antipsychotic therapy and short-term serious events in older adults with dementia. Arch Intern Med 2008;168(10):1090–6.

92. Schneider LS, Dagerman KS, Insel P. Risk of death with atypical antipsychotic drug treatment for dementia: meta-analysis of randomized placebo-controlled trials. JAMA 2005;294(15):1934–43.

93. Wang PS, Schneeweiss S, Avorn J, et al. Risk of death in elderly users of conventional vs. atypical antipsychotic medications. N Engl J Med 2005;353(22): 2335–41.

94. Flaherty JH, Rudolph J, Shay K, et al. Delirium is a serious and under-recognized problem: why assessment of mental status should be the sixth vital sign. J Am Geriatr Soc 2007;8(5):273–5.

95. Bergmann MA, Murphy KM, Kiely DK, et al. A model for management of delirious postacute care patients. J Am Geriatr Soc 2005;53(10):1817–25.

Impaired Consciousness and Herniation Syndromes

G. Bryan Young, MD, FRCP(C)

KEYWORDS

• Stupor • Coma • Herniation • Prognosis

This article reviews alterations in consciousness related to intracranial mass lesions. Such lesions can produce impairment of consciousness by their strategic location within components of the ascending reticular activating system (ARAS; see the article by Goldfine and Schiff elsewhere in this issue) or secondarily by compressing or distorting this system, interfering with its synaptic and neurochemical functions. This review concentrates principally on this secondary mechanism.

GRADATION OF IMPAIRMENT OF CONSCIOUSNESS

Consciousness is not a unitary entity, but is composed of two principal components: alertness and awareness. For practical purposes, the capacity for alertness is a prerequisite for awareness. As mentioned in two articles by Goldfine and Schiff; Hocher and Rabinstein elsewhere in this issue, alertness/arousal/awakening is dependent on the functional integrity of the ARAS, a network of neurons running from the midpontine tegmentum, through the dorsal midbrain and the thalamus (midline and intralaminar nuclei especially), and through to the cerebral cortex.

Classifying the degree of impairment of consciousness has traditionally used "coma scales," the most universal being the Glasgow Coma Scale; the most recent, and most useful, for intensive care unit patients appears to be the FOUR Score. These scales are discussed in detail, along with the assessment, in another article by Hocher and Rabinstein elsewhere in this issue.

Three commonly used terms to express progressively impaired consciousness are delirium, stupor, and coma. Even within these 3 entities there are various degrees of

The author has nothing to disclose.
Division of Neurology, Department of Clinical Neurological Sciences, University of Western Ontario, London Health Sciences Centre, 339 Windermere Road, London, Ontario N6A 5A5, Canada
E-mail address: bryan.young@lhsc.on.ca

Neurol Clin 29 (2011) 765–772
doi:10.1016/j.ncl.2011.07.008
0733-8619/11/$ – see front matter © 2011 Published by Elsevier Inc.

neurologic.theclinics.com

impairment, which makes clinical behavioral descriptions more useful than these "umbrella terms." These impairments are briefly discussed here.

Delirium

Delirium is well reviewed in the article by Angel and Young elsewhere in this issue. It is important to bear in mind that delirium is a type of impairment of consciousness, both the wakefulness and awareness components, and is characterized principally by problems with sustained attention. The other aspects, for example, impaired memory, poor sleep patterns, agitation or abulia, hallucinations, and autonomic changes, are varied "add-ons."

Stupor

Stupor means "stunned" in Latin, and refers to a state of unconsciousness from which the patient can be roused only by strong stimulation. There is clearly impairment in the function of the ARAS, but this network can be "activated" for brief periods. The patient tends to drift into a sleeplike state if unstimulated for even a few minutes.

Coma

Coma refers to unarousable unconsciousness, and represents a deeper state of impaired alertness than stupor. Typically the patient does not open the eyes to stimulation (with the exception of some cases of myoclonic seizures that are sometimes stimulus triggered). However, there is a gradation of motor responses that can occur in coma, ranging from no motor response to localizing the stimulus, for example, moving an upper limb toward the part of the body being stimulated.[1] Coma rarely lasts more than 3 weeks in patients who survive, as the redundancy of neurotransmitters and pathways in the ARAS allows for some degree of recovery of alerting responses.

Disorders of Awareness

Awareness is an integrated function of the cerebral cortex and thalamus. How awareness arises from the "complex system" that constitutes brain function is still not understood.[2] However, much can be learned of brain function from deficits, even though it is artificial to divide awareness into components that are affected by focal brain lesions. Perceptual tasks are heavily dependent on the posterior cerebrum, for example, processing of visual, auditory, and somatosensory information. Planning, motivation, and initiation and execution of motor tasks take place in the anterior cerebrum. Limbic structures are involved in memory and emotion and, of course, must tie in with both perceptual and executive functions. Further insights into deficits and the effects of "activation" of various brain regions are given in the three relevant articles by Goldfine and Schiff; Hocher and Rabinstein; Blumenfeld elsewhere in this issue.

HERNIATION SYNDROMES

A hernia is a protrusion or rupture. Medically the term was first used to describe gut herniation through a defect in the abdominal wall, diaphragm, or an abnormal opening, for example, an incisional hernia. However, with respect to brain tissue the term is used to describe a displacement of part of the brain from one compartment into another. The key concept is *compression* and displacement of brain structures from their normal anatomic location.

To produce impairment of alertness the displacement has to compress structures that form essential components of the ARAS (see the relevant article by Goldfine and Schiff elsewhere in this issue). In the classical view, based on the work of Plum and Posner,[3] unilateral, supratentorial mass lesions produce coma through downward displacement and compression of the diencephalon then brainstem or mesial temporal lobe structures, compressing the midbrain through the tentorial opening: "central" and "uncal" tentorial herniations, respectively. However, an alternative view is that the initial impairment of consciousness more commonly relates to lateral rather than downward herniation. This concept was initially proposed by Hasenjäger and Spatz[4] and by Fisher.[5] More recently, Ropper[6–9] has provided convincing evidence for subfalcial herniation with modern neuroimaging and careful postmortem examinations (**Table 1**). Indeed, there is a direct correlation between the shift of midline of the pineal gland in millimeters (mm) and the depth of impairment of consciousness (see **Table 1**). Most cases of coma show a lateral shift of 9 mm or greater.

The initial oculomotor nerve palsy that was earlier attributed to uncal herniation is more likely related to stretching of the third cranial nerve over the clivus, as part of the lateral supratentorial displacement.[9]

Transtentorial herniation does occur, but it is a relatively late event, is often terminal, and is associated with brainstem damage. The loss of reactivity of the contralateral pupil, oculomotor palsy on the side opposite the mass lesion, is usually due to intrinsic brainstem damage from compression.[10]

Other herniations are of somewhat less importance, as they are late and usually represent an advanced stage of brain swelling with a fatal outcome. Upward and downward cerebellar herniation fit into this category. Most often brainstem dysfunction from a rapidly enlarging cerebellar mass, for example, hemorrhage or infarct with swelling, is attributable to direct compression of the brainstem.

The advent of modern neuroimaging has provided better visualization of the early phases of herniation, obviating the need to rely on postmortem specimens that show the end result.

Subfalcial Herniation

There is a direct correlation between the number of millimeters of horizontal shift of the pineal gland (less precise correlation with the septum pellucidum shift) and the degree of impairment of alertness.[6] Shifts of 3 to 4 mm are not associated with any drowsiness, but greater shifts are accompanied by drowsiness, with stupor appearing between 6 and 9 mm and coma at greater than 9 mm (**Fig. 1**).[5,6] Compression of the pericallosal and callosomarginal arteries against the falx can lead to infarction of the medial surface of the frontal lobes, namely the cingulate gyrus, the medial portion of the superior frontal gyrus, and as far back as the precuneus. The edema that follows such infarction can lead to further mass effect.

Transtentorial Herniation

Transtentorial herniation has been divided into uncal and central types by Plum and Posner (**Fig. 2**).[3] In both types there is a downward displacement of brain through

Table 1 Horizontal pineal displacement and impaired consciousness	
Consciousness Level	**Distance from Midline (mm)**
Awake and alert	0–3
Drowsy	3–6
Stupor	6–9
Coma	>9

Data from Ropper AH. Lateral displacement of the brain and level of consciousness in patients with an acute hemispheral mass. N Engl J Med 1986;314:953–8.

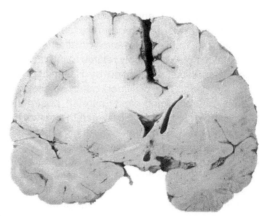

Fig. 1. Subfalcial herniation without uncal herniation. The patient had a meningioma overlying the right cerebral hemisphere, which produced cerebral edema and subfalcial herniation. Death occurred as a result of respiratory complications.

the tentorial opening. Both lateralized uncal and the more direct downward transtentorial herniation represent advanced stages of herniation. As already mentioned, the initial or "early third nerve stage" of uncal herniation (with an oculomotor nerve palsy ipsilateral to the mass) is more likely caused by stretching of the third nerve than compression by the uncus, and the decline in consciousness is more acutely related to the degree of lateral shift of supratentorial structures than to downward displacement (see earlier discussion). With advanced transtentorial herniation, the midbrain becomes compressed with loss of pupillary reactivity of the opposite pupil and shows decerebrate posturing. At this point the patient is usually unsalvageable, due to irreversible damage to the midbrain.[10] Neuroimaging and postmortem examination reveal ischemia and hemorrhage in the distribution of paramedian arteries of the midbrain and pons (Duret/crowsfoot hemorrhages: **Figs. 3** and **4**).

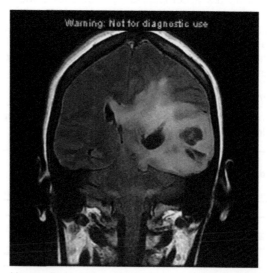

Fig. 2. Left temporal hemorrhagic lesion with both central and uncal herniation, with brainstem compression.

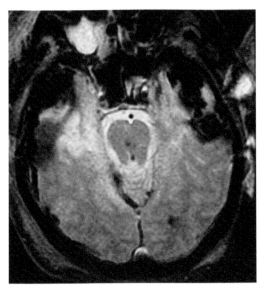

Fig. 3. Duret hemorrhage in the caudal midbrain from transtentorial herniation on magnetic resonance imaging.

Tonsillar Herniation

The herniation of the cerebellar tonsils through the foramen magnum in cases of mass effect relates to a pressure gradient between the posterior fossa and the upper spinal canal (**Fig. 5**). When this happens acutely there is compression of the caudal medulla, resulting in respiratory arrest. The obstruction to the outflow of the fourth ventricle causes an abrupt increase in intracranial pressure. Thus, tonsillar herniation is typically a terminal event, as the patient meets the clinical criteria for brain death. At postmortem the cerebellar tonsils are necrotic and hemorrhagic.

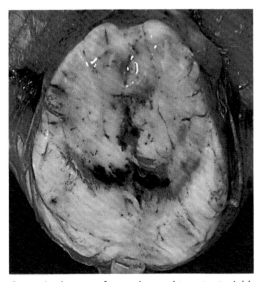

Fig. 4. Duret hemorrhages in the pons from advanced transtentorial herniation.

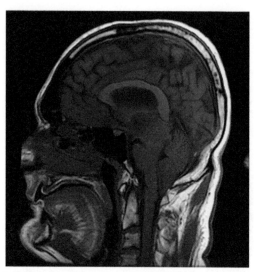

Fig. 5. Tonsillar herniation (due in this case to intracranial hypotension, rather than a mass lesion).

PREVENTION OF HERNIATION

It is vital to have a strong clinical suspicion that a patient may be at risk for a mass lesion that might expand and cause destructive herniation. Patients who are on anticoagulants or immunosuppressive drugs are at risk for such complications, and any complaint of headache or altered brain function should be taken very seriously: a careful examination and (usually) a computed tomography scan or magnetic resonance imaging (MRI) of the brain are indicated. Any history of progression of symptoms, including increasing headache, seizures, speech, cognitive dysfunction (eg, apraxia, neglect, disorientation), weakness, numbness, or visual disturbance, should prompt careful evaluation.

Once a mass lesion is discovered, it is best to deal with it as expeditiously as possible, especially if the lesion is likely to be rapidly growing or is in the posterior fossa. Debulking or removing the lesion surgically is often the logical and appropriate solution. This approach is almost always appropriate for extra-axial mass lesions such as subdural or epidural hematomas, empyemas, or meningiomas. Some lesions, for example, identified tumors that are radiosensitive or chemosensitive, might be treated nonsurgically. Multiple abscesses may respond to antimicrobial therapy, but large abscesses usually require surgical decompression.[11–13] Except for cerebellar hemorrhages, surgical removal of parenchymal bleeds has been shown to be ineffective.[14]

Decompressive craniectomy (DC) allows for an artificial hernia of the contents of an intracranial compartment though an expansion of the dura and an opening in the skull (see **Fig. 3** and the article by Sandrine de Ribaupierre on trauma elsewhere in this issue). DC can prevent the aforementioned life-threatening herniations and can reduce intracranial pressure. Three randomized controlled trials have established that DC for middle cerebral artery (MCA) territory ischemic strokes significantly lessened mortality and led to reasonably good outcomes in patients younger than 60 years when the operation was done within 48 hours of the stroke, regardless of which hemisphere was involved.[15–17] A meta-analysis confirmed this, and suggested that if more than half of MCA territory was ischemic or the volume on diffusion-weighted MRI was greater than 143 cm³ then surgery should be performed.[18] It has long been accepted that decompression of large cerebellar strokes is life-saving.[19–25] For trauma and aneurysmal subarachnoid hemorrhage there is still controversy, and such cases should probably be considered for craniectomy on a case-by-case basis.[26]

Measures to acutely lower intracranial pressure (ICP) can "buy time" to allow for swelling to subside, to allow for improved cerebral perfusion pressure (CPP; CPP = mean arterial blood pressure minus ICP) or for later surgical decompressive measures. If possible, it is desirable to monitor ICP to prompt such measures and to provide adequate cerebral perfusion.[27] These measures are most commonly implemented in cases of trauma, and are discussed in detail in the relevant article by Sandrine de Ribaupierre elsewhere in this issue.

ACKNOWLEDGMENTS

The author acknowledges the assistance of David Pelz and Lee-Cyn Ang in producing the figures.

REFERENCES

1. Fisher CM. The neurologic examination of the comatose patient. Acta Neurol Scand 1969;45(Suppl 36):1–56.
2. Nunez PL. Brain, mind and the structure of reality. New York: Oxford University Press; 2010.
3. Posner JB, Saper CB, Schiff ND, et al. Plum and Posner's diagnosis of stupor and coma. Oxford (UK): Oxford University Press; 2007. p. 88–118.
4. Hassenjäger T, Spatz H. Über örtliche veräderungern der Korfiguration des Gerhins beim Hindruck. Arch Psychiatr Nervenkr 1937;107:193–222 [in German].
5. Fisher CM. Acute brain herniation: a revised concept. Semin Neurol 1984;4: 417–21.
6. Ropper AH. Herniation. Handb Clin Neurol 2008;90:79–98.
7. Ropper AH. Lateral displacement of the brain and level of consciousness in patients with an acute hemispheral mass. N Engl J Med 1986;314:953–8.
8. Ropper AH. A preliminary MRI study of the geometry of brain displacement and level of consciousness with acute intracranial processes. Neurology 1989;39: 622–7.
9. Ropper AH, Gress DR. CT and clinical features of large cerebral hemorrhages. Cerebrovasc Dis 1991;1:38–42.
10. Ropper AH. The opposite pupil in herniation. Neurology 1990;40:1707–9.
11. Tessier JM, Scheld WM. Principles of antimicrobial therapy. Handb Clin Neurol 2010;96:17–29.
12. Honda H, Warren DK. Central nervous system infections: meningitis and brain abscess. Infect Dis Clin North Am 2009;23:609–23.
13. Hall WA, Truwit CL. The surgical management of infections involving the cerebrum. Neurosurgery 2008;62(Suppl 2):519–30.
14. Mendelow AD, Gregson BA, Fernandes HM, et al. Early surgery versus initial conservative treatment in patients with spontaneous supratentorial intracerebral haematomas in the International Surgical Trial in Intracerebral Haemorrhage (STICH): a randomised trial. Lancet 2005;365:387–97.
15. Vahedi K, Vicaut E, Mateo J, et al. A sequential-design, multicenter, randomized, controlled trial of early decompressive craniectomy in malignant middle cerebral artery infarction (DECIMAL Trial). Stroke 2007;38:2506–17.
16. Juttler E, Schwab S, Schmiedek P, et al. Decompressive Surgery for the Treatment of Malignant Infarction of the Middle Cerebral Artery (DESTINY): a randomized, controlled trial. Stroke 2007;38:2518–25.

17. Hofmeijer J, Kappelle LJ, Algra A, et al. HAMLET investigators. Surgical decompression for space-occupying cerebral infarction (the Hemicraniectomy After Middle Cerebral Artery infarction with Life-threatening Edema Trial [HAMLET]): a multicentre, open, randomised trial. Lancet Neurol 2009;8:326–33.

18. Vahedi K, Hofmeijer J, Juettler E, et al. Early decompressive surgery in malignant infarction of the middle cerebral artery: a pooled analysis of three randomised controlled trials. Lancet Neurol 2007;6:215–22.

19. Shenkin HA, Zavala M. Cerebellar strokes: mortality, surgical indications, and results of ventricular drainage. Lancet 1982;2:429–32.

20. Auer LM, Auer T, Sayama I. Indications for surgical treatment of cerebellar haemorrhage and infarction. Acta Neurochir (Wien) 1986;79:74–9.

21. Chen HJ, Lee TC, Wei CP. Treatment of cerebellar infarction by decompressive suboccipital craniectomy. Stroke 1992;23:957–61.

22. Heros RC. Cerebellar hemorrhage and infarction. Stroke 1982;13:106–9.

23. Heros RC. Surgical treatment of cerebellar infarction. Stroke 1992;23:937–8.

24. Hornig CR, Rust DS, Busse O, et al. Space-occupying cerebellar infarction. Clinical course and prognosis. Stroke 1994;25:372–4.

25. Jauss M, Krieger D, Hornig C, et al. Surgical and medical management of patients with massive cerebellar infarctions: results of the German-Austrian Cerebellar Infarction Study. J Neurol 1999;246:257–64.

26. Schirmer CM, Ackil AA Jr, Malek AM. Decompressive craniectomy. Neurocrit Care 2008;8:456–70.

27. Latorre JG, Greer DM. Management of acute intracranial hypertension: a review. Neurologist 2009;15:193–207.

The Vegetative and Minimally Conscious States: Diagnosis, Prognosis and Treatment

Ron Hirschberg, MD[a,b,c], Joseph T. Giacino, PhD[a,b,d],*

KEYWORDS

- Consciousness • Vegetative state • Traumatic brain injury
- Neuroimaging • Outcomes

Severe acquired brain injury has profound impact on alertness, cognition, and behavior. Among those who survive the initial injury, a significant minority fail to fully recover self and environmental awareness, and go on to experience prolonged disorders of consciousness (DOC) that can last a lifetime. Following emergence from coma, most individuals evolve into either a vegetative (VS) or minimally conscious state (MCS). Prevalence rates are difficult to estimate in the United States because of the lack of systematic surveillance procedures and range from 25,000 to 420,000[1,2] for VS and 112,000 to 280,000[3] for MCS. Patients, families, providers, and caregivers are all affected by the personal, financial, and societal consequences of prolonged VS and MCS. Although there are no standards of care to guide clinical management, a growing body of empirical evidence is beginning to accrue to inform clinical decision making. In this article, we review the state of the science as it pertains to diagnosis, prognosis, and treatment of patients with DOC.

The authors have nothing to disclose.
a Department of Physical Medicine and Rehabilitation, Harvard Medical School, 25 Shattuck Street, Boston, MA 02115, USA
b Department of Physical Medicine and Rehabilitation, Spaulding Rehabilitation Hospital, 125 Nashua Street, Boston, MA 02114, USA
c Department of Physical Medicine and Rehabilitation, Massachusetts General Hospital, 55 Fruit Street, Boston, MA 02114, USA
d Department of Psychiatry, Massachusetts General Hospital, 55 Fruit Street, Boston, MA 02114, USA
* Corresponding author. Department of Physical Medicine and Rehabilitation, Spaulding Rehabilitation Hospital, 125 Nashua Street, Boston, MA 02114.
E-mail address: jgiacino@partners.org

Neurol Clin 29 (2011) 773–786
doi:10.1016/j.ncl.2011.07.009
0733-8619/11/$ – see front matter © 2011 Elsevier Inc. All rights reserved.

neurologic.theclinics.com

HISTORICAL CONTEXT

In the 1890s, William James[4] construed consciousness as "awareness of the self and the environment." He viewed conscious awareness as the product of sensory and subjective experiences. For James, the "objects of our consciousness" included the environment and one's mental state. The evidence for consciousness was provided by "reactions" elicited by either internal or external events.[4] Three-quarters of a century later, Jennett and Plum[5] parsed arousal from awareness in considering consciousness, and proposed the term, "persistent vegetative state (PVS)" to refer to a state of "wakefulness without awareness." More than 2 decades after PVS was defined, the Multi-Society Task Force Report on PVS clarified that whereas "awareness requires wakefulness, wakefulness can be present without awareness."[1] The Task Force definition highlighted the preservation of sleep-wake cycles and concluded that PVS represents a wakeful state in which there is complete inability to experience the environment.[1]

In 1995, shortly after the release of the Multi-Society Task Force on PVS, the Aspen Neurobehavioral Workgroup was convened to reconcile disparities between diagnostic and prognostic recommendations proposed by the Task Force, and a position statement published a year later by the American Congress of Rehabilitation Medicine (ACRM).[6] The Aspen Workgroup included representatives from neurology, neurosurgery, neuropsychology, physical medicine and rehabilitation, nursing, allied health, and bioethics. After achieving consensus on the diagnostic and prognostic guidelines for VS, the Workgroup shifted its attention to the subpopulation of patients who showed minimal or inconsistent behavioral signs of consciousness. The term, "minimally responsive state (MRS)" had previously been proposed by the ACRM to differentiate patients who retained some definitive, albeit inconsistent, signs of conscious awareness from those in coma and VS.[6] The ACRM recommended to apply the term "MRS" when an "unequivocally meaningful" behavioral response was observed following a specific command, question, or environmental prompt on at least one occasion during a period of formal assessment. The Aspen Workgroup subsequently recommended to replace the term "MRS" by "MCS" to emphasize the partial preservation of consciousness that distinguishes this condition from coma and VS.[7]

DIAGNOSTIC ASSESSMENT
Vegetative State

A primary aim in clinical management of patients with DOC is to establish an accurate diagnosis. Critical decisions concerning prognosis and treatment rest heavily on the accurate determination of level of consciousness. The Multi-Society Task Force Report was pivotal to clinical practice, as it established operationally defined diagnostic criteria for the first time, proposed prognostic guidelines for recovery of consciousness and function, and evaluated the effectiveness of specific treatment interventions. The report also introduced the notion that VS usually exists as a transitional state between coma and higher levels of consciousness, and clarified that VS is considered "persistent" when this state lasts at least 4 weeks. The Task Force also proposed temporal parameters for the "permanent vegetative state" to establish the point at which the probability of subsequent recovery of consciousness is very low.[1] Relying on available outcome studies from around the world, the Task Force concluded that VS should be considered permanent after 3 months following hypoxic-ischemic, metabolic, and congenital causes, but not until 12 months after traumatic brain injury.

The diagnostic criteria for PVS recommended by the Task Force were met with broad consensus internationally and remain in force today. All of the following behavioral criteria must be met on bedside examination to establish the diagnosis of VS[1]:

- Intermittent wakefulness manifested by the presence of sleep/wake cycles (ie, periodic eye opening)
- No evidence of sustained, reproducible, purposeful, or voluntary behavioral responses to visual, auditory, tactile, or noxious stimuli
- No evidence of language comprehension or expression.

The development of behaviorally based criteria for detecting conscious awareness at the bedside has advanced research and clinical practice by constructing a common frame of reference from which to consider the boundary between consciousness and unconsciousness. Nonetheless, studies of diagnostic accuracy consistently suggest that 30% to 40% of patients unable to speak or follow commands are falsely diagnosed with VS.[8–10] Diagnostic error in DOC can have dramatic consequences given the influence of early diagnosis on decisions relating to continuation of life support, indications for neurorehabilitation, caretaker planning, and family adjustment.

Minimally Conscious State

After completing a systematic review of the literature, the Aspen Workgroup defined MCS as "a condition of severely altered consciousness in which there is *minimal but definite* behavioral evidence of conscious awareness." Behaviorally based diagnostic criteria were proposed and published in *Neurology* in 2002.[7] To establish the diagnosis of MCS, clearly discernible evidence of 1 or more of the following behaviors must be observed on bedside examination:

- Simple command-following
- Intelligible verbalization
- Recognizable verbal or gestural "yes/no" responses (without regard to accuracy)
- Movements or emotional responses that are triggered by relevant environmental stimuli and cannot be attributed to reflexive activity (eg, visual pursuit of a moving object).

The Aspen Workgroup recognized that as recovery of consciousness moves forward, an upper bound for MCS also needed to be established. Consequently, 2 behaviors were defined to mark "emergence from MCS" (EMCS): reliable demonstration of "interactive communication" (ie, accurate yes and no answers to situational orientation questions) and "functional object use" (ie, demonstration of 2 different familiar objects). Unlike the diagnosis of MCS, which requires evidence of *reproducible* goal-directed behavior, emergence from MCS requires *consistent* demonstration of volitional behavior.[7] **Table 1** lists the distinguishing behavioral features of coma, VS and MCS.

Neurobehavioral Rating Scales

In an effort to minimize diagnostic and prognostic error associated with assessment of patients with DOC, standardized neurobehavioral rating scales have been developed. The Glasgow Coma Scale (GCS), originally published in 1974, continues to be the standard for acute assessment of patients with DOC.[11] The longevity of the GCS is attributable to its strong inter-rater reliability, ease of administration, and well-established relationship to mortality and morbidity. The limitations of the GCS have also been well documented.[12] Among these, lack of sensitivity to subtle changes of

Table 1
Behavioral features of disorders of consciousness

Behavior	Coma	Vegetative State	Minimally Conscious State
Eye opening	None	Spontaneous	Spontaneous
Spontaneous movement	None	Reflexive/Patterned	Automatic/Object Manipulation
Response to pain	Posturing/None	Posturing/Withdrawal	Localization
Visual response	None	Startle/Pursuit (rare)	Object recognition/Pursuit
Affective response	None	Random	Contingent
Commands	None	None	Inconsistent
Verbalization	None	Random vocalization	Intelligible words
Communication	None	None	Unreliable

prognostic relevance has received the most attention. In response to this concern, a wide array of measures especially designed for long-term monitoring of patients with DOC have been developed.[13,14] Although many of these newer instruments offer a standardized approach to assessment, until recently, their psychometric underpinnings had not been empirically scrutinized.

In 2010, the Disorders of Consciousness Task Force of the ACRM completed an evidence-based review of behavioral assessment scales for patients with DOC.[15] Thirteen scales met the review criteria and were evaluated on their ability to differentiate VS, MCS, and EMCS; inter-rater reliability; diagnostic validity; and prognostic validity. The review concluded that among the scales reviewed, the Coma Recovery Scale—Revised (CRS-R)[16] received the most "acceptable" ratings in the categories investigated. The CRS-R is composed of 6 subscales addressing auditory, visual, motor, oromotor/verbal, communication, and arousal functions. Subscale items are hierarchically arranged with the lowest items reflecting brainstem-mediated functions and the highest items corresponding to cortical functions. CRS-R administration and scoring guidelines are manualized and the scale is intended for use by licensed medical and allied health professionals. The CRS-R was selected as the measure of choice for assessment of recovery of consciousness by the Interagency Traumatic Brain Injury Common Data Elements Outcomes Workgroup,[17] and has been used to investigate diagnostic accuracy,[8,18] the relationship between behavioral and neurophysiologic markers of consciousness,[19–21] outcome prediction,[22,23] and treatment effectiveness.[24,25] The scale is currently available in 12 languages (English, Spanish, Portuguese, Italian, French, Greek, German, Dutch, Norwegian, Danish, Swedish, Korean). **Fig. 1** shows the CRS-R Record Sheet.

Neuroimaging Applications in Diagnostic Assessment

The development of diagnostic applications of neuroimaging for patients with DOC has generated novel data that have begun to challenge conventional beliefs about the primacy of behavior in the assessment of level of consciousness. Detecting volitional behavior in patients with severe brain injury is often difficult, as fluctuations in arousal level, deficient drive, and sensory and motor impairments can mask signs of consciousness. Functional neuroimaging strategies provide a means of assessing cognition without reliance on verbal or motor behavior. Recent investigations have demonstrated the utility of functional neuroimaging paradigms designed to assess command-following ability in patients who lack the capacity for speech or active movement.[26,27]

Coma Recovery Scale – Revised ©2004
Record Sheet

This form should only be used in conjunction with the CRS-R Administration and Scoring Manual which defines guidelines for standardized application of the scale

Patient:	Diagnosis:	Etiology:
Date of onset:	Date of Examination:	

Date	Admission	2	3	4	5	6	7	8	9	10	11	12	13	14	15	16
Week																
AUDITORY FUNCTIONS																
4 Consistent Movement to Command *																
3 Reproducible Movement to Command *																
2 Localization to Sound																
1 Auditory Startle																
0 None																
VISUAL FUNCTIONS																
5 Object Recognition*																
4 Object Localization: Reaching*																
3 Visual Pursuit *																
2 Fixation*																
1 Visual Startle																
0 None																
MOTOR FUNCTIONS																
6 Functional Object Use**																
5 Automatic Motor Response*																
4 Object Manipulation*																
3 Localization to Noxious Stimulation*																
2 Flexion Withdrawal																
1 Abnormal Posturing																
0 None/Flaccid																
OROMOTOR/ VERBAL FUNCTIONS																
3 Intelligible Verbalization*																
2 Vocalization / Oral Movement																
1 Oral Reflexive Movement																
0 None																
COMMUNICATION SCALE																
2 Functional: Accurate**																
1 Non-functional: Intentional*																
0 None																
AROUSAL SCALE																
3 Attention																
2 Eye opening without stimulation																
1 Eye opening with stimulation																
0 no arousal response																
TOTAL SCORE																

Denotes emergence from MCS**
Denotes MCS*

Fig. 1. Record Sheet for the Coma Recovery Scale—Revised (CRS-R) excerpted from the CRS-R Administration and Scoring Manual (available from the authors by request). (*From* Giacino JT, Kalmar K. CRS-R Administration and Scoring Manual. Johnson Rehabilitation Instituion; with permission. Copyright © 2004.)

In a typical functional magnetic resonance imaging (fMRI) paradigm, the patient is instructed to perform a basic cognitive task while in the scanner. Regions of brain activity observed during task performance are compared with areas that are active during passive sensory stimulation and during periods of rest. Task-specific activation profiles are first acquired in healthy volunteers to serve as a normal referent for patient studies. A growing body of fMRI studies indicates that some patients who fail to show any behavioral evidence of response to commands administered at the bedside, produce activation profiles that are nearly indistinguishable from healthy volunteers performing similar command-following tasks while in the scanner.[26–28]

Owen and colleagues[26] identified a patient diagnosed with VS 5 months after sustaining a traumatic brain injury who was able to perform 2 different mental imagery tasks when instructed to do so during a series of fMRI scans. Selective activation was noted in the supplementary motor area in response to instructions to imagine playing tennis. In contrast, activation was noted in the parahippocampal gyrus and posterior parietal cortex when the patient was instructed to imagine walking around the rooms of her house. Although this patient was reportedly showing signs of visual fixation at the time of the study (suggesting transition from VS to MCS), this landmark study demonstrated the potential role of neuroimaging in detecting cognition in patients with underlying impairments unrelated to alterations in consciousness.

Rodriguez-Moreno and colleagues[28] developed a second fMRI-based command-following paradigm using a silent picture-naming task to capture internal speech in patients with varying degrees of impaired consciousness ranging from VS to the locked-in syndrome (LIS). In LIS, there is no speech and little to no active movement, although cognitive functions are well preserved. As expected, robust language network activation was observed in the patient with LIS, a patient who had emerged from MCS, and 2 patients in MCS. In addition, 1 patient in VS also evidenced widespread activation of the language network, including the superior temporal, inferior frontal, and medial frontal gyri. The investigators also found that patients with higher CRS-R scores showed more complete activation of language structures, suggesting that fMRI activation profiles may provide information concerning residual cognitive function that cannot be extracted at the bedside.

Monti and colleagues[29] developed passive listening and active auditory target detection tasks to evaluate executive functions in patients with no evidence of command-following on bedside testing. Healthy volunteers demonstrated activation of fronto-parietal networks in response to instructions to perform the target detection task. A similar activation pattern was observed in one patient in MCS suggesting compliance with the task demands.

An elegant follow-up study completed by Monti and colleagues[30] converted Owen and colleagues'[26] previously described imagery-based command-following paradigm into a yes-no signal system. Patients were instructed to imagine either playing tennis or walking around the rooms of their house when they wished to answer "yes," and to perform the opposite task when they wished to answer "no." Although 5 of the 54 patients (VS = 23; MCS = 31) were able to selectively trigger motor and spatial network activation on cue, 1 patient in MCS was able to use the imagery paradigms to reliably answer yes-no questions, despite the absence of this behavior on bedside examination.

These referenced studies indicate that at least some patients who appear unresponsive may retain higher levels of self and environmental awareness than would otherwise be suggested on bedside examination. As such, functional neuroimaging paradigms may eventually play an important role in reducing diagnostic error and improving prognostic accuracy.

PROGNOSIS

Duration of unconsciousness appears to be one of the strongest discrete predictors of subsequent recovery of consciousness.[1,31] Among patients who remain in VS for 3 months following traumatic brain injury, approximately 35% will recover consciousness by 1 year after injury. In nontraumatic VS lasting 3 months, the probability of recovery of consciousness at 1 year is substantially lower, dropping to approximately 5%. After 6 months in traumatic VS, there is still a 15% probability of recovery of consciousness as compared with near zero in nontraumatic VS.[1]

Regarding prognosis in MCS, Giacino and Kalmar[22] monitored the course of recovery across the first year after injury on the Disability Rating Scale (DRS) in 104 patients (MCS = 55; VS = 49) admitted to an inpatient rehabilitation program. Fifty percent of the MCS group fell within the "no to moderate disability" category on the DRS at the 12-month mark as compared with only 3% of those in VS. When the 2 diagnostic groups were further stratified by etiology, 38% of patients in traumatic MCS versus only 2% of those in nontraumatic VS had "no to moderate disability" at 12 months.

Although large group studies have identified clinical variables tied to outcome, there is no prognostic algorithm with high sensitivity and specificity at the single-case level. This is, in part, because of the lack of systematic study of the influence of mediating variables, such as quality of care on outcome. The existing prognostic guidelines for VS developed by the Multi-Society Task Force are almost 2 decades old and guidelines do not yet exist for MCS. In view of these circumstances, an expert panel jointly sponsored by the American Academy of Neurology, American Congress of Rehabilitation Medicine, and National Institute on Disability and Rehabilitation Research has been convened to conduct an evidence-based review of the literature and provide recommendations for practice. This initiative is expected to be completed in 2013.

Late Recovery in VS and MCS

The Multi-Society Task Force guidelines on PVS provided the first evidence-based guideline for permanent VS.[1] However, there were relatively few reports in the literature at the time of the Task Force review that included patients followed beyond 12 months after injury. Consequently, the number of potential recoveries occurring beyond the recommended temporal cutoffs for permanence was truncated. In addition, most of the available studies relied on "pooled" data that failed to distinguish outcomes between patients in VS and MCS. To avoid the risk of incorrectly inferring permanence, the Aspen Workgroup recommended abandoning the term, "permanent VS." Instead, the Workgroup recommended specifying the etiology (ie, traumatic or nontraumatic) and time since onset when diagnosing VS.[7]

Recent evidence suggests that the window for recovery of consciousness and function may extend well beyond 1 year in a substantial minority of patients.[32–34] Estraneo and colleagues[33] tracked recovery in 50 patients in traumatic and nontraumatic VS for an average of 26 months. The investigators reported that 20% of the sample recovered at least one sign of conscious awareness between 14 and 28 months after injury, and 24% emerged from MCS between 19 and 25 months after injury. Late recovery of consciousness was significantly associated with younger age at onset, traumatic etiology, and preserved pupillary response at the time of enrollment.

Lammi and colleagues[32] followed 18 patients who were in posttraumatic MCS at the time of discharge from inpatient rehabilitation for up to 5 years. Although outcomes were similar to those reported by Giacino and Kalmar[22] at 1 year after injury, more than one-third of the sample recovered to an independent level of cognitive or motor function between 2 and 5 years after injury. Interestingly, length of MCS was not significantly correlated with outcome on the DRS, suggesting that improvement to MCS may have been the critical variable in extending the recovery window.

Katz and colleagues[31] monitored outcomes in 36 patients who were admitted to a rehabilitation program at approximately 1 month following injury with a diagnosis of VS (n = 11) or MCS (n = 25). Seventy-two percent of the sample (VS = 5/11; MCS 20/25) emerged from MCS at an average of 9 weeks after injury, 58% (VS = 4/11; MCS = 17/25) recovered orientation at an average of 16 weeks after injury, and 28% (VS = 1/11; MCS = 9/25) regained household independence 33 weeks after injury on average. The investigators concluded that patients in VS who emerge to MCS within the first 8 weeks after injury are more likely to progress to higher levels of functional independence over the course of the next 1 to 4 years. Those who remained in MCS were more likely to have sustained a nontraumatic brain injury and to have been in VS longer than 8 weeks. These results support prior reports, suggesting that outcome from MCS is considerably more heterogeneous relative to VS.

Neuroimaging Applications in Prognosis

Neuroimaging studies may provide unique information to prognostic decision making in patients suspected or known to have neurologic impairments that confound bedside assessment. The so-called "default mode network (DMN)" has garnered attention in this regard given its structural and functional characteristics. Functional MRI studies have identified the DMN as a network of interconnected structures composed of the medial prefrontal cortex, temporo-parietal junction, and precuneus.[35] This circuit is believed to activate during periods of cognitive quiescence and deactivates in response to active cognitive processing. The DMN has been linked to conscious awareness in that it appears to have a role in scanning for salient environmental events and monitoring the interface between external events and the internal state.[36] Functional MRI studies indicate that the degree of DMN connectivity is greater in MCS relative to VS, and that severity of cognitive impairment appears to be proportional to the extent of the DMN connectivity.[37] Preserved DMN connectivity may be a harbinger of more favorable outcome.

In another series of fMRI studies, Coleman and colleagues[19] used a hierarchical language-processing paradigm to evaluate the integrity of the language network in 44 patients with DOC (VS: n = 22; MCS: n = 19). Subjects were exposed to linguistic material of variable semantic complexity to gauge the depth of processing. Activation profiles were categorized based on degree of impairment and outcomes compared across impairment categories. Results revealed a clear association between the integrity of the fMRI results and behavioral performance on the CRS-R at 6 months, suggesting a relationship between degree of language network activation and functional recovery.

Structural imaging studies may also play a role in informing prognosis in patients with DOC. Newcombe and colleagues[38] used diffusion tensor imaging (DTI) to evaluate the structural integrity of white matter pathways in a cohort of patients with traumatic (n = 7) and nontraumatic (n = 5) VS. The relationship between DTI abnormalities, language network fMRI activation profiles, and behavioral performance on the CRS-R was explored. DTI detected supratentorial white and gray matter changes in both groups that were not observed on conventional MRI sequences, and white matter abnormalities were more prevalent in the brainstem in patients with traumatic injuries. Correlation analyses indicated that patients with more extensive white matter abnormalities tended to perform more poorly on fMRI activation studies and received lower CRS-R scores. Early DTI may be useful in identifying characteristic lesion profiles associated with lower cognitive reserve and less favorable behavioral outcomes.

TREATMENT

Treatment interventions for patients with DOC should incorporate both preventive and restorative strategies. Immediately after injury, patients in VS and MCS are at risk for multiple complications arising from immobility. Muscle, tendon, and soft tissue contractures; skin breakdown; thrombo-embolic disease; and pulmonary or urinary tract infections are among the most common foci for prevention efforts. Despite the absence of a sufficient body of evidence to support definitive practice guidelines, restoration of sleep-wake cycles, nutritional balance, bowel and bladder regulation, and large joint passive mobilization should constitute basic clinical management aims.[39]

Restorative interventions are intended to promote arousal and drive goal-directed behavior. Centrally active medications, sensory stimulation, procedures, hyperbaric oxygen therapy, and deep brain stimulation have all been used to promote rate of recovery and reduce the severity of residual functional disability, although there is insufficient evidence to guide the selection of any particular intervention. In general, treatment-effectiveness studies have been compromised by small sample sizes, failure to mitigate examiner bias, and use of crude outcome measures.[39,40] In addition, caregivers are hesitant to provide consent for clinical trials that constrain the use of other potentially helpful medications.[41] Notwithstanding the limitations of the existing evidence base, clinicians are obligated to provide reasonable rehabilitative treatment options. In **Table 2** and in the following paragraphs, we briefly describe and review the results of some representative treatment studies.

Amantadine hydrochloride (AH) is commonly used in neurorehabilitation settings to enhance arousal and behavioral initiation in patients with DOC. A single-center randomized crossover trial conducted by Meythaler and colleagues[42] compared cognitive and motor changes in 35 patients with GCS scores of 10 or lower who received either AH or placebo for a period of 6 weeks. After the initial 6 weeks, patients were crossed to the alternate condition for an additional 6 weeks. Results suggested that patients treated with AH first showed faster gains on cognitive (ie, Mini Mental Status Examination) and functional status (ie, DRS) measures; however, there was no significant difference between the 2 groups when outcomes were reassessed at the 12-week mark. There was also evidence that the 2 groups were not equivalent with regard to injury severity.

Dramatic "awakenings" from states of unresponsiveness have been reported following administration of the soporific, zolpidem. The first case was described by Clauss and colleagues[43] in 2000 and additional case reports and case series have followed.[44–48] In the largest series reported to date, Whyte and Myers[45] monitored the response to zolpidem (10 mg) in 15 patients in traumatic and nontraumatic VS and MCS using a double-blind, placebo-controlled crossover design. Although only 1 of 15 subjects was considered a zolpidem "responder," behavioral changes were significant in that the responsive patient transitioned from VS to MCS following administration of the drug, and this effect was replicated over repeated trials. The paradoxic effect of zolpidem has been hypothesized to be related to "relaxation" of tonic inhibitory influences stemming from pallidal outflow to the thalamocortical system caused by striatal dysfunction.[49]

More definitive evidence regarding the effectiveness of amantadine and zolpidem in facilitating recovery in patients with DOC is likely to emerge from 2 recently launched double-blind prospective randomized placebo-controlled multicenter clinical trials. The first, a recently completed 10-site international trial of AH funded by the National Institute on Disability and Rehabilitation Research (NIDRR) is designed to determine whether short-term functional outcome is more favorable in posttraumatic VS and MCS patients exposed to amantadine versus placebo within 4 to 16 weeks of injury. The trial will also determine whether functional gains are maintained after drug washout (NIDRR Award #H133A031713). The second trial, also NIDRR funded, aims to determine the rate and mechanism of effect of zolpidem among individuals remaining in traumatic or nontraumatic VS and MCS for at least 4 months (NIDRR Award #H133G080066).

Nonpharmacologic treatment efforts in this population have historically focused on the use of sensorimotor stimulation. This strategy is premised, in part, on the notion

Table 2
Representative studies illustrating treatment interventions for patients with disorders of consciousness

Intervention	Rationale	Method	Aim	Representative Study	Results
Pharmacotherapy	Drug exposure may correct imbalance in inhibitory and facilitory neural systems responsive for symptom expression	Administration of dopaminergic, noradrenergic, and serotonergic medications	Improve arousal, initiation, and attention	Meythaler et al,[42] 2002	Rate of recovery significantly faster in patients treated with amantadine hydrochloride within 3 months of injury relative to placebo group.
Sensory stimulation	Information processing is dependent on calibration of stimulus intensity and response threshold	Administration of multimodal sensory stimuli (auditory, tactile, visual, olfactory)	Improve breadth and reliability of behavioral response repertoire	Mitchell et al,[50] 1990	Time to recovery of command-following and purposeful movement significantly shorter (mean difference = 5 days) in patients who received a structured sensory stimulation program for 1–2 hours/day over 7–12 days relative to no-treatment controls.
Deep Brain Stimulation (DBS)	Electro-physiologic stimulation of reticular-activating system produces physiologic changes associated with arousal	Chronic electrical stimulation of meso-diencephalic structures	Improved arousal and/or cognitive deficits associated with disruption of thalamo-cortical circuits	Schiff et al,[25] 2007	Improvement in arousal ratings, praxis, and swallowing on standardized assessments obtained during DBS-on vs -off periods.

that structured stimulation mitigates the risk of sensory deprivation in patients with severe disturbances in consciousness and may facilitate neuroplasticity.[43,44] Mitchell and colleagues[50] investigated the effect of a Coma Arousal Procedure (CAP) in which sensory stimuli were presented through all 5 modalities at "greatly heightened frequency, intensity, and duration." Subjects were 23 patients with severe traumatic brain injury who showed no purposeful movement and were unable to follow commands. Twelve subjects were assigned to the CAP treatment group. The remaining 12 subjects comprised the no-CAP control group and were matched according to age, sex, and type and location of injury. The CAP was administered 1 to 2 hours a day by trained family members for 7 to 12 days and the primary outcome was the time to recovery of command-following and purposeful movement. Coma duration was reported to be significantly shorter for the CAP group (mean difference = 5 days) in comparison with the control group. Because the sample was small and coma duration was not specified for either group, the shorter duration of coma noted in the CAP group may have been secondary to a few outlying scores in either group.

Thalamic deep brain stimulation (DBS) has been proposed as a method to improve arousal regulation in patients with DOC who retain functionally connected but downregulated or inconsistently active neural networks.[51] A double-blind alternating crossover study of DBS targeting central thalamic projections to the cortex demonstrated significant functional improvements in a 36-year-old man who remained in MCS for 6.5 years after sustaining severe traumatic brain injury during an assault. In this controlled study, performance on measures of arousal, motor control, and dysphagia was significantly better during periods in which DBS was turned on. Unexpectedly, performance remained well above baseline across all outcome measures after DBS was turned off, suggesting carryover effects.[25] Although the potential for deep brain stimulation and other neuromodulatory treatments to foster improvement beyond the period of spontaneous recovery is encouraging, additional large-scale trials are required to replicate preliminary findings, identify characteristics of responders versus nonresponders, and refine the technology.

SUMMARY

The pace of research on DOC has advanced rapidly over the past 15 years. The availability of clear, behaviorally defined differential diagnostic criteria has enabled clinicians and researchers to distinguish patients who retain some elements of conscious awareness (ie, MCS) from those who are completely unconscious (ie, VS). A growing body of evidence indicates that there are key pathophysiologic differences between VS and MCS that predispose to significant differences in functional outcome and probability of response to treatment. Standardized behavioral assessment strategies for detection of conscious awareness are improving the reliability and validity of bedside assessment but may be confounded by concomitant sensory and motor impairments. Specialized structural and functional neuroimaging technologies, including diffusion tensor imaging and fMRI activation paradigms, are beginning to provide novel information concerning the integrity of neural networks that mediate arousal and cognition. As these procedures enter the clinical mainstream, they are likely to improve diagnostic and prognostic precision and may help tie treatment interventions to underlying pathophysiologic profiles. The development of treatments for patients with DOC has lagged behind advances in assessment, leading to a proliferation of pharmacologic and nonpharmacologic interventions with uncertain efficacy and adverse event records. A clearer picture of the risks and benefits associated with particular treatments is expected to emerge over the next 5 years as the results of recently launched multicenter randomized controlled trials are made available.

REFERENCES

1. Medical aspects of the persistent vegetative state. The Multi-Society Task Force on PVS. N Engl J Med 1994;330:1499–508.
2. Spudis EV. The persistent vegetative state–1990. J Neurol Sci 1991;2:128–36.
3. Strauss DJ, Ashwal S, Day SM, et al. Life expectancy of children in vegetative and minimally conscious states. Pediatr Neurol 2000;23(4):312–9.
4. James W. The varieties of the religious experience. Lecture III: The reality of the unseen. In: Miller LL, editor. New Age, New Thought: William James and the Varieties of Religious Experience. Denver: Brooks Divinity School; 1999. p. 51–4.
5. Jennett B, Plum F. Persistent vegetative state after brain damage: a syndrome in search of a name. Lancet 1972;1:734–7.
6. American Congress of Rehabilitation Medicine. Recommendations for use of uniform nomenclature pertinent to persons with severe alterations in consciousness. Arch Phys Med Rehabil 2005;76:205–9.
7. Giacino JT, Ashwal S, Childs N, et al. The minimally conscious state: definition and diagnostic criteria. Neurology 2002;58:349–53.
8. Schnakers C, Vanhaudenhuyse A, Giacino J, et al. Diagnostic accuracy of the vegetative and minimally conscious state: clinical consensus versus standardized neurobehavioral assessment. BMC Neurol 2009;9:35.
9. Childs NL, Mercer WN, Childs HW. Accuracy of diagnosis of persistent vegetative state. Neurology 1993;43(8):1465–7.
10. Andrews K, Murphy L, Munday R, et al. Misdiagnosis of the vegetative state: retrospective study in a rehabilitation unit. BMJ 1996;7048:13–6.
11. Teasdale G, Jennett B. Assessment of coma and impaired consciousness. Lancet 1974;2:81–4.
12. Zafonte RD, Hammond FM, Mann NR, et al. Relationship between Glasgow Coma Scale and functional outcome. Am J Phys Med Rehabil 1996;75(5):364–9.
13. Giacino J, Malone R. The vegetative and minimally conscious states. (3rd series). Disorders of consciousness. In: Young GB, Wijdicks EF, editors, Handbook of clinical neurology, vol. 90. Elsevier; 2008. p. 99–111.
14. Giacino J, Smart C. Recent advances in behavioral assessment of individuals with disorders of consciousness. Curr Opin Neurol 2007;20:614–9.
15. Seel RT, Sherer M, Whyte J, et al. Assessment scales for disorders of consciousness: evidence-based recommendations for clinical practice and research. Arch Phys Med Rehabil 2010;91:1795–813.
16. Giacino JT, Kalmar K, Whyte J. The JFK coma recovery scale—revised: measurement characteristics and diagnostic utility. Arch Phys Med Rehabil 2004;85(12):2020–9.
17. Wilde EA, Whiteneck GG, Bogner J, et al. Recommendations for the use of common outcome measures in traumatic brain injury research. Arch Phys Med Rehabil 2010;91:1650–60.
18. Schnakers C, Majerus S, Giacino J, et al. A French validation study of the Coma Recovery Scale- Revised. Brain Inj 2008;22(10):786–92.
19. Coleman MR, Rodd JM, Davis MH, et al. Do vegetative patients retain aspects of language comprehension? Evidence from fMRI. Brain 2007;130:2494–507.
20. Vanhaudenhuyse A, Schnakers C, Brédart S, et al. Assessment of visual pursuit in post-comatose states: use a mirror. J Neurol Neurosurg Psychiatry 2008;79(2):223.

21. Smart C, Giacino J, Cullen T, et al. Locked-in syndrome complicated by central deafness: neuropsychological and neuroimaging findings. Nat Clin Pract Neurol 2008;4(8):448–53.
22. Giacino JT, Kalmar K. The vegetative and minimally conscious states: a comparison of clinical features and functional outcome. J Head Trauma Rehabil 1997; 12(4):36–51.
23. Vanhaudenhuyes A, Giacino J, Schnakers C, et al. Blink to visual threat does not herald consciousness in the vegetative state. Neurology 2008;71:1–2.
24. Schnakers C, Hustinx R, Vandewalle G, et al. Measuring the effect of amantadine in chronic anoxic vegetative state. J Neurol Neurosurg Psychiatry 2008;79(2):225–7.
25. Schiff ND, Giacino JT, Victor JD, et al. Behavioral improvements with thalamic stimulation after severe traumatic brain injury. Nature 2007;448:600–3.
26. Owen AM, Coleman MR, Boly M, et al. Detecting awareness in the vegetative state. Science 2006;313:1402.
27. Coleman MR, Davis MH, Rodd M, et al. Towards the routine use of brain imaging to aid the clinical diagnosis of disorders of consciousness. Brain 2009;132: 2541–52.
28. Rodriguez-Moreno D, Schiff ND, Giacino JG, et al. A network approach to assessing cognition in disorders of consciousness. Neurology 2010;75:1871–8.
29. Monti MM, Coleman MR, Owen AM. Executive functions in the absence of behavior: functional imaging of the minimally conscious state. Prog Brain Res 2009;177:249–60.
30. Monti MM, Vanhaudenhuyse A, Coleman MR, et al. Willful modulation of brain activity in disorders of consciousness. N Engl J Med 2010;362:579–89.
31. Katz DI, Polyak M, Coughlan D, et al. Natural history of recovery from brain injury after prolonged disorders of consciousness: outcome of patients admitted to inpatient rehabilitation with 1–4 year follow-up. Prog Brain Res 2009;177: 73–88.
32. Lammi MH, Smith VH, Tate RL, et al. The minimally conscious state and recovery potential: a follow-up study 2 to 5 years after traumatic brain injury. Arch Phys Med Rehabil 2005;86:746–54.
33. Estraneo A, Moretta P, Loreto V, et al. Late recovery after traumatic, anoxic, or hemorrhagic long-lasting vegetative state. Neurology 2010;75:239–45.
34. Luaute J, Maucort-Boulch D, Tell L, et al. Long-term outcomes of chronic minimally conscious and vegetative states. Neurology 2010;75:246–52.
35. Gusnard DA, Akbudak E, Shulman GL, et al. Medial prefrontal cortex and self-referential mental activity: relation to a default mode of brain function. Proc Natl Acad Sci U S A 2001;98(7):4259–64.
36. Vanhaudenhuyse A, Demertzi A, Schabus M, et al. Two distinct neuronal networks mediate the awareness of environment and of self. J Cogn Neurosci 2011;3:570–8.
37. Cruse D, Owen AM. Consciousness revealed: new insights into the vegetative and minimally conscious states. Curr Opin Neurol 2010;23(6):656–60.
38. Newcombe VF, Williams GB, Scoffings D, et al. Aetiological differences in neuroanatomy of the vegetative state: insights from diffusion tensor imaging and functional implications. J Neurol Neurosurg Psychiatry 2010;81:552–61.
39. Giacino JT. Rehabilitation of patients with disorders of consciousness. In: High W, Sander A, Struchen M, et al, editors. Rehabilitation for traumatic brain injury. New York: Oxford University Press; 2005. p. 305–37.
40. Lombardi F, Taricco M, De Tanti A. Sensory stimulation for brain injured individuals in coma or vegetative state (review). Cochrane Database Syst Rev 2007;2:1–11.

41. Whyte J. Treatments to enhance recovery from the vegetative and minimally conscious states: ethical issues surrounding efficacy studies. Am J Phys Med Rehabil 2007;86:86–92.
42. Meythaler JM, Brunner RC, Johnson A, et al. Amantadine to improve neurorecovery in traumatic brain injury-associated diffuse axonal injury: a pilot double-blind randomized trial. J Head Trauma Rehabil 2002;17(4):300–13.
43. Clauss RP, Güldenpfennig WM, Nel HW, et al. Extraordinary arousal from semi-comatose state on zolpidem. A case report. S Afr Med J 2000;90(1):68–72.
44. Singh R, McDonald C, Dawson K, et al. Zolpidem in a minimally conscious state. Brain Inj 2008 Jan;22(1):103–6.
45. Whyte J, Myers R. Incidence of clinically significant responses to zolpidem among patients with disorders of consciousness: a preliminary placebo controlled trial. Am J Phys Med Rehabil 2009;88(5):410–8.
46. Shames J, Ring R. Transient reversal of anoxic brain injury–related minimally conscious state after zolpidem administration: a case report. Arch Phys Med Rehabil 2008;89:386–8.
47. Cohen SI, Duong TT. Increased arousal in a patient with anoxic brain injury after administration of zolpidem. Am J Phys Med Rehabil 2008;87:229–31.
48. Brefel-Courbon C, Payoux P, Ory F. Evidence of zolpidem effect in hypoxic encephalopathy. Ann Neurol 2007;62:102–5.
49. Schiff ND. Recovery of consciousness after severe brain injury: the role of arousal regulation mechanisms and some speculation on the heart-brain interface. Cleve Clin J Med 2010;77:S27–33.
50. Mitchell S, Bradley VA, Welch JL, et al. Coma arousal procedure: a therapeutic intervention in the treatment of head injury. Brain Inj 1990;3:273–9.
51. Schiff ND, Purpura KP. Towards a neurophysiological basis for cognitive neuromodulation. Thalamus Relat Syst 2002;2:55–69.

Neurologic Determination of Death

Jeanne Teitelbaum, MD, FRCP[a],*, Sam D. Shemie, MD[b]

KEYWORDS

- Neurologic criteria • Brain death • Brain arrest
- Neurologic determination of death

Death determined by neurologic criteria or brain death is better understood as brain arrest or the final clinical expression of complete and irreversible neurologic failure. Baron and colleagues[1] recently published a review of the history of brain death. Despite widespread national, international, and legal acceptance of the concept, substantial variation exists in the standards and their application,[2–6] and there remains a need to clarify and standardize terminology (eg, ancillary and supplementary testing, brain death, or neurologic determination of death [NDD]). Appendix 1 contains the definitions of key words.

A 2002 survey by Wijdicks[2] explored the international practices for diagnosing brain death and found stunning, often troubling differences. Although there is relative consistency in brainstem reflex testing, there is surprising variation in the performance, methods, and targets of apnea testing; the number of physicians required; and the type and need for confirmatory testing.

In leading US hospitals, variations were found in prerequisites, acceptable core temperature, and the number of required examinations, among others.[7] Chart audits looking at patients diagnosed with brain death revealed incomplete documentation.[8] In an attempt to address the considerable practice variation, recent Canadian and American guidelines are available, and checklists greatly aid in the implementation of standardized practices.[9–11] Yet, despite this, considerable practice variation remains. Although the current evidence base for existing NDD guidelines is often inadequate, clear medical standards for NDD and defining qualifications of physicians performing NDD will augment the quality and rigor of the determination.

The aim of this article is to review the specific criteria and requirements of brain death, paying special attention to areas of controversy and practice inconsistency.

---

[a] Montreal Neurological Hospital, 3801 University Avenue, Room 364, Montreal, Quebec H3A2B4, Canada
[b] Montreal Children's Hospital, 2300 Rue Tupper, Montréal, Québec H3H 1P3, Canada
* Corresponding author.
E-mail address: jteitelbaum@hotmail.com

Neurol Clin 29 (2011) 787–799
doi:10.1016/j.ncl.2011.08.003
0733-8619/11/$ – see front matter © 2011 Elsevier Inc. All rights reserved.

CONCEPT AND DEFINITION OF THE NEUROLOGIC DETERMINATION OF DEATH/BRAIN DEATH

The Canadian forum on NDD defined neurologically determined death as the irreversible loss of the capacity for consciousness combined with the irreversible loss of all brain stem functions, including the capacity to breathe.[10] In the United States, the Uniform Determination of Death Act defines "brain death" as the irreversible cessation of all functions of the entire brain, including the brainstem.[12] In both countries, the determination is to be made according to accepted medical standards.

Of interest in the international context are the differences between whole brain–based and brainstem-based definitions. In most jurisdictions, brain death remains principally a clinical, bedside determination based on confirming the absence of brainstem function. In the United Kingdom, a brainstem-based definition of brain death is applied.[13] The Conference of Medical Royal Colleges and their Faculties in the United Kingdom stated that permanent functional death in the brainstem constitutes brain death. Irreversible loss of brainstem function is defined as the irremediable damage of all brainstem structures. However, it is determined in clinical terms, with the caveat that reversible causes of brainstem dysfunction have been excluded. Loss of ascending reticular activating system function would lead to the loss of consciousness and supplemental testing is not required. Yet, Pallis[14] includes the hypothalamus and interruption of the corticothalamic tract in his diagrams as an extended brainstem. Proof of the destruction of these areas cannot be met by the clinical tests required for the determination of brainstem death, and the UK Code of Practice requires no evidence that the brain stem (medullary) centers controlling heart rate and blood pressure have ceased to function.[13] Proponents of this theory have no problem with the whole brain criteria because the clinical determinants are fundamentally similar.

The important difference between the American and Canadian definitions is that the American definition requires the death of all areas of the brain. The Canadian definition is a clinical one that can be met by either whole brain or brainstem death and, therefore, may occur as a consequence of intracranial hypertension or primary direct brain stem injury or both. Unlike Pallis, the hypothalamus is not specifically identified in any Canadian description as being an integral part of the brainstem. However, there are currently no satisfactory ancillary tests for the confirmation of death in instances of isolated primary brain stem injury.

TIMING OF THE INITIAL ASSESSMENT AND EXAMINATION INTERVAL

There are 2 key timing issues regarding the declaration of brain death. The first relates to the timing of the first examination for brain death relative to the primary injury and the second relates to the time interval between examinations, should more than 1 examination be required.

Timing of the First Assessment

Pallis and Harley[14] of the United Kingdom define the time of the first assessment for brain death as the point when the preconditions for the diagnosis of brain death have been met; unresponsive apneic coma, a cause of coma capable of producing brain death, and a determination that the damage is irremediable.

The Australian and New Zealand Intensive Care Society guidelines[15] recommend that no fewer than 4 hours of documented coma should precede the first examination for brain death.

In the 1995 AAN guidelines and the 2010 review,[9] Wijdicks therefore does not recommend a specific time frame for the first assessment, stating only that a certain period of time must have passed (usually several hours) between the initial insult and the clinical examination for brain death. The Canadian forum also addressed this question at length. For the timing of the first examination, even though there was no compelling evidence, several practical factors were taken into consideration. First, neurologic assessment may be unreliable in the acute (24 hours) postresuscitation phase after cardiorespiratory arrest.[16] Indeed, initially absent pupillary and motor responses have returned in the first 24 hours after arrest.[17] Also, there are cases when cardiac arrest leads to brain death confirmed at 6 hours but with the return of some brainstem function by 24 hours.[18] Second, after severe metabolic or pure hypoxic injury (hypoglycemia, asphyxia, hypernatremia), it may be very difficult to know at what time the neurologic picture can be deemed irreversible. The recommendation is, therefore, as follows:

- The time of the first assessment for brain death is the point when the preconditions for the diagnosis of brain death have been met, with the following exceptions:
  - In cases of acute hypoxic-ischemic brain injury, clinical evaluation for NDD should be delayed for 24 hours after the cardiorespiratory arrest or when an ancillary test could be performed.
  - In cases of extreme metabolic insult, enough time should have passed for the clinician to think that the insult is permanent and there should be evidence of diffuse cerebral insult on imaging (magnetic resonance imaging [MRI]). If irreversibility remains an issue, an ancillary test should be performed in addition to the clinical examination.
  - For neonates younger than 30 days old, the minimum time from birth to the first determination is 48 hours.

Examiners are cautioned to review these factors in the context of the primary cause and examination. In addition, the evolving use of therapeutic hypothermia as a neuroprotective strategy after successful resuscitation from cardiac arrest may require a further delay.[19] When there is doubt, one should not proceed with NDD. Clinical judgment is the deciding factor.

Interval Time Between Examinations

The length of observation periods has varied extensively throughout the world and the United States.[20] Wijdicks provides a table of age-related interval times in his 1995 guidelines. In his 2010 update and review of the literature, he finds that there is no evidence-based answer. Indeed, recovery of neurologic function has not been reported after the clinical diagnosis of brain death using these criteria.

- Based on this evidence, the AAN guidelines state that a single examination suffices to establish the diagnosis but that US state statutes require 2 examinations, especially in the context of organ donation.
- The Canadian guidelines state that for the purposes of a postmortem transplant, the fact of death shall be determined by at least 2 physicians. The examinations may be performed concurrently. However, if the determinations are performed at different times, a full clinical examination, including apnea testing, must be performed at each determination. No fixed interval of time is recommended for the second determination except when age-related criteria apply.
  - For neonates to 1 year, a repeat examination at a different time is recommended to ensure independent confirmation by another qualified physician, regardless of the primary mechanism of the brain injury. It is prudent to have

an independent examination because of the lack of collective experience and research on brain death in this age group. There is no recommended minimum time interval between determinations. Should uncertainty or confounding issues arise that cannot be resolved, the time interval may be extended according to physician judgment or an ancillary test demonstrating the absence of intracerebral blood flow may be used.

○ For term newborns aged younger than 30 days, 2 determinations are required, with a minimum interval of 24 hours between examinations.

WHO IS QUALIFIED TO PERFORM THE ASSESSMENT?

Clear medical standards for NDD (brain death) and defining qualifications of physicians performing NDD augment the quality and rigor of the determination. Legally, all physicians are allowed to determine brain death. Brain death statutes in the United States differ by state and institution. Some US state or hospital guidelines require the examiner to have certain expertise; others specifically recommend that the assessment be done by a neurologist, neurosurgeon or intensive care physician. The AAN guidelines state: "Neurologists, neurosurgeons, and intensive care specialists may have specialized expertise, but it seems reasonable to require that all physicians making a determination of brain death be intimately familiar with brain death criteria and have demonstrated competence in this complex examination."[9] Recent Australian guidelines have included formal certification of competence.

The Canadian Forum thought that extensive clinical experience in treating patients with catastrophic brain injury was probably more important than the academic designations of those performing these evaluations. The Canadian recommendation is as follows:

The minimum level of physician qualification required to perform NDD should include full and current licensure for independent medical practice in the relevant Canadian jurisdiction, skill and knowledge in the management of patients with severe brain injury and NDD, and no association with the proposed recipient that might influence the physician's judgment. These qualifications exclude physicians who are only on an educational register.

CLINICAL EVALUATION

The requirements for the substantiation of brain death are quite uniform across guidelines and are cautious to exclude any potential diagnostic error or reversible conditions.

The prerequisite is that the clinical assessment for NDD cannot take place until blood pressure and temperature are normal. Exact values are not always stipulated and can vary between guidelines.

The minimum clinical criteria for NDD in adults (Appendix 2) includes the following:

1. Established cause capable of causing neurologic death with definite clinical or neuroimaging evidence of an acute central nervous system (CNS) event consistent with the irreversible loss of neurologic function and in the absence of reversible conditions capable of mimicking neurologic death.
2. Deep unresponsive coma with bilateral absence of motor responses, excluding spinal reflexes, which implies a lack of spontaneous movements and an absence of movement originating in the CNS, such as cranial nerve function, CNS-mediated motor response to pain in any distribution, seizures, and decorticate and decerebrate responses. Spinal reflexes or motor responses confined to spinal

distribution may persist and have been reported in up to 75% of patients progressing to brain death.[19] Several accepted spinal-originating movements in brain dead patients have been documented and described.[20]
3. Absent brain stem reflexes as defined by absent gag and cough reflexes and the bilateral absence of
    a. Corneal responses
    b. Pupillary responses to light, with pupils at midsize or greater
    c. Vestibuloocular responses (**Box 1**)
4. Absent respiratory effort based on the apnea test
5. Absent confounding factors.

For infants aged 30 days to 1 year (corrected for gestational age) (Appendix 3)

- The criteria include the oculocephalic reflex instead of the vestibule=ocular reflex in infants because of the unique anatomy of the external auditory canal (see Recommendation A.1).

For neonates from term (36 weeks' gestation) to 30 days (Appendix 4)

- Clinical criteria have primacy, as they do in the child and adult.
- Minimum clinical criteria include the absence of oculocephalic reflex and suck reflex.

CONFOUNDING FACTORS

Both the AAN and Canadian guidelines place the achievement of normal blood pressure and temperature in the prerequisites for clinical evaluation but the acceptable threshold values differ. The list of possible confounding factors is otherwise identical (**Box 2**).

When assessing for neurologic death, examiners are cautioned to review these confounding factors in the context of the primary cause and examination. If physicians are confounded by data, either absolutely or by differing perspectives, they should not proceed with NDD. Clinical judgment is the deciding factor.

There are key considerations that need to be specifically addressed.

- Unresuscitated shock: American guidelines require a systolic blood pressure more than 100 mm Hg before proceeding to brain death assessment. The

---

Box 1
Caloric testing (oculocephalic reflex)

Place the head of the bed at 30°.

Confirm the patency of the external auditory canal and remove excess wax and debris.

Check the tympanic membrane and rule out tears or perforation.

Prepare ice-cold water in a kidney basin.

The eyes should be held open.

Irrigate one ear at a time using a 50 or 60 mL syringe and a 20-gauge, 1.25 inch intravenous catheter.

Observe the eyes during and after irrigation for a full minute.

Allow 5 minutes between ears.

Full inhibition of the vestibular system requires 20 seconds of contact with a temperature of 0°C. The inhibition takes a minimum of 2 minutes to wear off after ice-water irrigation.

> **Box 2**
> **Confounding factors**
>
> *Conditions that can mimic brain death*
>
> Severe hypothermia, temperature (T) less than 32°C
>
> Hypotensive shock: systolic blood pressure too low to assure brain perfusion
>
> Peripheral nerve or muscle dysfunction or neuromuscular blockade
>
> Brainstem ischemia causing a locked-in syndrome
>
> Drug effect: paralyzing agent, barbiturate or benzodiazepine overdose, anesthetic agents
>
> *Conditions that affect the ability to confirm irreversibility*
>
> Hypothermia (core T <34°C)
>
> Severe metabolic disorders capable of causing a potentially reversible coma
>
> Severe metabolic abnormalities: glucose; electrolytes, including potassium, phosphate, calcium, and magnesium; inborn errors of metabolism; and liver and renal dysfunction may play a role in clinical presentation

Canadian guidelines do not specify the exact blood pressure value, although a systolic BP more than 90 mm Hg is usually chosen.

- Hypothermia
  - According to the Canadian guidelines, core temperature should be obtained through central blood, rectal, or esophageal-gastric measurement. Method of temperature measurement is not mentioned by the AAN.
  - The existing Canadian standard of 32.2°C was based on precedent.[10] The relevance of the scientific evidence and the application of this standard in the context of severe brain injury are uncertain, however.
  - Given that there is no evidence base, a decision was made by the Canadian Forum to adopt 34°C as a rational, safe, and attainable standard. This decision was based on the following rationale: ideally, temperature should be as close to normal as possible and this is the minimum temperature at which the test is valid; raising patients' temperature from 32.2°C to 34.0°C does not pose significant difficulty to the patients or the treating physician.
  - According to the AAN guidelines, core temperature should be raised and maintained at a minimum of 36°C.

Although clinically significant, drug intoxications (eg, alcohol, barbiturates, sedatives, hypnotics) are confounders that must be addressed before clinical assessment; therapeutic levels or therapeutic dosing of anticonvulsants, sedatives, and analgesics do not preclude the diagnosis of brain death.

The approach to the presence of medications (eg, sedation, analgesia, barbiturates) that may depress CNS function varies throughout the world. Variables to consider when considering the potential to confound the clinical evaluation are drug type, dosage, duration, and hepatorenal function. If uncertainty exists, drug levels should be monitored, drugs should be discontinued with time allowed for elimination, or an ancillary test should be performed.

APNEA TEST

The absence of a breathing drive is tested with a CO_2 challenge. North American guidelines usually recommend an apneic threshold $PaCO_2$ greater than or equal to

60 mm Hg. In contrast, the UK code requires a threshold $PaCO_2$ greater than or equal to 50 mm Hg. Documentation of an increase in $PaCO_2$ more than normal levels is typical practice.

Apnea testing requires normotension, normothermia, euvolemia, eucapnia ($PaCO_2$ 35–45 mm Hg), satisfactory oxygenation, and the absence of prior CO_2 retention (ie, chronic obstructive pulmonary disease, severe obesity).

The Canadian guidelines recommend that the thresholds at the completion of the apnea test be $PaCO_2$ greater than or equal to 60 mm Hg and greater than or equal to 20 mm Hg more than the preapnea test level and pH less than or equal to 7.28. These thresholds must be documented by arterial blood gas measurement. To interpret an apnea test correctly, the certifying physician must continuously observe patients for respiratory effort throughout the administration of the test. AAN apnea testing requires a postapnea $PaCO_2$ greater than or equal to 60 mm Hg or greater than or equal to 20 mm Hg more than the preapnea eucapnia.

For patients with severe lung disease, caution must be exercised in considering the validity of the apnea test. If there is a history suggestive of chronic respiratory insufficiency and responsiveness to only supranormal levels of carbon dioxide, or if patients depend on hypoxic drive, then the physician cannot be sure of the validity of the apnea test. In such conditions, an ancillary test should be administered.

The exact procedure for apnea testing is outlined in **Box 3**.

ANCILLARY TESTS

Sometimes clinical criteria cannot be applied reliably (eg, when the cranial nerves cannot be adequately examined, when neuromuscular paralysis or drug intoxication is present, in patients for whom the apnea test is precluded [respiratory instability or high cervical spine injury] or not valid [high CO_2 retainers], and when confounding factors remain unresolved). In these situations, ancillary tests are necessary. The different guidelines define when ancillary (sometimes called supplementary) testing should be done and the requirements that still need to be met before the testing.

At a minimum, unresuscitated shock and hypothermia must be corrected and 2 particular clinical criteria must be met before ancillary tests are performed: (1) there

---

Box 3
Apnea testing

Keep systolic blood pressure greater than or equal to 90 (or 100) mm Hg.

Preoxygenate for at least 10 minutes with 100% O_2.

Reduce ventilator frequency to obtain normocarbia (10 breaths per minute).

Baseline blood gas should have pCO_2 of 35 to 45 mm Hg, O_2 greater than or equal to 200 mm Hg, and pH greater than or equal to 7.3.

Disconnect the ventilator.

Place a catheter through the endotracheal tube to the level of the carina.

Deliver 100% O_2 at 6 L/min.

Observe for respiratory movements for 8 to 10 minutes.

Abort if systolic pressure is less than 90 mm Hg or SO_2 less than 85%.

Draw second blood gas after the 8 to 10 minutes of apnea.

Reconnect the ventilator and lower FiO_2.

must be an established cause capable of causing neurologic death in the absence of reversible conditions capable of mimicking neurologic death and (2) patients must be in a deep unresponsive coma.

In 2006, Young and colleagues[3,21] published a critical review of the various ancillary tests used to support the neurologic determination of death (brain death). Tests of brain perfusion were the only tests to satisfy the criteria, whereas electrophysiological and other tests were considered inadequate (Appendix 5). Although only 4-vessel cerebral angiography and radionuclide tests of blood flow/brain perfusion have been officially accepted as valid confirmatory tests, computed tomographic (CT) angiography and magnetic resonance (MR) angiography were subsequently found to be equally suitable. However, transcranial Doppler is not suitable because of frequent problems with insonation and the variability among operators.

The demonstration of the global absence of intracranial blood flow is presently considered the standard for NDD by ancillary testing.

Many guidelines still accept electroencephalogram (EEG) as an acceptable ancillary test to confirm brain death. The AAN guideline update[9] lists 4 acceptable tests, including EEG, and requires only 1 for validation. The English guidelines list the pros and cons of the various ancillary tests, and many guidelines still require an EEG as part of NDD despite the drawbacks.[2,3]

REFERENCES

1. Baron L, Shemie SD, Teitelbaum J, et al. Brief review: history, concepts and controversies in the neurological determination of death. Can J Anaesth 2006;53:602–8.
2. Wijdicks EF. Brain death worldwide: accepted fact but no global consensus in diagnostic criteria. Neurology 2002;58(1):20–5.
3. Shemie SD. Variability of brain death practices. Crit Care Med 2004;32(12):2564–5.
4. Powner DJ, Hernandez M, Rives TE. Variability among hospital policies for determining brain death in adults. Crit Care Med 2004;32(6):1284–8.
5. Mejia RE, Pollack MM. Variability in brain death determination practices in children. JAMA 1995;274(7):550–3.
6. Chang MY, McBride LA, Ferguson MA. Variability in brain death declaration practices in pediatric head trauma patients. Pediatr Neurosurg 2003;39(1):7–9.
7. Greer DM, Varelas PN, Haque S, et al. Variability of brain death determination guidelines in leading US neurologic institutions. Neurology 2008;70:284–9.
8. Wang M, Wallace P, Gruen JP. Brain death documentation: analysis and issues. Neurosurgery 2002;51:731–6.
9. Wijdicks EF, Varelas PN, Gronseth GS, et al. American Academy of Neurology evidence-based guideline update: determining brain death in adults: report of the Quality Standards Subcommittee of the American Academy of Neurology. Neurology 2010;74:1911–8.
10. Canadian Neurocritical Care Group. Guidelines for the diagnosis of brain death. Can J Neurol Sci 1999;26(1):64–6.
11. Shemie SD, Doig C, Dickens B, et al, Pediatric Reference Group and the Neonatal Reference Group. Severe brain injury to neurological determination of death: Canadian forum recommendations. CMAJ 2006;174(6):S1–30.
12. Uniform Determination of Death Act, 12 uniform laws annotated 589 (West 1993 and West Suppl 1997).
13. Diagnosis of brain death: statement issued by the honorary secretary of the conference of Medical Royal Colleges and their Faculties in the United Kingdom on the 11th October 1976. BMJ 1976;2:1187–8.

14. Pallis C, Harley DH. ABC of brainstem death. 2nd edition. London: BMJ publishing group; 1996.
15. Pearson IY. Australia and New Zealand Intensive Care Society statement and guidelines on brain death and model policy on organ donation. Anaesth Intensive Care 1995;23:140–8.
16. Booth CM, Boone RH, Tomlinson G, et al. Is this patient dead, vegetative, or severely neurologically impaired? Assessing outcome for comatose survivors of cardiac arrest. JAMA 2004;291(7):870–9.
17. Zanbergen EG, De Haan RJ, Stoutenbeek CP, et al. Systematic review of early prediction of poor outcome in anoxic-ischemic coma. Lancet 1998;352(9143):1808–12.
18. Webb AC, Samuels OB. Reversible brain death after cardiopulmonary arrest and induced hypothermia. Crit Care Med 2011;39(6):1538–42.
19. Shemie SD, Langevin S, Farrell C. Therapeutic hypothermia after cardiac arrest: another confounding factor in brain-death testing. Pediatr Neurol 2010;42(4):304.
20. Saposnik G, Basile VS, Young GB. Movements in brain death: a systematic review. Can J Neurol Sci 2009;26:154–60.
21. Young GB, Shemie SD, Doig CJ, et al. Brief review: the role of ancillary tests in the neurological determination of death. Can J Anaesth 2006;53:620–7.

APPENDIX 1: KEY TERMS: BRAIN DEATH

- Brain death is ubiquitous in medical, nursing, and lay literature. It is based on the concept of complete and irreversible loss of brain function. The Canadian Neurocritical Care guidelines[2] define brain death as "the irreversible loss of the capacity for consciousness combined with the irreversible loss of all brainstem functions, including the capacity to breathe. Brain death is equivalent to death of the individual, even though the heart continues to beat and spinal cord functions may persist."[10] This definition was adopted as the definition of neurologically determined death by the forum members see Recommendation A.7. The President's Commission for the Study of Ethical Problems in Medicine and Biomedical and Behavioral Research (United States)[14] defines brain death as "irreversible cessation of all functions of the entire brain, including the brainstem. The clinical diagnosis of brain death is equivalent to irreversible loss of all brainstem function."[10]

- Although brain death is an accepted concept, the definition lacks clarity in the Canadian context. Distinctions between brainstem death (UK definition) and whole brain death (US definition) are unclear in Canada.

- The actual process for determining brain death in Canada is legally stated as "according to accepted medical practice." A purpose of this forum was to clearly define and standardize "accepted medical practice."

Neurologic death

- Neurologic death is a term that is similar to brain death, but not commonly used.

Neurologic determination of death

- NDD is the process and procedure for determining death of an individual. NDD (see Recommendation A.7) is not a new definition of death. It is intended to be the end result of a clear and standardized process for the determination of death based on neurologic or brain-based criteria. For the purposes of this forum, the term brain death was replaced by NDD.

APPENDIX 2: CHECKLISTS FOR NEUROLOGIC DETERMINATION OF DEATH

Definitions and notes

Age definitions: children are those aged 1 to 18 years.

Infants are aged 30 days to 1 year (corrected for gestational age).

Term newborns are 36 weeks' gestation to 29 days old (corrected for gestational age).

Overarching principles: The legal time of death is marked by the first determination of death. Existing law states that for the purposes of postmortem donation, the fact of death shall be determined by 2 physicians. The physicians' determinations may be performed concurrently. If performed at different times, a full clinical examination, including the apnea test, must be performed without any fixed examination interval regardless of the primary cause. For infants and term newborns, the first and second physicians' determinations as defined by a full clinical examination, including the apnea test, must be performed at 2 different times. For infants, there is no fixed interval regardless of the primary cause. For term newborns, the first examination should be delayed 48 hours after birth and the interval should be greater than or equal to 24 hours, regardless of the primary cause.

Physicians declaring neurologic death

The minimum level of physician qualifications to perform NDD is full and current licensure for independent medical practice in the relevant Canadian jurisdiction. This qualification excludes physicians who are only on an educational register. The authority to perform NDD cannot be delegated. Physicians should have skill and knowledge in both the management of patients with severe brain injury and in the determination of neurologic death in the relevant age group. For the purposes of postmortem donation, a physician who has had any association with the proposed transplant recipient that might influence the physician's judgment shall not take part in the declaration of death.

Minimum clinical criteria

Established cause: Absence of clinical neurologic function with a known, proximate cause that is irreversible. There must be definite clinical or neuroimaging evidence of an acute CNS event that is consistent with the irreversible loss of neurologic function. NDD may occur as a consequence of intracranial hypertension, primary direct brainstem injury, or both.

Deep unresponsive coma: A lack of spontaneous movements and absence of movement originating in the CNS, such as cranial nerve function, CNS-mediated motor response to pain in any distribution, seizures, and decorticate and decerebrate responses. *Spinal reflexes*, or motor responses confined to spinal distribution, may persist.

Confounding factors

- Unresuscitated shock

- Hypothermia (core temperature <34°C and <36°C for newborns by central blood, rectal, or esophageal-gastric measurements)

- Severe metabolic disorders capable of causing a potentially reversible coma

If the primary cause does not fully explain the clinical picture and if in the treating physician's judgment that the metabolic abnormality may play a role, it should be corrected or an ancillary test should be performed.

- Peripheral nerve or muscle dysfunction or neuromuscular blockade potentially accounting for unresponsiveness

- Clinically significant drug intoxications (eg, alcohol, barbiturates, sedatives)

Therapeutic levels or therapeutic dosing of anticonvulsants, sedatives, and analgesics does not preclude the diagnosis.

Specific to cardiac arrest: Neurologic assessments may be unreliable in the acute postresuscitation phase after cardiorespiratory arrest. In cases of acute hypoxic-ischemic brain injury, clinical evaluation for NDD should be delayed for 24 hours or an ancillary test could be performed. Examiners are cautioned to review confounding issues in the context of the primary cause and examination. Clinical judgment is the deciding factor.

Apnea test

Optimal performance requires a period of preoxygenation followed by 100% O_2 delivered via the trachea on disconnection from mechanical ventilation. The certifying physician must continuously observe patients for respiratory effort. Thresholds at completion of the apnea test include the following: $PaCO_2$ greater than or equal to 60 mm Hg and greater than or equal to 20 mm Hg more than the preapnea test level and pH less than or equal to 7.28 as determined by arterial blood gases. Caution must be exercised in considering the validity in cases of chronic respiratory insufficiency or dependence on hypoxic respiratory drive.

Ancillary tests: Demonstration of the global absence of intracerebral blood flow is considered the standard for determination of death by ancillary testing. The following prerequisite conditions must be met before ancillary testing:

• Established cause

• Deep unresponsive coma

• Absence of unresuscitated shock and hypothermia

Currently validated techniques are 4-vessel cerebral angiogram or radionuclide cerebral blood flow imaging.
EEG is no longer recommended. NDD can be confirmed by ancillary testing when minimum clinical criteria cannot be completed or confounding factors cannot be corrected.

APPENDIX 3: CHECKLIST FOR ADULTS AND CHILDREN AGED 1 YEAR AND OLDER

a. Deep unresponsive coma with the following established etiology _____
b. Confounding factors precluding the diagnosis? Yes No
c. Temperature (core) _____
d. Brainstem reflexes:
Bilateral absence of motor responses (excluding spinal reflexes) Yes No
Absent cough Yes No
Absent gag Yes No
Bilateral absence of corneal responses Yes No
Bilateral absence of vestibulo-ocular responses Yes No
Bilateral absence of pupillary response to light (pupils ≥ mid-size) Yes No
e. Apnea Yes No
At completion of apnea test: pH _____ $PaCO_2$ _____ mm Hg
$PaCO_2$ ≥ 20 mm Hg above the pre-apnea test level Yes No
Ancillary tests
Ancillary tests, as defined by determination of the absence of intracerebral blood flow, should be performed when **any** of the minimum
clinical criteria cannot be established **or** unresolved confounding factors exist.
Ancillary testing has been performed Yes No
Date: _____Time: _____
Absence of intracerebral blood flow has been demonstrated by
Cerebral radiocontrast angiography
Radionuclide angiography

Other _____
Declaration and documentation
The first and second physicians' determinations may be performed concurrently. If performed at different times, a full clinical
examination including the apnea test must be performed, without any fixed examination interval, regardless of the primary etiology.
This patient fulfills the criteria for neurological determination of death
Physician (print name): _____ Signature: _____
Date: _____ Time: _____
Standard end-of-life care
Is this patient medically eligible for organ or tissue donation? Yes No
Has the option for organ or tissue donation been offered? Yes No
Has consent been obtained for donation? Yes No

APPENDIX 4: CHECKLIST FOR INFANTS AGED YOUNGER THAN 1 YEAR AND TERM NEWBORNS (36 WEEKS' GESTATION)

a. Deep unresponsive coma with the following established etiology _____

b. Confounding factors precluding the diagnosis? Yes   No

c. Temperature (core) _____

d. Brainstem reflexes:

Bilateral absence of motor responses (excluding spinal reflexes) Yes   No

Absent cough Yes   No

Absent gag Yes   No

Absent suck (newborn only) Yes   No   Not applicable

Bilateral absence of corneal responses Yes   No

Bilateral absence of vestibulo-ocular responses Yes   No

Bilateral absence of pupillary response to light (pupils ≥ mid-size) Yes   No

e. Apnea Yes   No

At completion of apnea test: pH _____ $PaCO_2$ _____ mm Hg

$PaCO_2 ≥ 20$ mm Hg above the pre-apnea test level Yes   No

Ancillary tests

Ancillary tests, as defined by determination of the absence of intracerebral blood flow, should be performed when **any** of the minimum

clinical criteria cannot be established **or** unresolved confounding factors exist.

Ancillary testing has been performed Yes   No

Date: _____Time: _____

Absence of intracerebral blood flow has been demonstrated by

Cerebral radiocontrast angiography

Radionuclide angiography

Other _____

Examination interval, declaration and documentation

The first and second physicians' determinations (a full clinical examination including the apnea test) should be performed at different

times. For infants, there is no fixed examination interval. For newborns, the first examination should be delayed until 48 h after birth

and the interval between examinations should be ≥ 24 h.

This patient fulfills the criteria for neurological determination of death

Physician (print name): _____ Signature: _____

Date: _____ Time: _____

Standard end-of-life care

Is this patient medically eligible for organ or tissue donation? Yes   No

Has the option for organ or tissue donation been offered? Yes   No

Has consent been obtained for donation? Yes   No

APPENDIX 5: ANCILLARY TESTING

The demonstration of the absence of intracerebral blood flow is considered the standard as an ancillary test for NDD. Currently validated imaging techniques are cerebral angiography[15] and radionuclide angiography.[16] The authors recognize that additional cerebral blood flow imaging technologies may further develop or evolve but they cannot be recommended at this time. EEG is no longer recommended as an ancillary test, in view of limitations, as discussed later.

Recommended ancillary tests

Cerebral angiography

A selective radiocontrast 4-vessel angiogram visualizing both the anterior and posterior cerebral circulation should be obtained. Cerebral-circulatory arrest occurs when intracerebral pressure exceeds arterial inflow pressure. External carotid circulation should be evident and filling of the superior sinus may be present. Angiography requires technical expertise and is performed in the radiology department, necessitating transport of potentially unstable patients. Arterial puncture and catheter-related complications have been described. Radiocontrast can produce idiosyncratic reactions and end-organ damage, such as renal dysfunction.

Radionuclide imaging techniques

Radionuclide angiography (perfusion scintigraphy) for brain death confirmation has been widely accepted for several years. In the last decade, radiopharmaceuticals, especially Tc99m hexamethylpropylene-amine oxime (Tc99m HMPAO), have been studied extensively and provide enhanced detection of intracerebral, posterior fossa, and brainstem blood flow.[16,17] Tc99m HMPAO is lipid soluble, crossing the blood-brain barrier, providing information on arterial cerebral blood flow and uptake of tracer within perfused brain tissue. The traditional gamma cameras used in this technique are immobile, necessitating patient transfer for study; but newer technologies are portable, allowing for studies to be performed at the bedside.

Ancillary tests in evolution*

Transcranial Doppler ultrasonography

Using a pulse Doppler instrument, the intracerebral arteries, including the vertebral or basilar arteries, are insonated bilaterally. Brain dead patients display either absent or reversed diastolic flow or small systolic spikes.[19] The noninvasiveness and portability of this technique are advantageous but the technology requires substantial clinical expertise for proper application and is not widely available. It has not been sufficiently validated at this time.

MRI

MRI-based angiography and imaging hold future promise but are not easily available and have not been sufficiently validated at this time.

EEG

EEG is readily available in most tertiary medical centers worldwide and has long been used as a supplementary test for brain death.[20] It can be performed at the bedside but has significant limitations.[3] The EEG detects cortical electrical activity but is unable to detect deep cerebral or brainstem function. The high sensitivity requirement for EEG recording may result in the detection of electric interference from many of the devices that are commonplace in the intensive care unit setting. EEG is also significantly affected by hypothermia, drug administration, and metabolic disturbances, thus, diminishing its clinical utility. It is no longer recommended as an ancillary test.

MR angiography

CT angiograph

Epilepsy and the Consciousness System: Transient Vegetative State?

Hal Blumenfeld, MD, PhD[a,b,c,*]

KEYWORDS

- Consciousness • Seizures • Absence seizures
- Temporal lobe epilepsy • Complex partial seizures
- Generalized tonic-clonic seizures • Thalamus • fMRI

Consciousness is an essential core feature of human life, so it is not surprising that disorders of consciousness have a major impact. Recent work has demonstrated that epilepsy shares many features with other disorders of consciousness. When patients lose consciousness during epileptic seizures they exhibit no meaningful responses to external stimuli; however, the eyes are usually open. In addition, although there is insufficient time to determine whether sleep-wake cycles are present, patients may exhibit orienting responses or other simple behaviors. Therefore, impaired consciousness during seizures resembles other disorders of consciousness such as vegetative state or minimally conscious state and, less so, coma. The major difference from these other disorders of consciousness is that (with the exception of status epilepticus) seizures typically last for minutes rather than days, months, or years. The transient nature of epileptic seizures provides a unique opportunity for determining the anatomic and physiologic basis of impaired consciousness and its recovery.

Seizures and other disorders of consciousness converge on a common set of cortical and subcortical structures. These structures constitute the "consciousness system," defined in the next section as the bilateral medial and lateral fronto-parietal

This work was supported by NIH (R01NS055829, R01NS066974, R01NS049307, R01MH67528, P30NS052519), a Donaghue Investigator Award, and the Betsy and Jonathan Blattmachr Family.
[a] Department of Neurology, Yale University School of Medicine, 333 Cedar Street, New Haven, CT 06520, USA
[b] Department of Neurobiology, Yale University School of Medicine, 333 Cedar Street, New Haven, CT 06520, USA
[c] Department of Neurosurgery, Yale University School of Medicine, 333 Cedar Street, New Haven, CT 06520, USA
* Department of Neurology, Yale University School of Medicine, 333 Cedar Street, New Haven, CT 06520-8018.
E-mail address: hal.blumenfeld@yale.edu

association cortex and subcortical arousal systems. Recent neuroimaging, intracranial EEG, and animal models demonstrate that the consciousness system forms a common anatomical substrate for all seizure types causing impaired consciousness. The main types of seizures causing transiently impaired consciousness include absence seizures, generalized tonic-clonic seizures, and temporal lobe complex partial seizures. This article will discuss the clinical and behavioral features, as well as recent neuroimaging and electrophysiology studies which have begun to shed light on the pathophysiology of impaired consciousness in these seizure types. The impact of impaired consciousness on quality of life in patients with epilepsy, and potential treatment strategies will also be discussed.

THE CONSCIOUSNESS SYSTEM

Following the tradition of Plum and Posner,[1] it has been useful to separate consciousness into systems that are important for the *content* of consciousness, and those that control the *level* of consciousness. The content of consciousness can be thought of as the subject matter or substrate on which systems controlling the level of consciousness act. Thus, the content of consciousness includes all the information encoded in our hierarchically organized sensory and motor systems, as well as in the systems dedicated to memory and emotions. The level of consciousness is controlled by a specialized system of cortical and subcortical structures, which regulate alertness, attention, and awareness (mnemonic: AAA).[2,3] In analogy to other nervous system networks serving specialized functions such as the motor, sensory, and limbic systems, the networks regulating the level of consciousness should logically be referred to as the "consciousness system."[3,4]

The consciousness system comprises cortical regions important for higher-order integration including the lateral frontal and parietal association cortex, as well as the medial frontal, anterior, and posterior cingulate, and medial parietal (precuneus, retrosplenial) cortex (**Fig. 1**). Subcortical structures participating in the consciousness

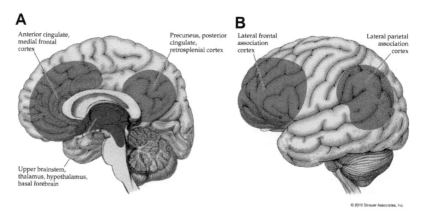

Fig. 1. The consciousness system. Anatomic structures involved in regulating the level of alertness, attention, and awareness. (*A*) Medial view showing cortical (*blue*) and subcortical (*red*) components of the consciousness system. (*B*) Lateral cortical components of the consciousness system. Note that other circuits not pictured here, such as the basal ganglia and cerebellum, may also play a role in attention and other aspects of consciousness. (*Reproduced from* Blumenfeld H. Neuroanatomy through clinical cases. 2nd edition. Sunderland (MA): Sinauer Associates; 2010; with permission.)

system include the activating systems of the upper pons and midbrain, the thalamus, hypothalamus, and basal forebrain (see **Fig. 1**). Numerous studies have shown that these structures are crucial for normal alertness, attention, and awareness.[5,6] In addition, disorders of consciousness including coma, vegetative state, and minimally conscious state are known to be associated with dysfunction in these cortical and subcortical brain networks[7,8] (see also articles by N. Schiff and J. Giacino elsewhere in this issue). The sections that follow will provide evidence that 3 types of epileptic seizures—namely absence, generalized tonic-clonic, and temporal lobe complex partial seizures—all converge on the consciousness system when they cause impaired consciousness (see **Fig. 1**). Although the anatomic regions causing impaired consciousness in these 3 seizure types appear to be the same, the physiologic mechanisms may differ. Thus, different patterns of abnormal increases or decreases in activity can occur in different seizure types, but they all lead to impaired consciousness by affecting the same set of anatomic structures.

ABSENCE SEIZURES

Absence (petit mal) seizures are typically brief 5- to 10-second events consisting of staring and unresponsiveness. Electroencephalography (EEG) during absence seizures shows widespread bilateral 3- to 4-Hz spike-wave discharges (**Fig. 2**A). Absence seizures usually last 5 to 10 seconds, with abrupt onset and end of EEG changes and behavioral deficits. Seen most commonly in children as part of childhood absence epilepsy, absence seizures occur less often in adolescents and adults. Before the initiation of treatment, seizures can recur up to hundreds of times per day, causing significant impairment in school and work performance.

Behavioral changes during absence seizures consist of arrest of ongoing movements, and lack of response to questions and commands. Absence seizures appear as if someone has "pushed the pause button" on the patient's behavior and responsiveness. Episodes are commonly accompanied by minor eyelid, mouth, or finger movements, but more significant motor activity is not part of typical absence seizures. The eyelids may droop but remain open; in fact if the eyes are closed before onset they tend to open during seizures.[9] Onset and end are usually abrupt, and patients do not usually show significant postictal deficits, although subtle impairment has been reported in some studies for a few seconds after seizures end.[10–14] The usual duration of absence seizures is 5 to 10 seconds, and some classify episodes lasting less than 3 seconds as interictal epileptiform activity rather than seizures.[15,16] However, this arbitrary cutoff is not fully supported by the available data, because even very brief episodes of spike-wave activity lasting a second or less may cause behavioral deficits when evaluated by careful testing.[10,17–19] The time course of impairment during absence seizures exhibits a "trough" (see **Fig. 2**B) with maximal deficits occurring within about a second of seizure onset, and performance then gradually improving toward the end of the seizure.[18,20–25] It has been reported that task performance is relatively spared during the last 2 to 3 seconds of longer seizures,[18,22,25–27] although the exact ending time of longer seizures may be difficult to determine electrographically because the spike-wave pattern often gradually merges into a period of generalized slowing without spikes. Memory for new information presented to patients during absence seizures is usually (but not always) lost, and some studies have reported a short period of anterograde amnesia during which information from a few seconds before the seizure also cannot be retrieved.[21,23,28–32]

Many patients retain the capacity to perform simple tasks such as repetitive finger tapping during absence seizures.[17,18,20,32–34] In general, tasks that require greater

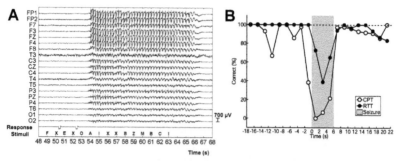

Fig. 2. Electroencephalography (EEG) and behavior during typical absence seizures. (*A*) EEG showing typical 3- to 4-Hz spike-wave discharge during an absence seizure. Amplitude is maximal in frontal electrodes (FP1, FP2, F7, F3, FZ, F4, F8) and lower in more posterior occipital regions (O1, O2). A series of letters were presented to the patient (Stimuli) in a continuous performance task. Prior to the seizure the patient pushed the button (Response, voltage deflections) correctly to each target letter (X). However, when the target letter X occurred during the seizure, the patient was unable to respond. Linked-ears referential EEG recording. Functional magnetic resonance imaging (fMRI) changes for this seizure are shown in **Fig. 3**. (*B*) Average behavioral impairment during absence seizures. Percent correct responses are shown over time (2-second time bins) before, during, and after seizures (shaded region, normalized to mean seizure duration of ~6 seconds). Results are shown for 2 different tasks: in the continuous performance task (CPT) random letters appeared once per second and patients were instructed to push a button each time the target letter X appeared (see also *A*); in the repetitive tapping task (RTT) patients were instructed to push the button for every letter regardless of its identity. Performance on the more difficult CPT task declined rapidly for letters presented just before seizure onset and recovered quickly after seizure end. Impaired performance on the RTT task was more transient than on CPT, did not begin until after seizure onset, and was less severely impaired during seizures than the CPT task ($F = 15.3$, $P = .017$; analysis of variance). Results are based on a total of 53 seizures in 8 patients; 41 seizures in 5 patients during CPT and 12 seizures in 4 patients during RTT. ([*A*] *Reproduced from* Berman R, Negishi M, Vestal M, et al. Simultaneous EEG, fMRI, and behavioral testing in typical childhood absence seizures. Epilepsia 2010;51(10):2011–22; with permission; and [*B*] Bai X, Vestal M, Berman R, et al. Dynamic time course of typical childhood absence seizures: EEG, behavior, and functional magnetic resonance imaging. J Neurosci 2010;30:5884–93; with permission.)

decision making, such as selecting a particular letter on visual presentation or responding to verbal questions, are most severely impaired during absence seizures, whereas simpler more automatic tasks may be relatively spared (reviewed in Ref.[35]) (see **Fig. 2B**). One patient reported that she could continue to play the violin during absence seizures as long as the passage was not very difficult or new to her, and another reported that if he had an absence seizure while swimming he would come to the surface and tread water until it was over. In addition to variations in the severity of impairment depending on the task, there is a large degree of variability in impairment on the same task both between patients and from one seizure to the next within the same patient.[35] The cause of this variability is not known. Therefore, investigating the relationship between variable task performance and variable EEG and neuroimaging involvement of specific brain regions may provide crucial insights into the mechanisms of impaired consciousness in absence seizures.

Absence seizures electrographically are accompanied by 3- to 4-Hz spike-wave discharges that have a widespread distribution, but tend to have a larger amplitude in more anterior head regions (see **Fig. 2A**).[36–38] The frequency and amplitude of the discharges gradually decreases toward the end of seizures. Recent source localization studies using high-density EEG recordings or magnetoencephalography (MEG) have reported maximal involvement of focal regions of the medial frontal, or bilateral lateral frontal cortex.[39–42] Along with measurements from animal models also showing focal involvement in bilateral cortical and subcortical structures,[43–46] these findings support the growing notion that "generalized" seizures are not truly generalized.[47,48] Rather, absence seizures appear to involve focal brain regions most intensely while sparing others.

A few aspects of the EEG signal have been investigated in relation to behavioral impairment during absence seizures. First, as already noted, some studies report that longer EEG duration is related to more severe behavioral impairment in absence seizures.[22,32,49,50] However, others have described deficits even with very brief spike-wave discharges on careful testing.[10,17] Several studies have examined other features of the EEG and have found that spike-wave amplitude, rhythmicity, frontocentral distribution, or "generalization" predicted more severe behavioral impairment during absence seizures.[10,32,33,51,52] Of importance, some of the variable performance from one seizure to the next may also be related to the timing of tasks relative to spike-wave onset and end because, as already noted, impairment may be maximal shortly after spike-wave onset and less severe toward the end of seizures.

Neuroimaging of absence seizures has been greatly facilitated in the past 10 years by use of functional magnetic resonance imaging (fMRI), which has better spatial and temporal resolution than methods used in earlier studies (reviewed in Ref.[53]). Combining EEG with fMRI has allowed the analysis of fMRI changes during absence seizures, demonstrating mainly increases in the thalamus, whereas cortical areas have shown a mixture of fMRI increases and decreases (**Fig. 3**). Cortical fMRI decreases during absence seizures involve mainly the so-called default mode network including the posterior cingulate/precuneus, lateral parietal, and medial frontal cortex.[54–57] Meanwhile, cortical fMRI increases are variably seen mainly in primary cortical areas including primary visual, primary auditory, and primary sensorimotor cortex, as well as in the frontal association cortex (see **Fig. 3**).[17] Recent work has demonstrated that conventional fMRI analysis methods do not adequately capture the true time course of fMRI signals during absence seizures,[20,58–61] which in addition to the aforementioned areas also show biphasic fMRI changes in the lateral frontal association cortex.[20] Also of note, the relationship between fMRI changes and neuronal activity is not fully known during absence seizures. Studies from animal models suggest that fMRI increases are related to increased neuronal activity.[44,45,62] However, the underlying neuronal activity in regions (including the default mode network) showing decreased fMRI signals during absence seizures is not known, and will require further investigation with better models.

To summarize, fMRI studies have revealed a complex sequence of fMRI changes in absence seizures including the main structures of the consciousness system (see **Fig. 1**). Thus, the thalamus shows mainly fMRI increases, the medial frontoparietal and lateral parietal cortex mainly decreases, and lateral frontal cortex biphasic changes.[20] Changes in primary cortical areas may also contribute to impaired consciousness during absence seizures.

fMRI has the potential to explain the anatomic basis of the variable behavioral performance from one seizure to the next, which could provide crucial insights into the specific structures involved in impaired consciousness. Variability in the fMRI pattern has been observed in different seizures and different patients.[17,63] However, very few studies have directly investigated the relationship between variable performance and fMRI. Studying variable ictal behavior and fMRI in children presents

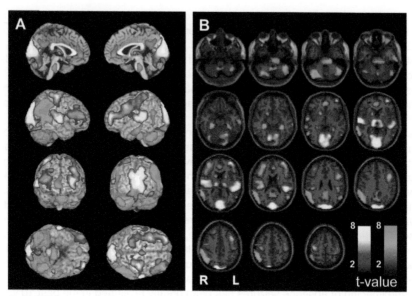

Fig. 3. fMRI changes during a typical absence seizure involve the consciousness system and primary cortices. Blood oxygen level dependent (BOLD) fMRI changes are shown from a 12-second seizure in a 14-year-old girl with childhood absence epilepsy (EEG for this seizure is shown in **Fig. 2A**). The consciousness system demonstrates BOLD fMRI increases in the thalamus, decreases in the interhemispheric regions (anterior cingulate, precuneus), decreases in the lateral parietal cortex, and increases in the lateral frontal cortex. In addition, fMRI increases are present in the primary cortices including the primary visual (occipital), primary auditory (superior temporal), and primary sensorimotor (Rolandic) cortex. fMRI decreases are also seen in the pons, basal ganglia, and cerebellum. Results were analyzed in SPM2 (http://www.fil.ion.ucl.ac.uk/SPM) using a t-test to compare seizure versus baseline with uncorrected height threshold ($P = .001$) and extent threshold (k = 3 voxels). (Unpublished data *Courtesy of* R. Berman).

substantial challenges, and many subjects are needed to obtain sufficient seizures for meaningful analysis. To date, two studies have shown that absence seizures with impaired responsiveness tend to have more fMRI changes in the cortex and thalamus than seizures without impaired responsiveness.[17,64] However, both studies were limited by relatively small sample sizes, and by the lack of specific changes in defined anatomic regions to explain the impairment. An additional single case was reported with relatively spared function during absence seizures and asymmetric fMRI changes affecting the right hemisphere more strongly.[65] Finally, another recent study examined the timing of behavioral impairment relative to EEG and fMRI and found that fMRI changes appeared to both precede and outlast the more transient behavioral and EEG changes.[20] Despite the inherent challenges, additional work is clearly needed to relate behavior and fMRI in absence epilepsy.

Overall, the behavioral impairment and anatomic regions involved in absence seizures are similar to other more chronic disorders of consciousness.[7,8] Like the minimally conscious state,[66,67] patients have their eyes open and are variably capable of simple responses at times, but do not show consistent evidence of functional interactive communication or object use. Anatomic regions affected during absence seizures also resemble other disorders of consciousness, because there is dysfunction in the bilateral association cortex and upper brainstem/diencephalic arousal systems comprising the consciousness system (see **Fig. 1**). However, further work will be needed to identify the specific anatomic and physiologic differences between absence seizures with complete behavioral arrest and those that leave some behavioral responses intact.

GENERALIZED TONIC-CLONIC SEIZURES

Generalized tonic-clonic (grand mal) seizures are dramatic convulsive episodes. Patients exhibit sustained tonic limb extension, followed by rhythmic clonic jerking of all limbs and deep unresponsiveness both during seizures and in the postictal period. Generalized tonic-clonic seizures can occur in primary generalized epilepsy or can arise when partial seizures spread and secondarily generalize. These seizures are also provoked by a variety of physiologic derangements (electrolyte imbalance, hypoglycemia, toxin exposure, electrical shock, and so forth) in patients who do not have habitual seizures.

The behavior in generalized tonic-clonic seizures usually includes complete lack of responsiveness to questions, commands, or other stimuli, and amnesia for the both the ictal and postictal periods. As in the vegetative state, the eyes are open during generalized tonic-clonic seizures, but in most other ways the lack of meaningful response to external stimuli is similar to coma. Postictally the eyes close, and the patient is often in an unresponsive sleeplike state for a variable period of time. The motor activity in tonic-clonic seizures typically lasts about 2 minutes. This period includes a tonic phase lasting about 30 seconds, which gives way to a "vibratory" phase, followed by more discrete jerks in the clonic phase.[68–71] It is interesting that many seizures do not exhibit the classic pattern of tonic followed by clonic activity. Instead patients may initially have clonic jerks then tonic activity, followed by another phase of clonic jerks, or the tonic phase may be incompletely expressed or not occur at all. These observations suggest that, like absence seizures, "generalized" tonic-clonic seizures do not homogeneously involve the whole nervous system; rather, selective networks may be most intensely involved while others are relatively spared. Work from animal models also supports relatively intense involvement of specific brain regions during generalized tonic-clonic seizures.[72]

Consciousness is spared in a minority of patients who have episodes that are otherwise behaviorally indistinguishable from generalized tonic-clonic seizures.[73–75] Tonic-clonic seizures with spared consciousness are often described as being quite unpleasant or painful by patients unfortunate enough to experience these episodes. The mechanism for spared consciousness in these patients is not known, but it has been speculated that their seizures may arise from bilateral motor or supplementary motor regions while largely sparing the association cortex.[73]

The scalp EEG during generalized tonic-clonic seizures shows high-frequency polyspike activity during the tonic phase, which gives way to rhythmic polyspike and slow-wave activity in the clonic phase. Postictally, while patients usually lie flaccid and unresponsive, the EEG shows generalized suppression, consisting of relatively low-amplitude EEG activity. Of interest, intracranial EEG recordings have shown that generalized tonic-clonic seizures do not involve the whole brain, and that some regions can be relatively spared.[76] One important study that has not yet been done, to the author's knowledge, would be to examine the intracranial EEG of the rare patients who have preserved consciousness in generalized tonic-clonic seizures, and to determine how the anatomic distribution of the discharges differs from patients with impaired consciousness.

Neuroimaging of generalized tonic-clonic seizures cannot readily be done with fMRI because convulsions require close clinical attention and induce significant movement artifacts. Instead, insights have been gained from ictal single-photon emission computed tomography (SPECT) as well as positron emission tomography (PET).[77] PET cerebral blood flow imaging also requires imaging during the convulsion. With SPECT, on the other hand, injection of radiopharmaceutical during the seizure is taken up within 20 to 30 seconds by the brain, providing a map of relative blood flow at the time of the injection. Therefore, imaging can be done later when the patient is clinically stable and no longer moving. Ictal SPECT is analyzed by comparison with baseline interictal SPECT in the same patients.[78,79] SPECT imaging of generalized tonic-clonic seizure has been done in both electroconvulsive therapy–induced seizures[80–85] and in spontaneous secondarily generalized seizures,[68,71,82,86–88] with similar results.

Electroconvulsive therapy–induced seizures have the advantage of controlled timing and relatively consistent seizure onset. Seizures are induced by placement of electrodes in fixed locations either in the bilateral frontotemporal, bilateral frontal, or right unilateral regions.[84] Early cerebral blood flow (CBF) increases occur near the region of the electrodes, presumably reflecting seizure onset.[83] CBF maps of the whole seizure show changes that overlap with the consciousness system, including increases in the lateral frontal and mediolateral parietal cortex, decreases in the interhemispheric medial frontal and cingulate cortex, and increases in deep structures including the thalamus (**Fig. 4**).[81–84] Similar regional changes were also found in a study using PET CBF imaging.[77]

SPECT imaging in epilepsy patients during secondarily generalized tonic-clonic seizures has also shown involvement of the consciousness system (see **Fig. 1**), including increases in the lateral frontoparietal cortex, upper brainstem, and thalamus,

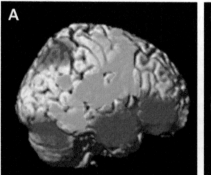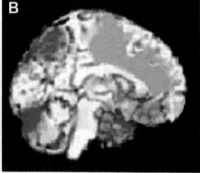

Fig. 4. Generalized tonic-clonic seizure induced by bilateral frontotemporal electroconvulsive therapy. Ictal single-photon emission computed tomography (SPECT) image for a single generalized tonic-clonic seizure compared with interictal baseline (*red* = cerebral blood flow [CBF] increases; *green* = CBF decreases). (*A*) Lateral view. (*B*) Medial view. Changes in the consciousness system include CBF increases in lateral frontotemporal cortex, lateral parietal and medial parietal cortex. CBF increases were also present in the thalamus (best seen in cross sections, not shown), as well as in the cerebellum. CBF decreases were present in the medial frontal and cingulate cortex, as well as in lateral cortical regions. SPM extent threshold k = 125 voxels; height threshold: P = .01. (*Modified from* Blumenfeld H, McNally KA, Ostroff RB, et al. Targeted prefrontal cortical activation with bifrontal ECT. Psychiatry Res 2003;123:165–70; with permission.)

and decreases in the interhemispheric regions.[68,71,82] As in absence seizures, these so-called generalized tonic-clonic seizures produce changes that are not homogeneous throughout the brain, but rather affect some regions more intensely than others.

Of note, some brain regions show relative CBF decreases during both spontaneous and induced generalized tonic-clonic seizures, particularly in the interhemispheric frontal and cingulate regions (see **Fig. 4**). In the postictal period, when patients remain deeply unresponsive, these CBF decreases become more pronounced and also include the medial and lateral frontoparietal association cortex.[68] Our group has observed that there are CBF increases in the cerebellum that progressively increase at late times during generalized tonic-clonic seizures and into the postictal period (**Fig. 5**).[68] This increased CBF in the cerebellum is correlated with CBF increases in the thalamus and upper brainstem, as well as with CBF decreases in the medial and lateral frontoparietal association cortex (see **Fig. 5**). These findings suggest that, in agreement with prior work in animal models,[89] strong activation of inhibitory cerebellar Purkinje cells late in seizures may inhibit thalamocortical networks, contributing to seizure termination as well as to impaired cortical function and suppressed consciousness in the postictal period.

In summary, generalized tonic-clonic seizures usually cause complete unresponsiveness but the eyes are open, making the behavior resemble a transient vegetative state. Anatomic involvement of the consciousness system includes abnormal increased activity in the upper brainstem and diencephalon, decreases in the medial frontal and cingulate cortex, and increases in the lateral frontal and mediolateral parietal association cortex. Postictal depressed cortical function may have a functional relationship with increased activity in the cerebellum. Further investigations are needed to better understand the mechanisms of selective network involvement in generalized tonic-clonic seizures, and the cortical-subcortical interactions governing postictal suppression of physiology and behavior.

TEMPORAL LOBE COMPLEX PARTIAL SEIZURES: NETWORK INHIBITION HYPOTHESIS

Impaired consciousness is classically seen in disorders that involve bilateral cortical-subcortical networks.[1] It is therefore not entirely surprising that absence seizures and generalized tonic-clonic seizures cause impaired consciousness, perhaps through bilateral involvement of the consciousness system as already noted. However, why focal temporal lobe seizures should so often cause impaired consciousness is more puzzling. During temporal lobe seizures, patients are typically unresponsive to questions and commands for 1 to 2 minutes, and then remain confused for a variable period of time postictally. Scalp EEG recordings during seizures show rhythmic theta frequency discharges usually of greatest amplitude over one temporal lobe. The "network inhibition hypothesis," described in greater detail in the discussion that follows, proposes that focal temporal lobe seizures inhibit subcortical arousal systems, leading to depressed cortical function and impaired consciousness.

Onset of a temporal lobe seizure may be heralded by an aura or warning consisting of a fearful premonition, rising feeling in the stomach, or other unusual sensations such as déjà vu. Patients usually retain normal responses to question or commands, at least initially. In terminology that was adopted in 1981 and remains widely used, if consciousness is spared throughout the seizure it is called simple partial, whereas if consciousness is impaired it is called a complex partial seizure.[90] (See also Ref.[91] for a more recent discussion of epilepsy classification.) In complex partial temporal lobe seizures there is typically behavioral arrest, staring, and automatic repetitive behaviors called automatisms including lip smacking, chewing, and picking or rubbing

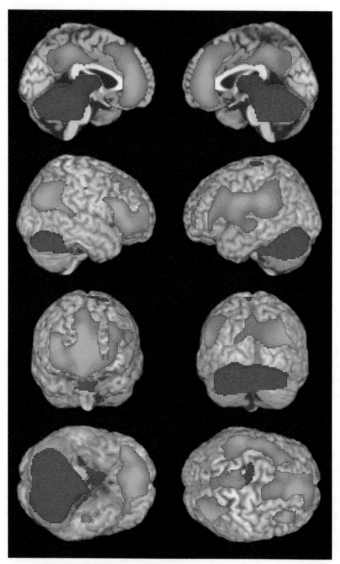

Fig. 5. Frontoparietal CBF decreases and thalamic increases are correlated with increased CBF in the cerebellum during and following generalized tonic-clonic seizures. Network correlations are shown for spontaneous secondarily generalized tonic-clonic seizures imaged with ictal SPECT in epilepsy patients during video/EEG monitoring. Positive (*red*) and negative (*green*) correlations are shown between CBF changes in the cerebellum and the rest of the brain across patients (n = 59 seizures in 53 patients). Significant positive correlations were found between the cerebellum and the upper brainstem tegmentum and thalamus. Negative correlations were found with the bilateral frontoparietal association cortex, anterior and posterior cingulate, and precuneus. Images were analyzed with SPM extent threshold k = 125 voxels, and height threshold *P* = .01. (*Reproduced from* Blumenfeld H, Varghese G, Purcaro MJ, et al. Cortical and subcortical networks in human secondarily generalized tonic-clonic seizures. Brain 2009;132:999–1012; with permission.)

movements of the hands. During this time the eyes remain open and patients do not respond to questions or commands. However, they may show simple responses to stimuli including orienting or grasping responses called reactive automatisms.[92] After the seizure ends, patients usually have a period of continued decreased responsiveness, confusion, and amnesia for events around the time of the seizure. The lack of meaningful responses during complex partial seizures, but with preserved eye opening and simple orienting movements, resembles a transient form of vegetative state.[93–95] However, the presence of manual automatisms may be considered more similar to behaviors seen in the minimally conscious state.[66,67]

Like tonic-clonic seizures, SPECT imaging has been a more practical way of performing neuroimaging in patients than fMRI during temporal lobe complex partial seizures. As expected, in temporal lobe seizures SPECT imaging shows increased CBF in the temporal lobe on the side of seizure onset.[79,87,96] However, there is also decreased CBF in bilateral regions of the lateral and medial frontoparietal association cortex (**Fig. 6**A, B).[97–101] In addition, increased CBF in the upper brainstem and medial diencephalon has been observed in temporal lobe seizures (see **Fig. 6**B).[97,102–105] Of

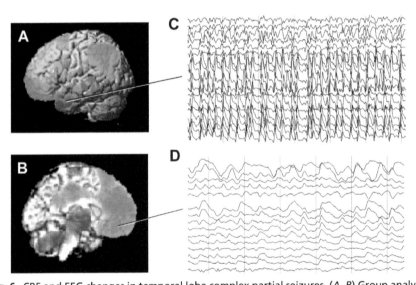

Fig. 6. CBF and EEG changes in temporal lobe complex partial seizures. (*A*, *B*) Group analysis of SPECT ictal-interictal difference imaging during temporal lobe seizures. CBF increases are present in the temporal lobe (*A*) and in the medial thalamus (*B*). Decreases are seen in the lateral frontoparietal association cortex (*A*) and in the interhemispheric regions (*B*). (*C*, *D*) Intracranial EEG recordings from a patient during a temporal lobe seizure. High-frequency polyspike-and-wave seizure activity is seen in the temporal lobe (*C*). The orbital and medial frontal cortex (and other regions, EEG not shown) do not show polyspike activity, but instead large-amplitude, irregular slow rhythms resembling coma or sleep (*D*). Vertical lines in *C* and *D* denote 1-second intervals. Note that the EEG and SPECT data were from similar patients, but were not simultaneous, and are shown together here for illustrative purposes only. ([*A*, *B*] *Modified from* Blumenfeld H, McNally KA, Vanderhill SD, et al. Positive and negative network correlations in temporal lobe epilepsy. Cerebral Cortex 2004;14:892–902; with permission; and [*C*, *D*] Blumenfeld H, Rivera M, McNally KA, et al. Ictal neocortical slowing in temporal lobe epilepsy. Neurology 2004;63:1015–21; with permission.)

importance, it has been found that the CBF decreases in the frontoparietal association cortex, as well as CBF increases in the upper brainstem and medial diencephalon, are associated with impaired consciousness in partial seizures.[97,103] Simple partial seizures, in which consciousness is spared, tend to exhibit more limited CBF changes confined to the temporal lobe. In addition, increased CBF in the medial thalamus was found to be correlated with decreased CBF in bilateral medial and lateral frontoparietal association cortex,[97] suggesting a mechanistic link between cortical and subcortical changes in temporal lobe epilepsy. Of note, the midline subcortical structures as well as the medial and lateral frontoparietal cortex regions affected in temporal lobe complex partial seizures again correspond to the same anatomic regions involved in absence and tonic-clonic seizures, namely the consciousness system (see **Fig. 1**).

Intracranial EEG recordings are often performed as part of surgical planning in patients with temporal lobe epilepsy, and provide an opportunity to more directly study the physiologic changes in the association cortex during temporal lobe seizures. Although the temporal lobe shows high-frequency alpha (8–12 Hz), beta (13–25 Hz), and higher-frequency polyspike-and-wave discharges during temporal lobe seizures (see **Fig. 6**C), the frontoparietal association cortex shows delta (1–4 Hz) and slower oscillations (see **Fig. 6**D).[106,107] These neocortical slow waves more closely resemble the EEG of coma, encephalopathy, or slow-wave sleep than ictal patterns on intracranial EEG.[108–110] The anatomic distribution of ictal neocortical slow waves in temporal lobe seizures includes the bilateral lateral frontal, orbital frontal, medial frontal, cingulate, and lateral parietal cortex, corresponding to the same regions in which decreased CBF is observed on SPECT imaging.[97,106,107] Slow wave activity and CBF decreases in the frontoparietal association cortex were significantly greater in complex partial than in simple partial seizures.[97,107] Both the neocortical slow waves and CBF decreases in frontoparietal association cortex persist into the postictal period, during which time patients often remain confused.

These findings support the network inhibition hypothesis for impaired consciousness in temporal lobe epilepsy (**Fig. 7**).[3,107,108,111–115] The network inhibition hypothesis proposes that temporal lobe seizures propagate to subcortical structures, leading to inhibition (through mechanisms still being investigated) of subcortical arousal systems (see **Fig. 7**A–C). This in turn removes the normal activation of the frontoparietal association cortex, leading to depressed neocortical function and impaired consciousness (see **Fig. 7**D). Of note, in the network inhibition hypothesis the neocortex enters a sleep-like (or minimally conscious-like) state, not due to direct seizure propagation but because of remote network effects on subcortical arousal systems. Another way of describing these long-range effects of seizures on other parts of the brain is "ictal diaschesis."[114,115]

The fundamental changes occurring in neocortical, subcortical, and limbic networks have recently been investigated in rodent models of hippocampal seizures. As in human temporal lobe epilepsy, rats with spontaneous limbic seizures following pilocarpine-induced status epilepticus as well as acute seizures induced by hippocampal stimulation exhibit fast activity in the hippocampus but slow 1- to 3-Hz activity in the frontoparietal cortex, associated with behavioral arrest.[112] This neocortical slow activity differs fundamentally from seizure activity measured in the same animals. Seizure activity in the hippocampus or neocortex is associated with increased neuronal action potential firing, CBF, cerebral blood volume, blood oxygen level–dependent fMRI signal, and cerebral metabolic rate of oxygen consumption.[112] By contrast, neocortical slow activity during hippocampal seizures is associated with decreases in all of these parameters, closely resembling slow-wave activity in deep anesthesia.[109,110,112]

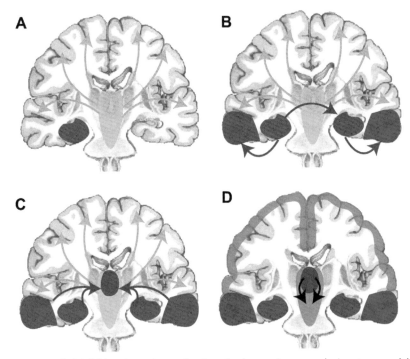

Fig. 7. Network inhibition hypotheses for impaired consciousness during temporal lobe complex partial seizures. (*A*) Under normal conditions, the upper brainstem-diencephalic activating systems interact (*yellow arrows*) with the cerebral cortex to maintain normal consciousness. A focal seizure involving the mesial temporal lobe begins unilaterally (*red region*). If it remains unilateral then a simple-partial seizure will occur without impairment of consciousness. (*B*) Propagation (*red arrows*) of seizure activity from the mesial temporal lobe to the ipsilateral lateral temporal lobe and the contralateral temporal lobe. (*C*). Spread of seizure activity from bilateral temporal lobes to midline subcortical structures. (*D*). Inhibition (*blue arrows*) of the midline subcortical structures, together with the resulting depressed activity in bilateral frontoparietal association cortex in complex-partial seizures, leads to loss of consciousness. (*Reproduced from* Englot DJ, Yang L, Hamid H, et al. Impaired consciousness in temporal lobe seizures: role of cortical slow activity. Brain 2010;133(Pt 12): 3764–77; with permission.)

The rat model has also begun to shed important insights into the network mechanisms of ictal neocortical slow waves. High-field fMRI mapping during hippocampal seizures demonstrated increased fMRI signal in the hippocampus, decreases in orbital frontal, anterior cingulate, and retrosplenial cortex, and subcortical increases in the medial thalamus and lateral septal nuclei.[112,113] Because the lateral septal nuclei contain a large population of γ-aminobutyric acid (GABA)ergic inhibitory neurons, it was hypothesized that activation of the lateral septal nuclei and other GABAergic subcortical structures during seizures could inhibit the subcortical arousal systems (network inhibition hypothesis). In support of this, local stimulation of the lateral septal nuclei produced neocortical slow waves and behavioral arrest mimicking the effects of hippocampal seizures.[113] In addition, animals in which the hippocampus was disconnected from the lateral septal nuclei (by cutting the fornix) had focal seizures in the hippocampus without neocortical slow activity and without behavioral arrest.[113] These findings further support the network inhibition hypothesis, and suggest that hippocampal seizures produce neocortical slow activity and impaired consciousness through network effects critically involving subcortical structures.[108]

In summary, temporal lobe complex partial seizures cause unresponsiveness with the eyes open and some automatic repetitive movements, most similar to a transient vegetative or minimally conscious state. Like absence and generalized tonic-clonic seizures, abnormal brain activity again converges on the anatomic structures of the consciousness system (see **Fig. 1**). Thus, temporal lobe complex partial seizures are associated with abnormal increased activity in the upper brainstem and diencephalon, and decreased activity in the medial frontal, cingulate, precuneus, and lateral frontoparietal association cortex, which persists into the postictal period. Both human data and animal models support a network inhibition hypothesis in which limbic seizures propagate to subcortical structures, which inhibit subcortical arousal networks, in turn causing neocortical slow waves and impaired consciousness. Additional mechanistic studies are needed to determine in greater detail how subcortical structures are inhibited during temporal lobe seizures to produce the impaired consciousness seen in temporal lobe seizures.

IMPACT OF IMPAIRED CONSCIOUSNESS ON QUALITY OF LIFE IN EPILEPSY

Impaired consciousness has a major negative impact on quality of life in patients with epilepsy. In large patient series the major factors that determined impaired quality of life in epilepsy were frequency and severity of seizures.[116,117] Impaired consciousness is a crucial determinant of seizure severity and can have numerous adverse consequences including motor vehicle accidents, burns, falls, drowning, other accidental injuries, loss of productivity at work or school, and social stigmatization. One of the more challenging aspects of the sudden impaired consciousness in epilepsy is the unpredictable times at which this can occur, disrupting ongoing activities and producing fear that a seizure could happen at any time.[118,119]

Because many adults depend on driving to reach work or other daily activities, loss of driving privileges has a large effect on quality of life. Though laws vary based on location, in most places patients are prohibited from driving if they have uncontrolled seizures associated with impaired consciousness. Several studies have looked at the risk of driving in patients with epilepsy, and have found variable results. Risk of motor vehicle accidents in patients with epilepsy may not be higher than in other patients with chronic illnesses such as diabetes.[120,121] Although more limited, there are data to suggest that patients with uncontrolled seizures are at greater risk of motor vehicle accidents,[120,122–124] and that certain seizure types such as generalized tonic-clonic or complex partial seizures may pose a greater risk than simple partial or myoclonic, or perhaps absence, seizures.[125,126] In examining these seizure types, it is likely that several factors including impaired consciousness, seizure duration, and motor deficits could affect driving safety. A recent study used a computer game–based driving simulator to prospectively evaluate driving performance during seizures.[127] Patients were instructed to play a realistic driving game using a steering wheel and gas/brake pedal controllers during inpatient video/EEG monitoring while performance metrics were collected continuously. Collisions and other evidence of loss of control (sustained decrease in steering-wheel velocity, gas pedal use, or car velocity) were most evident for generalized tonic-clonic seizures, whereas no significant deficits were observed in subclinical seizures.[127] Partial seizures (including both simple partial and complex partial seizures) and absence seizures caused impairment of driving in some but not all seizures. Additional prospective data of this kind may make it possible to determine specifically which patients are at greatest risk of motor vehicle accidents during seizures, and could be useful for advising patients and physicians.

TREATMENT STRATEGIES

Although the best way to prevent impaired consciousness in epilepsy would be to stop all seizures, in patients with medically refractory epilepsy this cannot always be achieved. For these patients it would be a welcome improvement in lifestyle to at least prevent impaired consciousness during seizures. Several treatment modalities could be considered for preventing or reducing impaired consciousness in epilepsy. For example, because cortical slow oscillations in complex partial seizures are similar to slow-wave sleep, medications that promote the awake state, such as modafinil,[128,129] could be tested to determine whether they improve alertness during and following seizures. Deep brain stimulation is being investigated for the prevention of seizures,[130–134] but stimulation of thalamic arousal circuits has also been used to improve alertness in disorders of consciousness,[135,136] so could potentially be tested for this purpose in epilepsy as well. Disconnection procedures were found in rodent models to prevent neocortical slow waves and to improve responsiveness in limbic seizures.[113] The specific disconnection procedure used was fornix transection, which may not be feasible in humans because of potential memory side effects[137,138] (although see also Ref.[139]). However, this at least demonstrates that in principle a procedure of this kind could ultimately prevent epileptic unconsciousness when the underlying circuits and mechanisms are better understood.

Finally, it will be important to study behavioral interventions that may increase awareness by patients and families of impaired consciousness during seizures. This approach could help in the development of practical strategies for improving quality of life. In addition to impaired consciousness during seizures, patients with epilepsy commonly are unaware of the fact that they have had seizures and tend to underreport them.[140–144] Improved prospective measures are needed to determine and evaluate impaired consciousness during seizures,[145] and to relate impaired consciousness or other variables to patient recognition and report.[146] Behavioral or educational interventions may be particularly helpful in increasing seizure recognition and report by patients, which could be highly valuable in improving their clinical care.

SUMMARY AND FUTURE DIRECTIONS

Recent human neuroimaging studies, intracranial EEG analysis, and animal model investigations have greatly increased our understanding of the fundamental mechanisms of impaired consciousness in epilepsy. The 3 seizure types causing impaired consciousness, namely absence, generalized tonic-clonic, and complex partial seizures, all converge on a final common set of anatomic structures we refer to as the consciousness system, consisting of medial and lateral frontoparietal association cortex and subcortical activating networks. These same anatomic structures in the consciousness system are also affected in other states of impaired consciousness, including sleep, anesthesia, coma, vegetative state, and minimally conscious state.[7,8]

In behavioral terms absence or complex partial seizures often resemble a transient vegetative state, in which patients exhibit no meaningful behavioral responses, yet have open eyes and maintain some rudimentary postural tone and orienting responses. Other absence or complex partial seizures more closely resemble a transient minimally conscious state, because patients may show automatisms or variable simple responses yet do not demonstrate consistent functional interactive communication or object use. Generalized tonic-clonic seizures resemble coma because orienting responses and postural stability are lost, yet unlike most cases of coma, the eyes do remain open.

The anatomic and physiologic changes in the consciousness system associated with seizures can be summarized as follows. Absence seizures exhibit fMRI signal increases in the thalamus, decreases in the anterior cingulate, medial frontal cortex, and precuneus, and a mixture of increases and decreases in the lateral frontoparietal association cortex. Generalized tonic-clonic seizures produce CBF increases in lateral frontal and mediolateral parietal cortex, decreases in medial frontal and cingulate cortex, and increases in the thalamus and upper brainstem during seizures. Postictally after generalized tonic-clonic seizures there is decreased CBF in medial and lateral frontoparietal association cortex. Temporal lobe complex partial seizures show increased activity in the medial diencephalon, with decreased activity in the medial frontal, cingulate, precuneus, and lateral frontoparietal association cortex.

Work to date has provided some insights into the fundamental network mechanisms for these changes, but there is much that remains to be done. For example, an elegant temporal sequence of cortical and subcortical fMRI changes are seen beginning 5 to 10 seconds before and continuing over 20 seconds after absence seizures,[20,58,61] but the neurophysiologic basis of these changes is not known. In generalized tonic-clonic seizures, cerebellar CBF increases continue into the postictal period and are correlated with CBF decreases in the forebrain,[68] but the role of these networks in seizure termination or postictal depression has not been thoroughly investigated. In temporal lobe seizures, evidence from human patients and animal models support the network inhibition hypothesis in which disruption of subcortical arousal systems leads to depressed neocortical function,[107,112,113] but the exact cellular and neurotransmitter mechanisms for these changes require further investigation.

Additional work is also needed to relate variable deficits in consciousness with specific regions involved or spared during seizures. For example, it is not clear why profound deficits in consciousness occur in some absence seizures and some generalized tonic-clonic seizures but not in others. Further work with behavioral tasks and neuroimaging during absence seizures or intracranial recordings during tonic-clonic seizures may help clarify these unresolved questions.

Finally, improved treatments are needed to prevent impaired consciousness in epilepsy, particularly for patients in whom seizures cannot be stopped. Advances in understanding the fundamental mechanisms of impaired consciousness in epilepsy will be crucial for developing novel treatments targeting this major source of patient disability. Further work in this field will, it is hoped, lead to medications, surgical procedures, and behavioral interventions to reduce impaired consciousness and greatly improve the quality of life of patients with epilepsy.

REFERENCES

1. Plum F, Posner JB. The diagnosis of stupor and coma. 3rd edition. Philadelphia: Davis; 1982.
2. Blumenfeld H. Neuroanatomy through clinical cases. Sunderland (MA): Sinauer Assoc. Publ., Inc; 2002.
3. Blumenfeld H. Epilepsy and consciousness. In: Laureys S, editor. The neurology of consciousness: cognitive neuroscience and neuropathology. New York: G Tononi Academic Press; 2009. p. 15–30. Chapter 2.
4. Blumenfeld H. Neuroanatomy through clinical cases. 2nd edition. Sunderland (MA): Sinauer Assoc Publ Co; 2010.

5. Steriade M, Jones EG, McCormick DA, editors. Thalamus. Amsterdam: Elsevier Science; 1997.

6. Steriade MM, McCarley RW. Brain control of wakefulness and sleep. 2nd edition. New York: Springer; 2010.

7. Laureys S, Tononi G. The neurology of consciousness: cognitive neuroscience and neuropathology. Amsterdam: Academic Press; 2008.

8. Laureys S, Schiff ND. Disorders of consciousness. Annals of the New York Academy of Sciences. Hoboken: Wiley-Blackwell; 2009.

9. Sadleir LG, Scheffer IE, Smith S, et al. Factors influencing clinical features of absence seizures [see comment]. Epilepsia 2008;49:2100–7.

10. Browne TR, Penry JK, Porter RJ, et al. Responsiveness before, during and after spike-wave paroxysms. Neurology 1974;24:659–65.

11. Goldie L, Green JM. Spike and wave discharges and alterations of conscious awareness. Nature 1961;191:200–1.

12. Grisell JL, Levin SM, Cohen BD, et al. Effects of subclinical seizure activity on overt behavior. Neurology 1964;14:133–5.

13. Lehmann HJ. Weckreaktionen bei pyknoleptischen absenzen. Arch Psychiatr Nervenkr 1963;204:417–26.

14. Mallin U, Stefan H, Penin H. Psychopathometrische Studien zum Verlauf epileptischer Absencen. Z EEG EMG 1981;12:45–9.

15. Daly D, Pedley TA. Current practice of clinical electroencephalography. 2nd edition. New York: Raven Press; 1990.

16. Sadleir LG, Scheffer IE, Smith S, et al. EEG features of absence seizures in idiopathic generalized epilepsy: impact of syndrome, age, and state. Epilepsia 2009;50:1572–8.

17. Berman R, Negishi M, Vestal M, et al. Simultaneous EEG, fMRI, and behavioral testing in typical childhood absence seizures. Epilepsia 2010;51(10):2011–22.

18. Shimazono Y, Hirai T, Okuma T, et al. Disturbance of consciousness in petit mal epilepsy. Epilepsia 1953;2:49–55.

19. Tuvo F. Contribution a l'etude des niveaux de conscience au cours des paroxysmes epileptiques infraclinique. Electroencephalogr Clin Neurophysiol 1958;10:715–8.

20. Bai X, Vestal M, Berman R, et al. Dynamic time course of typical childhood absence seizures: EEG, behavior, and functional magnetic resonance imaging. J Neurosci 2010;30:5884–93.

21. Bates JA. A technique for identifying changes in consciousness. Electroencephalogr Clin Neurophysiol 1953;5:445–6.

22. Goode DJ, Penry JK, Dreifuss FE. Effects of paroxysmal spike-wave on continuous visual-motor performance. Epilepsia 1970;11:241–54.

23. Jus A, Jus C. Etude electro-clinique des alterations de conscience dans le petit mal. Studii si cercetari de Neurol 1960;5:243–54.

24. Panayiotopoulos CP, Obeid T, Waheed G. Differentiation of typical absence seizures in epileptic syndromes: a video-EEG study of 124 seizures in 20 patients. Brain 1989;112:1039–56.

25. Tizard B, Margerison JH. Psychological functions during wave-spike discharges. Br J Soc Clin Psychol 1963;3:6–15.

26. Fernandez H, Robinson R, Taylor RR. A device for testing consciousness. Am J EEG Technol 1967;7:77–8.

27. Mirsky AF, Rosvold HE. Behavioral and physiological studies in impaired attention. In: Zea V, editor. Psychopharmacological methods: proceedings of a symposium on the effects of psychotropic drugs on higher nervous activity. Oxford: Pergamon Press; 1963. p. 302–15.

28. Boudin G, Barbizet J, Masson S. Etude de la dissolution de la conscience dans 3 cas de petit mal avec crises prolongees. Rev Neurol 1958;99:483–7.
29. Geller MR, Geller A. Brief amnestic effects of spike wave discharges. (Section on Child Neurology, abstract CN1). Neurology 1970;20:380–1.
30. Hutt SJ, Gilbert S. Effects of evoked spike-wave discharges upon short term memory in patients with epilepsy. Cortex 1980;16:445–57.
31. Jus A, Jus K. Retrograde amnesia in petit mal. Arch Gen Psychiatry 1962;6: 163–7.
32. Mirsky AF, Van Buren JM. On the nature of the "absence" in centrencephalic epilepsy: a study of some behavioral, electroencephalographic, and autonomic factors. Electroencephalogr Clin Neurophysiol 1965;18:334–48.
33. Courtois GA, Ingvar DH, Jasper HH. Nervous and mental defects during petit mal attacks. Electroencephalogr Clin Neurophysiol 1953;(Suppl 3):87.
34. Gastaut H. The brain stem and cerebral electrogenesis in relation to consciousness. In: Delafresnaye JF, editor. Brain mechanisms and consciousness. Springfield (IL): Thomas; 1954. p. 249–83.
35. Blumenfeld H. Consciousness and epilepsy: why are patients with absence seizures absent? Prog Brain Res 2005;150:271–86.
36. Coppola R. Topographic display of spike-and-wave discharges. In: Mysobodsky MS, Mirsky AF, editors. Elements of petit mal epilepsy. New York: Peter Lang; 1988. p. 105–30.
37. Rodin E, Ancheta O. Cerebral electrical fields during petit mal absences. Electroencephalogr Clin Neurophysiol 1987;66:457–66.
38. Weir B. The morphology of the spike-wave complex. Electroencephalogr Clin Neurophysiol 1965;19:284–90.
39. Holmes MD, Brown M, Tucker DM. Are "generalized" seizures truly generalized? Evidence of localized mesial frontal and frontopolar discharges in absence. Epilepsia 2004;45:1568–79.
40. Sakurai K, Takeda Y, Tanaka N, et al. Generalized spike-wave discharges involve a default mode network in patients with juvenile absence epilepsy: a MEG study. Epilepsy Res 2010;89(2–3):176–84.
41. Stefan H, Paulini-Ruf A, Hopfengartner R, et al. Network characteristics of idiopathic generalized epilepsies in combined MEG/EEG. Epilepsy Res 2009;85: 187–98.
42. Westmijse I, Ossenblok P, Gunning B, et al. Onset and propagation of spike and slow wave discharges in human absence epilepsy: a MEG study. Epilepsia 2009;50(12):2538–48.
43. Meeren HK, Pijn JP, Van Luijtelaar EL, et al. Cortical focus drives widespread corticothalamic networks during spontaneous absence seizures in rats. J Neurosci 2002;22:1480–95.
44. Nersesyan H, Hyder F, Rothman D, et al. Dynamic fMRI and EEG recordings during spike-wave seizures and generalized tonic-clonic seizures in WAG/Rij rats. J Cereb Blood Flow Metab 2004;24:589–99.
45. Nersesyan H, Herman P, Erdogan E, et al. Relative changes in cerebral blood flow and neuronal activity in local microdomains during generalized seizures. J Cereb Blood Flow Metab 2004;24:1057–68.
46. Vergnes M, Marescaux C, Depaulis A. Mapping of spontaneous spike and wave discharges in Wistar rats with genetic generalized non-convulsive epilepsy. Brain Res 1990;523:87–91.
47. Blumenfeld H. Cellular and network mechanisms of spike-wave seizures. Epilepsia 2005;46(Suppl 9):21–33.

48. Meeren H, van Luijtelaar G, Lopes da Silva F, et al. Evolving concepts on the pathophysiology of absence seizures: the cortical focus theory. Arch Neurol 2005;62:371–6.

49. Guey J, Tassinari CA, Charles C, et al. Variations du niveau d'efficience en relation avec des descharges epileptiques paroxystiques. Rev Neurol 1965;112: 311–7.

50. Schwab RS. Method of measuring consciousness in attacks of petit mal epilepsy. (Society Transactions: Boston Society of Psychiatry and Neurology, presented May 19, 1938). Arch Neurol Psychiatry 1939;41:215–7.

51. Porter RJ, Penry JK. Responsiveness at the onset of spike-wave bursts. Electroencephalogr Clin Neurophysiol 1973;34:239–45.

52. Sellden U. Psychotechnical performance related to paroxysmal discharges in EEG. Clin Electroenceph 1971;2.

53. Motelow JE, Blumenfeld H. Functional neuroimaging of spike-wave seizures. Methods Mol Biol 2009;489(9):189–209.

54. Archer JS, Abbott DF, Waites AB, et al. fMRI "deactivation" of the posterior cingulate during generalized spike and wave. Neuroimage 2003;20:1915–22.

55. Danielson NB, Guo JN, Blumenfeld H. The default mode network and altered consciousness in epilepsy. Behav Neurol 2011;24(1):55–65.

56. Gotman J, Grova C, Bagshaw A, et al. Generalized epileptic discharges show thalamocortical activation and suspension of the default state of the brain. Proc Natl Acad Sci U S A 2005;102:15236–40.

57. Salek-Haddadi A, Lemieux L, Merschhemke M, et al. Functional magnetic resonance imaging of human absence seizures. Ann Neurol 2003;53:663–7.

58. Carney PW, Masterton RA, Harvey AS, et al. The core network in absence epilepsy. Differences in cortical and thalamic BOLD response. Neurology 2010;75:904–11.

59. Moeller F, Siebner HR, Wolff S, et al. Simultaneous EEG-fMRI in drug-naive children with newly diagnosed absence epilepsy. Epilepsia 2008;49(9): 1510–9.

60. Moeller F, Siebner HR, Wolff S, et al. Changes in activity of striato-thalamo-cortical network precede generalized spike wave discharges. Neuroimage 2008;39(4):1839–49.

61. Rathakrishnan R, Moeller F, Levan P, et al. BOLD signal changes preceding negative responses in EEG-fMRI in patients with focal epilepsy. Epilepsia 2010;51(9):1837–45.

62. Mishra AM, Ellens DJ, Schridde U, et al. Where fMRI and electrophysiology agree to disagree: corticothalamic and striatal activity patterns in the WAG/Rij rat. J Neurosci 2011. [Epub ahead of print].

63. Moeller F, LeVan P, Muhle H, et al. Absence seizures: individual patterns revealed by EEG-fMRI. Epilepsia 2010;51:2000–10.

64. Li Q, Luo C, Yang T, et al. EEG-fMRI study on the interictal and ictal generalized spike-wave discharges in patients with childhood absence epilepsy. Epilepsy Res 2009;87:160–8.

65. Moeller F, Muhle H, Wiegand G, et al. EEG-fMRI study of generalized spike and wave discharges without transitory cognitive impairment. Epilepsy Behav 2010; 18(3):313–6.

66. Giacino J, Whyte J. The vegetative and minimally conscious states: current knowledge and remaining questions. J Head Trauma Rehabil 2005;20:30–50.

67. Giacino JT, Ashwal S, Childs N, et al. The minimally conscious state: definition and diagnostic criteria [see comment]. Neurology 2002;58:349–53.

68. Blumenfeld H, Varghese G, Purcaro MJ, et al. Cortical and subcortical networks in human secondarily generalized tonic-clonic seizures. Brain 2009;132:999–1012.
69. Jobst BC, Williamson PD, Neuschwander TB, et al. Secondarily generalized seizures in mesial temporal epilepsy: clinical characteristics, lateralizing signs, and association with sleep-wake cycle. Epilepsia 2001;42:1279–87.
70. Theodore WH, Porter RJ, Albert P, et al. The secondarily generalized tonic-clonic seizure: a videotape analysis. Neurology 1994;44:1403–7.
71. Varghese G, Purcaro MJ, Motelow JE, et al. Clinical use of ictal SPECT in secondarily generalized tonic-clonic seizures. Brain 2009;132(8):2102–13.
72. DeSalvo MN, Schridde U, Mishra AM, et al. Focal BOLD fMRI changes in bicuculline-induced tonic-clonic seizures in the rat. Neuroimage 2010;50:902–9.
73. Bell WL, Walczak TS, Shin C, et al. Painful generalised clonic and tonic-clonic seizures with retained consciousness. J Neurol Neurosurg Psychiatry 1997;63:792–5.
74. Botez MI, Serbanescu T, Stoica I. The problem of focal epileptic seizures on both parts of the body without loss of consciousness. Psychiatr Neurol Neurochir 1966;69:431–7.
75. Weinberger J, Lusins J. Simultaneous bilateral focal seizures without loss of consciousness. Mt Sinai J Med 1973;40:693–6.
76. Schindler K, Leung H, Lehnertz K, et al. How generalised are secondarily "generalised" tonic clonic seizures? J Neurol Neurosurg Psychiatry 2007;78:993–6.
77. Takano H, Motohashi N, Uema T, et al. Changes in regional cerebral blood flow during acute electroconvulsive therapy in patients with depression: positron emission tomographic study. Br J Psychiatry 2007;190:63–8.
78. Kim SH, Zubal IG, Blumenfeld H. Epilepsy localization by ictal and interictal SPECT. In: Van Heertum RL, Ichise M, Tikofsky RS, editors. Functional cerebral SPECT and PET imaging 2009. Philadelpia: Lippincott Williams & Wilkins; 2009. p. 131–48. Chapter 10.
79. McNally KA, Paige AL, Varghese G, et al. Localizing value of ictal-interictal SPECT analyzed by SPM (ISAS). Epilepsia 2005;46:1450–64.
80. Bajc M, Medved V, Basic M, et al. Acute effect of electroconvulsive therapy on brain perfusion assessed by Tc99m-hexamethylpropyleneamineoxim and single photon emission computed tomography. Acta Psychiatr Scand 1989;80:421–6.
81. Blumenfeld H, McNally KA, Ostroff RB, et al. Targeted prefrontal cortical activation with bifrontal ECT. Psychiatry Res 2003;123:165–70.
82. Blumenfeld H, Westerveld M, Ostroff RB, et al. Selective frontal, parietal and temporal networks in generalized seizures. Neuroimage 2003;19:1556–66.
83. Enev M, McNally KA, Varghese G, et al. Imaging onset and propagation of ECT-induced seizures. Epilepsia 2007;48:238–44.
84. McNally KA, Blumenfeld H. Focal network involvement in generalized seizures: new insights from electroconvulsive therapy. Epilepsy Behav 2004;5:3–12.
85. Vollmer-Haase J, Folkerts HW, Haase CG, et al. Cerebral hemodynamics during electrically induced seizures. Neuroreport 1998;9:407–10.
86. Lee BI, Markand ON, Wellman HN, et al. HIPDM single photon emission computed tomography brain imaging in partial onset secondarily generalized tonic-clonic seizures. Epilepsia 1987;28:305–11.
87. Rowe CC, Berkovic SF, Sia ST, et al. Localization of epileptic foci with postictal single photon emission computed tomography. Ann Neurol 1989;26:660–8.
88. Shin WC, Hong SB, Tae WS, et al. Ictal hyperperfusion patterns according to the progression of temporal lobe seizures. Neurology 2002;58:373–80.

89. Salgado-Benitez A, Briones R, Fernandez-Guardiola A. Purkinje cell responses to a cerebral penicillin-induced epileptogenic focus in the cat. Epilepsia 1982; 23:597–606.

90. ILAE. Proposal for revised clinical and electroencephalographic classification of epileptic seizures. From the Commission on Classification and Terminology of the International League Against Epilepsy. Epilepsia 1981;22:489–501.

91. Berg AT, Berkovic SF, Brodie MJ, et al. Revised terminology and concepts for organization of seizures and epilepsies: report of the ILAE Commission on Classification and Terminology, 2005-2009. Epilepsia 2010;51:676–85.

92. Escueta AV, Kunze U, Waddell G, et al. Lapse of consciousness and automatisms in temporal lobe epilepsy: a videotape analysis. Neurology 1977;27: 144–55.

93. American Congress of Rehabilitation Medicine. Recommendations for use of uniform nomenclature pertinent to patients with severe alterations in consciousness. American Congress of Rehabilitation Medicine [see comment] [erratum appears in Arch Phys Med Rehabil 1995 Apr;76(4):397]. Arch Phys Med Rehabil 1995;76:205–9.

94. Blumenfeld H. The neurologic examination of consciousness. In: Laureys S, editor. The neurology of consciousness. G Tononi Elsevier, Ltd; 2008. p. 15–30. Chapter 2.

95. Majerus S, Gill-Thwaites H, Andrews K, et al. Behavioral evaluation of consciousness in severe brain damage. Prog Brain Res 2005;150:397–413.

96. Devous MD Sr, Thisted RA, Morgan GF, et al. SPECT brain imaging in epilepsy: a meta-analysis. J Nucl Med 1998;39:285–93.

97. Blumenfeld H, McNally KA, Vanderhill SD, et al. Positive and negative network correlations in temporal lobe epilepsy. Cereb Cortex 2004;14:892–902.

98. Chang DJ, Zubal IG, Gottschalk C, et al. Comparison of statistical parametric mapping and SPECT difference imaging in patients with temporal lobe epilepsy. Epilepsia 2002;43:68–74.

99. Menzel C, Grunwald F, Klemm E, et al. Inhibitory effects of mesial temporal partial seizures onto frontal neocortical structures. Acta Neurol Belg 1998;98:327–31.

100. Rabinowicz AL, Salas E, Beserra F, et al. Changes in regional cerebral blood flow beyond the temporal lobe in unilateral temporal lobe epilepsy. Epilepsia 1997;38:1011–4.

101. Van Paesschen W, Dupont P, Van Driel G, et al. SPECT perfusion changes during complex partial seizures in patients with hippocampal sclerosis. Brain 2003;126:1103–11.

102. Hogan RE, Kaiboriboon K, Bertrand ME, et al. Composite SISCOM perfusion patterns in right and left temporal seizures. Arch Neurol 2006;63:1419–26.

103. Lee KH, Meador KJ, Park YD, et al. Pathophysiology of altered consciousness during seizures: subtraction SPECT study [comment]. Neurology 2002;59: 841–6.

104. Mayanagi Y, Watanabe E, Kaneko Y. Mesial temporal lobe epilepsy: clinical features and seizure mechanism. Epilepsia 1996;37(Suppl 3):57–60.

105. Tae WS, Joo EY, Kim JH, et al. Cerebral perfusion changes in mesial temporal lobe epilepsy: SPM analysis of ictal and interictal SPECT. Neuroimage 2005; 24:101–10.

106. Blumenfeld H, Rivera M, McNally KA, et al. Ictal neocortical slowing in temporal lobe epilepsy. Neurology 2004;63:1015–21.

107. Englot DJ, Yang L, Hamid H, et al. Impaired consciousness in temporal lobe seizures: role of cortical slow activity. Brain 2010;133(Pt 12):3764–77.

108. Englot DJ, Blumenfeld H. Consciousness and epilepsy: why are complex-partial seizures complex? Prog Brain Res 2009;177:147–70.
109. Haider B, Duque A, Hasenstaub AR, et al. Neocortical network activity in vivo is generated through a dynamic balance of excitation and inhibition. J Neurosci 2006;26:4535–45.
110. Steriade M, Contreras D, Curro Dossi R, et al. The slow (<1 Hz) oscillation in reticular thalamic and thalamocortical neurons: scenario of sleep rhythm generation in interacting thalamic and neocortical networks. J Neurosci 1993;13:3284–99.
111. Blumenfeld H, Taylor J. Why do seizures cause loss of consciousness? Neuroscientist 2003;9:301–10.
112. Englot DJ, Mishra AM, Mansuripur PK, et al. Remote effects of focal hippocampal seizures on the rat neocortex. J Neurosci 2008;28(36):9066–81.
113. Englot DJ, Modi B, Mishra AM, et al. Cortical deactivation induced by subcortical network dysfunction in limbic seizures. J Neurosci 2009;29(41):13006–18.
114. Norden AD, Blumenfeld H. The role of subcortical structures in human epilepsy. Epilepsy Behav 2002;3:219–31.
115. Yu L, Blumenfeld H. Theories of impaired consciousness in epilepsy. Ann N Y Acad Sci 2009;1157:48–60.
116. Sperling MR. The consequences of uncontrolled epilepsy. CNS Spectr 2004;9: 98–101.
117. Vickrey BG, Berg AT, Sperling MR, et al. Relationships between seizure severity and health-related quality of life in refractory localization-related epilepsy. Epilepsia 2000;41:760–4.
118. Elliott IM, Lach L, Smith ML. I just want to be normal: a qualitative study exploring how children and adolescents view the impact of intractable epilepsy on their quality of life. Epilepsy Behav 2005;7:664–78.
119. Morrell MJ. Stigma and epilepsy. Epilepsy Behav 2002;3(6 S 2):21–5.
120. Hansotia P, Broste SK. The effect of epilepsy or diabetes mellitus on the risk of automobile accidents [see comment]. N Engl J Med 1991;324:22–6.
121. Lossius R, Kinge E, Nakken KO. Epilepsy and driving: considerations on how eligibility should be decided. Acta Neurol Scand Suppl 2010;190:67–71.
122. Krauss GL, Krumholz A, Carter RC, et al. Risk factors for seizure-related motor vehicle crashes in patients with epilepsy [see comment]. Neurology 1999;52: 1324–9.
123. Sheth SG, Krauss G, Krumholz A, et al. Mortality in epilepsy: driving fatalities vs other causes of death in patients with epilepsy [summary for patients in Neurology. 2004 Sep 28;63(6):E12–3; PMID: 15452331]. Neurology 2004;63: 1002–7.
124. Taylor J, Chadwick D, Johnson T. Risk of accidents in drivers with epilepsy. J Neurol Neurosurg Psychiatry 1996;60:621–7.
125. Berkovic SF. Epilepsy syndromes: effects on cognition, performance and driving ability. Med Law 2000;19:757–61.
126. Gastaut H, Zifkin BG. The risk of automobile accidents with seizures occurring while driving: relation to seizure type. Neurology 1987;37:1613–6.
127. Yang L, Morland TB, Schmits K, et al. A prospective study of loss of consciousness in epilepsy using virtual reality driving simulation and other video games. Epilepsy Behav 2010;18:238–46.
128. Arias-Carrión O, Palomero-Rivero M, Millán-Aldaco D, et al. Infusion of modafinil into anterior hypothalamus or pedunculopontine tegmental nucleus at different time-points enhances waking and blocks the expression of recovery sleep in rats after sleep deprivation. Exp Neurol 2011;229(2):358–63.

129. Ballon JS, Feifel D. A systematic review of modafinil: potential clinical uses and mechanisms of action. J Clin Psychiatry 2006;67:554–66.
130. Fisher R, Salanova V, Witt T, et al. Electrical stimulation of the anterior nucleus of thalamus for treatment of refractory epilepsy. Epilepsia 2010;51:899–908.
131. Jobst BC, Darcey TM, Thadani VM, et al. Brain stimulation for the treatment of epilepsy. Epilepsia 2010;51(Suppl 3):88–92.
132. Kahane P, Depaulis A. Deep brain stimulation in epilepsy: what is next? Curr Opin Neurol 2010;23:177–82.
133. Morrell M. Brain stimulation for epilepsy: can scheduled or responsive neurostimulation stop seizures? Curr Opin Neurol 2006;19:164–8.
134. Theodore WH, Fisher RS. Brain stimulation for epilepsy [erratum appears in Lancet Neurol. 2004 Jun;3(6):332]. Lancet Neurol 2004;3:111–8.
135. Schiff ND, Giacino JT, Kalmar K, et al. Behavioural improvements with thalamic stimulation after severe traumatic brain injury [see comment] [erratum appears in Nature. 2008 Mar 6;452(7183):120 Note: Biondi, T [added]]. Nature 2007;448: 600–3.
136. Yamamoto T, Katayama Y. Deep brain stimulation therapy for the vegetative state. Neuropsychol Rehabil 2005;15:406–13.
137. Easton A, Zinkivskay A, Eacott MJ. Recollection is impaired, but familiarity remains intact in rats with lesions of the fornix. Hippocampus 2009;19:837–43.
138. Heilman KM, Sypert GW. Korsakoff's syndrome resulting from bilateral fornix lesions. Neurology 1977;27:490–3.
139. Garcia-Bengochea F, Friedman WA. Persistent memory loss following section of the anterior fornix in humans. A historical review. Surg Neurol 1987;27:361–4.
140. Blum DE, Eskola J, Bortz JJ, et al. Patient awareness of seizures. Neurology 1996;47:260–4.
141. Cavanna AE, Mula M, Servo S, et al. Measuring the level and content of consciousness during epileptic seizures: the Ictal Consciousness Inventory. Epilepsy Behav 2008;13:184–8.
142. Hoppe C, Poepel A, Elger CE. Epilepsy: accuracy of patient seizure counts. Arch Neurol 2007;64:1595–9.
143. Kerling F, Mueller S, Pauli E, et al. When do patients forget their seizures? An electroclinical study. Epilepsy Behav 2006;9:281–5.
144. Tatum WO, Winters L, Gieron M, et al. Outpatient seizure identification: results of 502 patients using computer-assisted ambulatory EEG. J Clin Neurophysiol 2001;18:14–9.
145. Yang L, Shklyar I, Lee HW, et al. Impaired consciousness in epilepsy investigated by a prospective responsiveness in epilepsy scale (RES). Epilepsia, In review. 2011.
146. Detyniecki K, Yang L, Enamandram S, et al. Seizure recognition during inpatient Video/EEG Monitoring. AES meeting. San Antonio, TX, December 3–7, [abstracts 1382]. 2010. Available at: http://www.aesnet.org/.

Anoxic-Ischemic Encephalopathy and Strokes Causing Impaired Consciousness

Miguel Bussière, MD, PhD[a],*, G. Bryan Young, MD, FRCP(C)[b]

KEYWORDS

• Anoxic-ischemic encephalopathy • Ischemic stroke
• Intracerebral hemorrhage • Subarachnoid hemorrhage

In this article, the authors review coma due to global ischemia (cardiac arrest or severe hypotension) or focal ischemia or hemorrhage. Hypoxemia by itself rarely causes neuronal death unless the arterial partial pressure of oxygen decreases to less than 25 mm Hg[1]; however, lesser degrees of hypoxemia can contribute to damage in the presence of severe hypotension.

ANOXIC-ISCHEMIC ENCEPHALOPATHY

Within 1 minute of cardiac arrest, phosphocreatine, a major source of high-energy phosphate, is depleted. The sodium-potassium membrane pump rapidly fails as a result of an inadequate supply of adenosine triphosphate, causing an influx of sodium into neurons and glia accompanied by potassium ion efflux. With energy failure in the mitochondria, lactate production increases, and without oxygen the excess electrons allow the formation of destructive superoxide free radicals.[2] Glutamate, released into the extracellular fluid caused by a failure of the glutamate buffering mechanism, binds to and activates N-methyl-D-aspartate receptors. The resultant influx of sodium and calcium ions adds to osmotic swelling (cytotoxic edema) and activates proteinases (calpains that break down elements of the cytoskeleton) and phospholipases,

---

The authors have nothing to disclose.
[a] Division of Neurology and Interventional Neuroradiology, Department of Medicine, University of Ottawa, The Ottawa Hospital, Civic Campus, C-2174, 1053 Carling Avenue, Ottawa, ON K1Y 4E9, Canada
[b] Division of Neurology, Department of Clinical Neurological Sciences, University of Western Ontario, London Health Sciences Centre, 339 Windermere Road, London, ON N6A 5A5, Canada
* Corresponding author.
E-mail address: mbussiere@toh.on.ca

Neurol Clin 29 (2011) 825–836
doi:10.1016/j.ncl.2011.07.001
0733-8619/11/$ – see front matter © 2011 Elsevier Inc. All rights reserved.

producing arachidonic acid and causing the release of cytochrome c. With reperfusion, that is, when the heart is restarted, there is increased free radical production, including peroxynitrate, which inactivates superoxide dismutase (a free radical scavenging enzyme) and damages complexes I and II of the mitochondrial respiratory chain, leading to further membrane damage.[2] Calcium influx into the mitochondria triggers additional phospholipase activation (digesting membrane phospholipids) and turns on apoptotic mechanisms. Incremental ischemic damage with reperfusion relates, at least in part, to eicosanoids (generated by arachidonic acid) that cause increased adhesion of white blood cells and platelets to capillary walls, contributing to the no-reflow phenomenon. Edema and microhemorrhages caused by leaky damaged blood vessels can further impair perfusion and worsen ischemia.

Coma occurs quickly with global ischemia because of widespread metabolic, neuronal, and glial failure, leading to loss of membrane potential and synaptic function. Sedating drugs and paralyzing agents used in patients treated with the hypothermic protocol can prolong the period of unresponsiveness, but the established neuroprotective benefit of hypothermia justifies their use.[3,4]

Advances have been made in the prognostic determination of patients with anoxic-ischemic encephalopathy. In 2006, the American Academy of Neurology published practice parameters for determining the neurologic prognosis of patients who had been resuscitated from cardiac arrest (**Fig. 1**).[5] However, the articles used in formulating these guidelines preceded the advent of the hypothermic protocol, which has

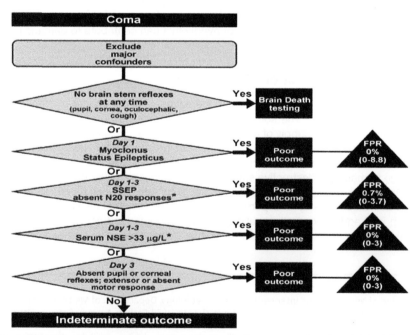

Fig. 1. The American Academy of Neurology practice parameters for determining the neurologic prognosis of patients resuscitated from cardiac arrest. FPR, false-positive rate; NSE, neuron-specific enolase; SSEP, somatosensory evoked potential. (*From* Wijdicks EF, Hijdra A, Young GB, et al. Practice parameter: prediction of outcome in comatose survivors after cardiopulmonary resuscitation (an evidence based review): report of the Quality Standards Subcommittee of the American Academy of Neurology. Neurology 2006;67:204; with permission.)

been shown to have a neuroprotective effect and is now a standard of care in most centers. Studies on patients with cardiac arrest treated with the hypothermic protocol are showing that some of the guidelines may not be valid. Rossetti and colleagues[6] and Al Thenayan and colleagues[7] both showed that the motor response is unreliable at 3 days and that 6 days or more may be necessary to use the motor response as a prognostic criterion for poor outcome.[7] Similarly, the presence of myoclonic status epilepticus may not be sufficient on its own to be reliably predictive.[6] It would seem that the absence of the pupillary and corneal reflexes and the N20 somatosensory evoked potential response remains valid at the timelines suggested by the American Academy of Neurology, but further clinical research is needed to refine the practice parameters for patients who have been treated with the hypothermic protocol.[6,7]

ISCHEMIC AND HEMORRHAGIC STROKE

Strokes, either ischemic or hemorrhagic, typically cause acute onset of focal neurologic deficits such as hemiparesis, hemisensory or hemivisual loss, or aphasia.[8] Impairment of consciousness, at least acutely, is an uncommon symptom of stroke. However, consciousness may be affected by ischemia or hemorrhage if damage occurs to specific brain structures involved in alertness, with widespread hemispheric or bihemispheric damage, or as a result of secondary complications such as hemorrhagic transformation of an ischemic infarct, malignant edema, mass effect, or cerebrospinal fluid outflow obstruction causing raised intracranial pressure or as a result of seizures. Superimposed metabolic disturbances, infection, and adverse effects of medications may also contribute to impaired alertness in patients with stroke.

Ischemic Stroke

Thromboemboli from large vessel atherosclerotic disease or of cardiac origin are responsible for up to half of ischemic strokes.[8–10] Small vessel or penetrating artery disease (lacunar) represents the third most common cause of ischemic stroke. Patients with penetrating artery disease typically present with classic clinical syndromes without impaired consciousness because of small infarcts in the deep regions of the brain or brainstem.[11,12] Approximately, 15% to 20% of strokes remain cryptogenic in origin despite extensive investigation.[9,10] Various uncommon causes account for the remainder of ischemic strokes (<5%), including hypoperfusion, arterial dissection, vasculitis, thrombophilias, and cortical vein or venous sinus thrombosis. The symptoms and severity of deficits caused by ischemic stroke vary depending on the site of arterial occlusion and the degree of collateral blood flow.

Anterior circulation ischemia
Anterior cerebral artery Unilateral anterior cerebral artery (ACA) infarction typically causes contralateral leg weakness and sensory loss but does not impair consciousness. Bilateral ACA territory ischemia affecting the mesiofrontal structures (orbitofrontal cortex, anterior cingulate gyri, and anterior limbs of the internal capsule) may cause akinetic mutism, a state in which patients are awake but mute and make little voluntary movement but may fixate and track with their eyes.[12] Infarcts affecting the supplementary motor areas, even unilaterally, may produce abulia or profound lack of spontaneity.[12]

Middle cerebral artery Patients with extensive middle cerebral artery (MCA) territory infarction due to proximal MCA occlusion usually only have mild decreased responsiveness and alertness at onset. Aphasia due to dominant hemisphere involvement should not be confused with impaired alertness. Early impairment of the level of consciousness at or shortly after stroke onset, however, is a strong predictor of poor outcome.[13] Patients with extensive MCA territory infarction may develop malignant cerebral edema (see later).

Anterior choroidal artery Unilateral anterior choroidal artery infarcts may cause contralateral weakness and sensory loss and hemianopsia due to injury to the posterior limb of the internal capsule and lateral geniculate nucleus. Bilateral anterior choroidal infarction, although exceedingly uncommon, can cause akinetic mutism and bilateral hemiparesis or hemiplegia.[12]

Internal carotid artery Internal carotid artery (ICA) occlusion can result in extensive unilateral hemispheric infarction. The term total anterior circulation stroke has been used to describe complete infarction of both the ACA and MCA territories. These large strokes carry a poor prognosis with a high mortality rate (about 60%). Patients present with profound hemiplegia, hemisensory and visual loss, and global aphasia if the dominant hemisphere is involved, in addition to decreased alertness and responsiveness. Bilateral ICA occlusion, a very rare occurrence, can cause sudden coma with preservation of brainstem reflexes.[14]

Posterior circulation ischemia

Many nuclei and ascending projections in the rostral brainstem and thalami play key roles in the maintenance and modulation of wakefulness, including the reticular formation, noradrenergic nuclei such as the locus coeruleus, serotonergic nuclei such as the dorsal raphe, as well as rostrally directed cholinergic, adrenergic, and serotonergic projections.[15–17] Perforating vessels arising from the basilar artery, proximal posterior cerebral arteries, and posterior communicating arteries supply blood to the brainstem and diencephalon. Occlusion of these vessels caused by cardioembolism, atheroembolism, or in situ atherothrombosis can disrupt these pathways and nuclei and cause alterations in the state of consciousness.

Bilateral thalamic infarction, especially if it involves the paramedian regions, can cause decreased levels of consciousness (**Fig. 2**).[18,19] Akinetic mutism, vertical gaze paresis, amnesia, and altered behavior or personality may also be a consequence of medial thalamic injury but may only become apparent when alertness improves.[18,19] The top of the basilar syndrome, most often caused by an embolus, is a manifestation of ischemic injury, usually bilateral, to the rostral midbrain and thalamus. Patients

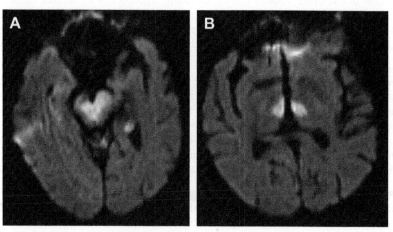

Fig. 2. Axial diffusion-weighted magnetic resonance images of the brain showing bilateral rostral midbrain (*A*) and paramedian thalamic (*B*) infarctions.

develop pupillary and eye movement abnormalities and a depressed level of consciousness and may or may not have visual field, motor, and sensory abnormalities.

Basilar artery occlusion carries a grave prognosis with a mortality rate as high as 90%.[20] Patients may present with abrupt loss of consciousness or with transient or progressive brainstem and cerebellar symptoms, such as vertigo, ataxia, dysarthria, diplopia, or visual field loss, often followed by an abrupt neurologic decline. Basilar occlusion occurs as a result of an embolus in the basilar artery from the heart or proximal vertebrobasilar system or thrombosis of an atherosclerotic and stenotic basilar artery.[20]

Strokes in multiple arterial territories

Infarctions in multiple vascular territories are often accompanied by impairment in alertness. Strokes associated with cardiac surgery, as an example, are commonly multiple and occur because of embolism, hypoperfusion, or both.[21,22] Patients with watershed or borderzone infarcts tend to have longer periods of unconsciousness after cardiac surgery compared with patients with embolic infarcts.[21] In another study, widespread ischemic brain injury was documented on neuroimaging in several patients with postoperative coma, most frequently associated with cardiovascular surgery and/or the occurrence of intraoperative hypotension.[23]

Malignant edema after ischemic stroke

Cerebral edema, mostly cytotoxic in nature, develops and progresses over the first 3 to 5 days after an ischemic stroke and generally begins to subside within 1 to 2 weeks. In approximately 1% to 10% of MCA territory strokes, malignant edema can develop with rapid and severe tissue swelling causing mass effect, raised intracranial pressure, and risk of lateral tentorial herniation (**Fig. 3**).[24,25] Direct compression and distortion of the rostral brainstem and thalami lead to impairment in consciousness. Patients with malignant edema after large anterior circulation infarcts typically exhibit a progressive decline in the level of consciousness over the first 24 to 48 hours.[24,25] A mortality rate as high as 80% is associated with this condition. The most consistent factor associated with the development of malignant edema after a hemispheric stroke is the extent or size of the baseline infarction. Patients with anterior circulation infarcts involving less than 50% of the hemisphere are at an increased risk of developing malignant edema.[26]

Severe edema can also complicate 10% to 20% of cerebellar infarcts (**Fig. 4**).[27,28] The posterior fossa is contained by the skull and tentorial dura and has a limited capacity to accommodate increases in volume. Thus, cerebellar tonsil herniation may be the consequence of unrecognized and untreated severe edema after a large

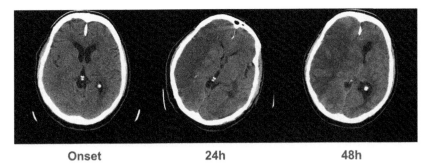

Onset   24h   48h

Fig. 3. Serial axial computed tomographic scan of the head demonstrating the development of malignant edema in the first 48 hours after a large right MCA infarct.

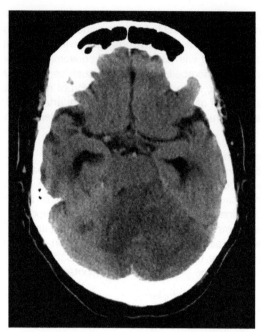

Fig. 4. Axial computed tomographic scan of the head showing brainstem and fourth ventricle compressions due to severe edema developing after a large left cerebellar infarct.

cerebellar hemisphere infarct. Clinical symptoms at presentation include vertigo, nausea and vomiting, dysarthria, and ataxia. Patients may become increasingly drowsy over the first 2 to 3 days before abrupt respiratory and cardiovascular compromise or arrest occurs.[29]

Venous sinus thrombosis

Thrombosis of the deep cerebral veins can result in profound impairment of consciousness. The internal cerebral veins drain blood from the thalami and rostral midbrain into the vein of Galen and straight sinus.[30] Venous congestion due to thrombosis of the deep cerebral veins can cause severe edema in these structures leading to venous infarction and hemorrhage (**Fig. 5**).[31]

Hemorrhagic Stroke

Intracranial hemorrhage is the cause of about 20% of all strokes.[8–10] These spontaneous nontraumatic intracranial bleeds can be subclassified into intracerebral hemorrhage (ICH) or subarachnoid hemorrhage (SAH).

There are no clinical features at symptom onset that are of sufficient specificity to reliably distinguish patients with hemorrhagic stroke and those with ischemic stroke.[32] This is the primary reason why neuroimaging is required before consideration of thrombolysis for ischemic stroke.[33] Coma at onset, however, increases the probability of a hemorrhagic stroke.[32]

ICH

Primary ICHs are caused by hypertension or amyloid angiopathy and account for 78% to 88% of all ICHs.[34] Secondary ICHs can occur due to various causes, including coagulopathy, vascular malformations, tumor, venous thrombosis, vasculitis, or reversible

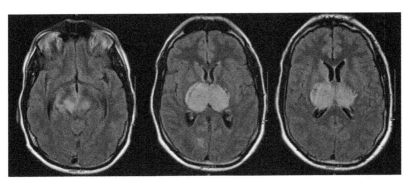

Fig. 5. Axial fluid-attenuated inversion recovery magnetic resonance images of the brain in a patient with deep cerebral vein thrombosis demonstrating bilateral thalamic and rostral midbrain hyperintensity due to venous congestion.

cerebral vasoconstriction syndromes. Hypertensive bleeds occur most commonly in the basal ganglia, pons, thalamus, and cerebellum.[34] Large hemorrhages in the basal ganglia or thalamus may extend or decompress into the ventricular system. ICHs caused by amyloid angiopathy occur in a lobar distribution. These patients often have evidence of numerous previous microbleeds on magnetic resonance imaging (MRI) using gradient echo or susceptibility-weighted sequences.[35,36]

ICHs may impair consciousness by several mechanisms. ICH that occurs in the rostral brainstem may disrupt the ascending reticular activating system, as described previously (see section on Posterior Circulation Ischemia). Large supratentorial lobar hemorrhages may cause mass effect, raised intracranial pressure leading to herniation, and compression of the diencephalon and brainstem. Large ICHs centered in the thalamus or basal ganglia may extend into the ventricular system and thus impair cerebrospinal fluid outflow, and cause hydrocephalus and raise intracranial pressure. Large infratentorial bleeds, similarly, may exert mass effect, leading to obstruction of the ventricular system, hydrocephalus, and elevated intracranial pressure or pressure within the posterior fossa leading to upward, central, or downward cerebellar tonsil herniation. Sudden or progressive neurologic decline after ICH is often caused by hematoma enlargement.[34]

SAH

SAH is the underlying cause of 5% of all strokes and up to 20% of hemorrhagic strokes. Rupture of an intracranial saccular aneurysm is the cause of nontraumatic SAH in up to 85% of cases.[37,38] Other causes include perimesencephalic bleeds, vascular malformations, mycotic aneurysms, arterial dissection, coagulopathy, venous thrombosis, vasculitis, and reversible cerebral vasoconstriction syndromes.

The classic clinical presentation of a patient with SAH is a very sudden severe headache associated with photophobia and neck stiffness. About 10% to 20% of patients with SAH, however, arrive at the hospital in a coma or with depressed level of consciousness.[39,40] Sudden severe pain may precipitate a vasovagal response in some patients, leading to syncope. In most patients, however, the abrupt loss of consciousness is believed to occur secondary to a sudden increase in intracranial pressure because of rapid expansion of the volume of the subarachnoid space or acute hydrocephalus. Patients with aneurysms arising from the MCA bifurcation may develop large clots in the Sylvian fissure and surrounding brain parenchyma, which may also exert mass effect. Hemorrhage from anterior communicating artery complex aneurysms or ICA terminus aneurysms may extend into the ventricular system and further obstruct cerebrospinal fluid outflow. Anterior communicating artery complex aneurysms may also rupture into and damage both frontal lobes causing an akinetic mute state. Rupture of basilar tip aneurysms may cause injury to structures critical to the maintenance of consciousness in the rostral brainstem or diencephalon (see section on Posterior Circulation Ischemia).

Vasospasm or narrowing of the lumen of intracranial arteries is detectable in up to 70% of patients with SAH on angiography within 3 to 12 days after an SAH. Up to half of these patients develop delayed cerebral ischemia as a consequence of severe vasospasm.[41] New focal deficits may develop that correlate with the progression of severe vasospasm in affected intracranial vessels. Frequently, however, confusion or somnolence is the only symptom of delayed cerebral ischemia.

Poststroke Seizures and Coma

Seizures causing impaired consciousness are discussed in the article by Blumenfeld elsewhere in this issue. Strokes cause focal lesions and therefore may cause partial seizures. Impairment of consciousness occurs when seizures become secondarily generalized or less commonly with complex partial seizures that involve limbic structures. Various more isolated impairments, for example, speech or perception, can occur with seizures that spread into various brain regions.

The most sensitive method of detecting seizures in the acute phase (within the first 24 hours) of stroke is the use of continuous electroencephalographic (EEG) monitoring.[42] One continuous EEG study of 232 patients with stroke found seizures in 6.5%, mostly as focal status epilepticus or with periodic lateralized epileptiform discharges. Seizures following either ischemic or hemorrhagic stroke have been reported from 2% to 32%.[42] The variation relates to different case mixes, varied methods of detection, small series, and duration of follow-up. A follow-up questionnaire study of 372 patients with stroke in Thailand found an incidence of 15.6%, higher than most studies.[43] Most seizures occurred within 2 weeks of the stroke and were more likely if the stroke was hemorrhagic and involved the cerebral cortex. Imaging studies with MRI confirm that cerebral cortical involvement is a significant risk factor for the development of late seizures after ischemic stroke.[44]

Diagnosis and Management of Strokes Causing Impaired Consciousness

Rapid and accurate diagnosis of stroke subtype, either ischemic or hemorrhagic, relies on parenchymal brain and vascular imaging. A noncontrast computed tomographic (CT) scan of the head and CT angiogram are the initial imaging studies of choice for patients clinically suspected of having a stroke in most centers.[45,46] Diffusion-weighted imaging is more sensitive to detect early ischemic infarct but MRI is not as readily accessible in most centers. Vascular imaging with a CT or magnetic resonance angiogram can demonstrate occluded vessels in the setting of an ischemic stroke, rule out secondary causes of ICH, or locate the presence of intracranial aneurysms in the setting of SAH.[39,40,45,46] CT angiography demonstrating contrast extravasation (spot sign) within an ICH identifies patients at high risk of hematoma enlargement and neurologic deterioration.[47] Perfusion imaging is a technique that shows promise in the near future to improve patient selection and extend the time window for thrombolysis for acute ischemic stroke[45,46] and in the early detection of ischemia due to vasospasm from aneurysm-related SAH.[48]

Patients who present with an ischemic stroke within 4.5 hours of onset are potential candidates for thrombolysis with intravenous recombinant tissue plasminogen activator.[49,50] Direct intra-arterial thrombolysis, mechanical clot disruption, thrombectomy, or thromboaspiration[51] can be considered where available for select patients with large vessel occlusions to increase the chance of recanalization. The safety and efficacy of endovascular therapies for ischemic stroke are currently under investigation in large randomized studies.[52,53]

Close observation and management of patients with stroke in a stroke unit improves outcomes.[54] Further investigations are aimed at determining the cause of the stroke to prevent recurrent events. Patients with large cerebral or cerebellar hemisphere strokes are at risk of developing malignant edema, herniation, and death. Decompressive craniectomy can be lifesaving and result in acceptable outcomes in select patients.[24,25,29]

Management of patients with ICH remains primarily supportive.[55] Coagulation deficiencies or abnormalities should be corrected as appropriate. A modest reduction in blood pressure is recommended in the setting of severe hypertension while maintaining adequate cerebral perfusion. Although early administration of recombinant factor VIIa may limit hematoma expansion, no clear benefit was demonstrated in recent trials in an unselected population.[56] Surgical decompression is not routinely recommended but should be considered in patients with cerebellar ICH who are deteriorating or in patients with large superficial lobar clots.[55]

After ensuring hemodynamic and respiratory stability, the initial step in the management of patients with aneurysmal SAH is to prevent aneurysm rebleeding. The decision to treat a ruptured aneurysm by endovascular coiling or surgical clipping depends on many factors, including available local expertise, the location and morphology of the aneurysm, as well as patient comorbidities.[37,39,40] Further management is aimed at the prevention, detection, and treatment of potential complications of SAH such as hydrocephalus and cerebral vasospasm. Administration of nimodipine,[57] and possibly oral statins[58] and intravenous magnesium[59] may help reduce the risk of delayed cerebral ischemia and improve outcomes. Serial transcranial Doppler ultrasonography and noninvasive vascular imaging are used to screen for arterial narrowing due to vasospasm.[39,40] Patients with suspected delayed cerebral ischemia are treated with volume expansion and vasopressors.[37,39,40] Early intra-arterial administration of vasodilatory drugs such as milrinone or nicardipine or angioplasty of proximal arterial segments may be required to prevent stroke in patients who do not improve despite aggressive medical therapy.[37,39,40]

Treatment of seizures or status epilepticus in the acute phase of stroke should follow standard procedure. In choosing a drug for secondary prevention of poststroke seizures, the physician should consider the age of the patient, comedications (drug interactions), and affordability. A recent Cochrane review of the use of antiepileptic drugs found no randomized controlled trials comparing antiepileptic drugs with placebo for either primary or secondary prevention of seizures after stroke.[60] Three studies compared various drugs for their effectiveness in secondary prevention of seizures in older patients.[61–63] The studies were somewhat conflicting and 2 of the 3 included causes other than stroke. Although no conclusion can be reached, it seems that lamotrigine and levetiracetam are promising and deserve further study. Levetiracetam is supported by 1 observational study.[64] Treatment with tissue plasminogen activator is not in itself associated with an increased risk of acute phase seizures and can reduce the risk of poststroke seizures by ameliorating stroke severity.[65]

REFERENCES

1. Miyamoto O, Auer RN. Hypoxia, hyperoxia, ischemia, and brain necrosis. Neurology 2000;25(54):362–71.

2. Busl KM, Greer DM. Hypoxic-ischemic brain injury: pathophysiology, neuropathology and mechanisms. NeuroRehabilitation 2010;26:5–13.
3. The Hypothermia after Cardiac Arrest Study Group. Mild therapeutic hypothermia to improve neurologic outcome after cardiac arrest. N Engl J Med 2002;346: 549–56.
4. Bernard SA, Gray TW, Buist MD, et al. Treatment of comatose survivors of out-of-hospital cardiac arrest with induced hypothermia. N Engl J Med 2002;346: 557–63.
5. Wijdicks EF, Hijdra A, Young GB, et al. Practice parameter: prediction of outcome in comatose survivors after cardiopulmonary resuscitation (an evidence based review): report of the Quality Standards Subcommittee of the American Academy of Neurology. Neurology 2006;67:203–10.
6. Rossetti AO, Oddo M, Logroscino G, et al. Prognostication after hypothermia and cardiac arrest: a prospective study. Ann Neurol 2010;67:301–7.
7. Al Thenayan E, Savard M, Sharpe M, et al. Predictors of poor neurologic outcome after induced mild hypothermia following cardiac arrest. Neurology 2008;71: 1535–7.
8. Donnan GA, Fisher M, Macleod M, et al. Stroke. Lancet 2008;371:1612–23.
9. Grau AJ, Weimar C, Buggle F, et al. Risk factors, outcome, and treatment in subtypes of ischemic stroke: the German stroke data bank. Stroke 2001;32: 2559–66.
10. Foulkes MA, Wolf PA, Price TR, et al. The stroke data bank: design, methods, and baseline characteristics. Stroke 1988;19:547–54.
11. Arboix A, Marti-Vilalta JL. Lacunar stroke. Expert Rev Neurother 2009;9:179–96.
12. Kumral E, Topcuoglu MA, Onal MZ. Anterior circulation syndromes. Handb Clin Neurol 2008;93:485–536.
13. Cucchiara BL, Kasner SE, Wolk DA, et al. Early impairment in consciousness predicts mortality after hemispheric ischemic stroke. Crit Care Med 2004;32:241–5.
14. Kwon SU, Lee SH, Kim JS. Sudden coma from acute bilateral internal carotid artery territory infarction. Neurology 2002;58:1846–9.
15. Parvisi J, Damasio AR. Neuroanatomical correlates of brainstem coma. Brain 2003; 126:1524–36.
16. Parvisi J, Damasio AR. Consciousness and the brainstem. Cognition 2001;79: 135–9.
17. Plum F, Posner JB. The diagnosis of stupor and coma. 3rd edition. Philadelphia: F.A. Davis; 1980.
18. Carrera E, Bogousslavsky J. The thalamus and behavior: effects of anatomically distinct strokes. Neurology 2006;66:1817–23.
19. Schmahmann JD. Vascular syndromes of the thalamus. Stroke 2003;34:2264–78.
20. Baird TA, Muir KW, Bone I. Basilar artery occlusion. Neurocrit Care 2004;1:319–29.
21. Salazar JD, Wityk RJ, Grega MA, et al. Stroke after cardiac surgery: short- and long-term outcomes. Ann Thorac Surg 2001;72:1195–201.
22. McKhann GM, Grega MA, Borowicz LM Jr, et al. Stroke and encephalopathy after cardiac surgery: an update. Stroke 2006;37:562–71.
23. Gootjes EC, Wijdicks EF, McClelland RL. Postoperative stupor and coma. Mayo Clin Proc 2005;80:350–4.
24. Huttner HB, Schwab S. Malignant middle cerebral artery infarction: clinical characteristics, treatment strategies, and future perspectives. Lancet Neurol 2009;8: 949–58.
25. Vahedi K, Hofmeijer J, Juettler E, et al, DECIMAL, DESTINY, and HAMLET investigators. Early decompressive surgery in malignant infarction of the middle

cerebral artery: a pooled analysis of three randomised controlled trials. Lancet Neurol 2007;6:215–22.

26. Hofmeijer J, Algra A, Kappelle LJ, et al. Predictors of life-threatening brain edema in middle cerebral artery infarction. Cerebrovasc Dis 2008;25:176–84.

27. Koh MG, Phan TG, Atkinson JL, et al. Neuroimaging in deteriorating patients with cerebellar infarcts and mass effect. Stroke 2000;31:2062–7.

28. Hornig CR, Rust DS, Busse O, et al. Space-occupying cerebellar infarction. Clinical course and prognosis. Stroke 1994;25:372–4.

29. Sykora M, Diedler J, Jüttler E, et al. Intensive care management of acute stroke: surgical treatment. Int J Stroke 2010;5:170–7.

30. Leach JL, Fortuna RB, Jones BV, et al. Imaging of cerebral venous thrombosis: current techniques, spectrum of findings, and diagnostic pitfalls. Radiographics 2006;26(Suppl 1):S19–41.

31. Stam J. Thrombosis of the cerebral veins and sinuses. N Engl J Med 2005;352:1791–8.

32. Runchey S, McGee S. Does this patient have a hemorrhagic stroke? Clinical findings distinguishing hemorrhagic stroke from ischemic stroke. JAMA 2010;303:2280–6.

33. Adams HP Jr, del Zoppo G, Alberts MJ, et al. Guidelines for the early management of adults with ischemic stroke: a guideline from the American Heart Association/American Stroke Association Stroke Council, Clinical Cardiology Council, Cardiovascular Radiology and Intervention Council, and the Atherosclerotic Peripheral Vascular Disease and Quality of Care Outcomes in Research Interdisciplinary Working Groups: the American Academy of Neurology affirms the value of this guideline as an educational tool for neurologists. Stroke 2007;38:1655–711.

34. Qureshi AI, Tuhrim S, Broderick JP, et al. Spontaneous intracerebral hemorrhage. N Engl J Med 2001;344:1450–60.

35. Greenberg SM, Vernooij MW, Cordonnier C, et al, Microbleed Study Group. Cerebral microbleeds: a guide to detection and interpretation. Lancet Neurol 2009;8:165–74.

36. Cordonnier C. Brain microbleeds: more evidence, but still a clinical dilemma. Curr Opin Neurol 2011;24:69–74.

37. Brisman JL, Song JK, Newell DW. Cerebral aneurysms. N Engl J Med 2006;355:928–39.

38. van Gijn J, Kerr RS, Rinkel GJ. Subarachnoid haemorrhage. Lancet 2007;369:306–18.

39. Rabinstein AA, Lanzino G, Wijdicks EF. Multidisciplinary management and emerging therapeutic strategies in aneurysmal subarachnoid haemorrhage. Lancet Neurol 2010;9:504–19.

40. Diringer MN. Management of aneurysmal subarachnoid hemorrhage. Crit Care Med 2009;37:432–40.

41. Weyer GW, Nolan CP, Macdonald RL. Evidence-based cerebral vasospasm management. Neurosurg Focus 2006;21:E8.

42. Mecarelli O, Pro S, Randi F, et al. EEG patterns and epileptic seizures in acute phase stroke. Cerebrovasc Dis 2010;31:191–8.

43. Panitchote A, Tiamkao S. Prevalence of post-stroke seizures in Srinagarind Hospital. J Med Assoc Thai 2010;93:1037–42.

44. Chiang IH, Chang WN, Lin WC, et al. Risk factors for seizures after first-time ischemic stroke by magnetic resonance imaging. Acta Neurol Taiwan 2010;19:26–32.

45. Butcher K, Emery D. Acute stroke imaging I. Can J Neurol Sci 2010;37:4–16.

46. Butcher K, Emery D. Acute stroke imaging II. Can J Neurol Sci 2010;37:17–27.

47. Wada R, Aviv RI, Fox AJ, et al. CT angiography "spot sign" predicts hematoma expansion in acute intracerebral hemorrhage. Stroke 2007;38:1257–62.

48. Wintermark M, Sincic R, Sridhar D, et al. Cerebral perfusion CT: technique and clinical applications. J Neuroradiol 2008;35:253–60.

49. NINDS investigators. Tissue plasminogen activator for acute ischemic stroke. The National Institute of Neurological Disorders and Stroke rt-PA Stroke Study Group. N Engl J Med 1995;333:1581–7.

50. Hacke W, Kaste M, Bluhmki E, et al. Thrombolysis with alteplase 3 to 4.5 hours after acute ischemic stroke. N Engl J Med 2008;359:1317–29.

51. Nogueira RG, Yoo AJ, Buonanno FS, et al. Endovascular approaches to acute stroke, part 2: a comprehensive review of studies and trials. AJNR Am J Neuroradiol 2009;30:859–75.

52. Khatri P, Hill M, Palesch Y, et al. Methodology of the interventional management of stroke III trial. Int J Stroke 2008;3:130–7.

53. Kidwell CS. MR and recanalization of stroke clots using embolectomy. Available at: ClinicalTrials.gov. NCT00094588, Accessed February 22, 2011.

54. Stroke Unit Trialists' Collaboration. Organised inpatient (stroke unit) care for stroke. Cochrane Database Syst Rev 2007;4:CD000197.

55. Morgenstern LB, Hemphill JC 3rd, Anderson C, et al. Guidelines for the management of spontaneous intracerebral hemorrhage: a guideline for healthcare professionals from the American Heart Association/American Stroke Association. Stroke 2010;41:2108–29.

56. Mayer SA, Brun NC, Begtrup K, et al. Efficacy and safety of recombinant activated factor VII for acute intracerebral hemorrhage. N Engl J Med 2008;358:2127–37.

57. Dorhout Mees SM, Rinkel GJ, Feigin VL, et al. Calcium antagonists for aneurysmal subarachnoid haemorrhage. Cochrane Database Syst Rev 2007;3:CD000277.

58. Sabri M, Macdonald RL. Statins: a potential therapeutic addition to treatment for aneurysmal subarachnoid hemorrhage? World Neurosurg 2010;73(6):646–53.

59. Westermaier T, Stetter C, Vince GH, et al. Prophylactic intravenous magnesium sulfate for treatment of aneurysmal subarachnoid hemorrhage: a randomized, placebo-controlled, clinical study. Crit Care Med 2010;38:1284–90.

60. Kwan J, Wood E. Antiepileptic drugs for the primary and secondary prevention of seizures after stroke. Cochrane Database Syst Rev 2010;1:CD005398.

61. Rowan AJ, Ramsay RE, Collins JF, et al. New onset geriatric epilepsy: a randomized study of gabapentin, lamotrigine and carbamazepine. Neurology 2005;64:1868–73.

62. Gilad R, Sadeh M, Rapoport A, et al. Monotherapy of lamotrigine versus carbamazepine in patients with poststroke seizure. Clin Neuropharmacol 2007;30:189–95.

63. Marson AG, Al-Kharusi AM, Alwaidh M, et al. The SANAD study of effectiveness of valproate, lamotrigine, or topiramate for generalized and unclassifiable epilepsy: an unblinded randomised controlled trial. Lancet 2007;369:1016–26.

64. Daniele O, Didato G, Fierro B, et al. Early post-stroke seizures treated with levetiracetam. J Neurol Sci 2005;238(Suppl 1):S112.

65. De Reuck J, Van Maele G. Acute ischemic stroke treatment and the occurrence of seizures. Clin Neurol Neurosurg 2010;112:328–31.

Metabolic Encephalopathies

Michael J. Angel, MD, PhD, FRCP(C)[a],*, G. Bryan Young, MD, FRCP(C)[b]

KEYWORDS

- Metabolic encephalopathy • Altered consciousness
- Neurodegeneration • Neuroimaging

Kinnier Wilson coined the term metabolic encephalopathy to describe a clinical state of global cerebral dysfunction induced by systemic stress that can vary in clinical presentation from mild executive dysfunction to deep coma with decerebrate posturing; the causes are numerous. Some mechanisms by which cerebral dysfunction occurs in metabolic encephalopathies include focal or global cerebral edema, alterations in transmitter function, the accumulation of uncleared toxic metabolites, postcapillary venule vasogenic edema, and energy failure. Such varied mechanisms reflect the heterogeneous etiology that produces this condition of altered consciousness. Metabolic encephalopathy is therefore not a diagnosis, but rather a clinical state. Differentiating this from progressive neurodegenerative dementing processes may be at times obvious. For example, the patient with delirium, headache, vomiting, and a seizure with serum sodium of 102 mmol/L clearly qualifies as an acute hyponatremia encephalopathy. On the other hand, situations may arise whereby the clinical signs of inattention, myoclonus, and confusion clearly overlap with other diagnoses such as corticobasal ganglionic degeneration, Creutzfeld-Jacob disease, or Alzheimer disease with a superimposed septic encephalopathy. Establishing the presence of a metabolic encephalopathy as opposed to a dementing process is clearly of paramount importance, as the prognoses and responses to treatment are vastly different.

This article focuses on common causes of metabolic encephalopathy, and reviews common causes, clinical presentations and, where relevant, management. An exhaustive inventory and discussion of the pathophysiology that is beyond the scope of this article, and the reader is referred to the article by Angel and colleagues.[1]

HEPATIC ENCEPHALOPATHY

Hepatic encephalopathy (HE) can be classified temporally as acute or chronic, as the etiology, clinical features, and treatments differ. Acute HE can be a florid neuropsychiatric presentation caused by hepatocellular dysfunction and cerebral edema.

[a] Division of Neurology, Department of Medicine, University of Toronto, Toronto, ON, Canada
[b] Division of Neurology, Department of Clinical Neurological Sciences, University of Western Ontario, London Health Sciences Centre, 339 Windermere Road, London, ON N6A 5A5, Canada
* Corresponding author.
E-mail address: mike.angel@utoronto.ca

Neurol Clin 29 (2011) 837–882
doi:10.1016/j.ncl.2011.08.002
0733-8619/11/$ – see front matter © 2011 Elsevier Inc. All rights reserved.

neurologic.theclinics.com

Common causes of acute liver failure include viral hepatitides, drugs (eg, acetaminophen, Ecstasy, idiopathic drug reaction), toxins, vascular disease (eg, ischemia, Budd-Chiari syndrome, heat stroke, malignant hyperthermia), as well as Wilson disease, lymphoma, Reye syndrome, and the acute fatty liver of pregnancy. HE associated with chronic liver failure is more insidious and is due to portosystemic shunting; causes commonly include alcoholic cirrhosis; nonalcoholic cirrhosis (eg, Wilson disease, viral hepatitis), transjugular intrahepatic portosystemic shunt (TIPS), and urea acid cycle impairment (although the latter may also have an acute presentation with cerebral edema).

Clinical Findings

The clinical presentation of acute and fulminant liver failure may resemble drug intoxication or a condition of primary psychiatric etiology. The initial stages (stages I–II) are hyperkinetic and agitated, and may be followed within hours by stupor with preservation of arousal (stage III), then coma (stage IV), and is summarized in **Table 1**. By stage IV, cerebral edema is typically present, and patients often have widened pulse pressure, bradycardia, and decorticate or decerebrate posturing.

The classification of HE associated with portosystemic shunting is subdivided into minimal HE and overt (grade I–IV) HE (see **Table 1**). Minimal HE is characterized by impaired attention and visuomotor skills. Minimal HE was previously called "subclinical hepatic encephalopathy," a term that should be abandoned, as it falsely implies

Table 1
Neurologic and neuropsychiatric abnormalities related to severity of cirrhosis-induced hepatic encephalopathy

	Grade 1	Grade 2	Grade 3	Grade 4
Consciousness	Alert; mild inattention	Blunting	Stuporous but rousable	Coma
Behavior	Reversal of sleep pattern; irritable; depressed	Apathy; lethargy; disinhibition; anxious	Paranoia	—
Affect	Labile	Labile	Blunted	—
Cognition	Impaired visuomotor skills	Delirium	Too impaired to test	—
Neurologic examination	Postural-action tremor, asterixis, multifocal myoclonus;			
	↑Deep tendon reflexes	Frontal release signs (grasp; sucking); gegenhalten; dysarthria; ataxic gait; Parkinsonism	Dilated pupils; nystagmus	Spasticity; clonus extensor plantar responses; decorticate; decerebrate, abnormal eye movements

Data from Lockwood AH. Toxic and metabolic encephalopathies. In: Bradley WG, Daroff RB, Fenichel G, et al, editors. Neurology in clinical practice. Philadelphia: Elsevier; 2004.

a functionally intact nervous system when in fact the clinical features may have implications on fitness to drive or operate heavy machinery. The transition from grades I to IV of HE associated with chronic liver failure is more gradual than in acute liver failure, and can be relapsing-remitting or fluctuating according to intercurrent infection, protein load, gastrointestinal bleeds, constipation, or sedative use, for example.

Imaging

Bilateral excessive deposition of manganese in the globus pallidus can be present in liver disease, and viewed as T1 hyperintensities on magnetic resonance imaging (MRI).[2,3] Beyond supporting a clinical diagnosis of liver disease, these imaging characteristics are of questionable clinical usefulness, as they lack specificity and there is no clear relationship between the MRI characteristics and the clinical severity of HE. In acute HE, computed tomography (CT) imaging is a useful tool in grading cerebral edema.[4]

Neurophysiological Tests

Electroencephalography

The triphasic wave represents the hallmark electroencephalography (EEG) finding in well-developed forms of HE. Milder degrees of HE include a slowing of the dominant posterior rhythm (alpha slowing), with increased presence of theta (>4 but <8 Hz) and delta (4 Hz or less) frequencies. The most severe abnormality consists of delta waves alone, variably associated with epileptiform activity or epochs of suppression. The EEG pattern does not strictly correlate with ammonia levels.[5] Quantification of the various frequency bands is an effective way to classify the severity of encephalopathy.[6]

Evoked potentials

In fulminant hepatic failure, absence of the N70 wave from median nerve somatosensory evoked potentials may be used to differentiate those patients whose clinical outcome is poor and who therefore need a transplant, from those who may respond to medical management.[7] In chronic HE, both somatosensory evoked potentials and brainstem evoked potentials may be objective markers of disease severity. For example, a delay and prolongation of the N20, P25, N35, P45, N65, and P90 waves of the median nerve somatosensory evoked potential correlates with clinical severity.[8] The P300 wave is an event-related brainstem auditory evoked potential and relies on discriminative ability of the brain. In chronic HE there is an increase in the latency of this wave. The P300 is a sensitive test for grade I HE[9] but not for minimal HE.[10]

Pathophysiology

The pathophysiology of HE is not known with certainty. Central to the current theory is raised arterial and brain ammonia.[11] Ammonia is absorbed in the gut, and via portal circulation is delivered to the liver for detoxification. Hepatocellular dysfunction (acute liver failure) or portocaval shunting (chronic liver failure) can increase arterial ammonia. As ammonia passes through the blood-brain barrier it is taken up by astrocytes and metabolized into glutamine, via the adenosine triphosphatase–dependent glutamine synthase. Ammonia may enhance γ-aminobutyric acid (GABA) transmission by at least 3 independent ways. The first is by ammonia-induced enhancement of GABA$_A$ receptor activation. The second involves increasing the availability of GABA at the synaptic cleft. The third involves ammonia-induced expression of astrocytic peripheral-type benzodiazepine receptor (PTBR).[12] Activation of PTBR promotes synthesis and release of the neurosteroids, tetrahydroprogesterone (THP), and tetrahydrodeoxycorticosterone (THDOC), which are agonists of the GABA receptor complex, and in animal models induce clinical and cytopathological characteristics of HE.[13] Other chemical and structural changes that contribute to the clinical presentation of HE include astrocytic cell volume dysregulation, reactive oxygen species generation/oxidative stress, and protein tyrosine nitration of astrocytes.

Treatment

The management of acute and fulminant liver failure is orthotopic liver transplantation when treatment of the underlying disease (eg, infection, drug overdose) or emergency measures to lower intracranial pressure (ICP) (hyperosmolar therapy and hypothermia) prove unsuccessful. Management of the encephalopathy associated with chronic liver failure should target (1) treatment of any intercurrent infection, (2) addressing and reversing any inciting triggers, eg, treating active gastrointestinal bleed or discontinuation of sedative medication, (3) restriction of subsequent dietary protein, and (4) lowering blood ammonia. Dietary protein intake of 1 to 2 g/kg per day is enough to maintain adequate nitrogen balance, while reducing the risk of recurrent HE.[14] The nonabsorbable disaccharide lactulose reduces ammonia production within the gut by (1) acidification of gut lumen thus reducing the uptake of ammonia, (2) increasing uptake of ammonia by gut flora that is subsequently passed in the stool, and (3) catharsis. L-Ornithine-L-aspartate (OA) lowers arterial ammonia with clinical improvement in cognitive test scores in patients with HE.[15] The definitive treatment for advanced, medically refractory encephalopathy from chronic liver failure is orthotopic liver transplantation.[16]

Other Treatments

Flumazenil, an antagonist of the benzodiazepine recognition site located on the GABA$_A$ receptor, has been shown to produce a small clinical improvement possibly by the reversal of action of endogenous benzodiazepine molecules (endozepines), which are thought to have a contributory role in the pathogenesis of HE.[17]

Neomycin and rifaximin are antibiotics that target urease-producing bacteria. Both are considered effective at lowering serum ammonia[18] but are no more effective than lactulose. Rifaximin alone[19] or together with lactulose[20] reduces risk of developing HE and shortens hospitalization due to HE.[20] Branch chain amino acids (BCAA) have been shown to improve minimal HE but have no effect on recurrence of HE.[21] In rare cases, neomycin can cause ototoxicity or nephrotoxicity.

UREMIC ENCEPHALOPATHY

Uremia is caused by excessive accumulation of products of protein metabolism, and loss of intrinsic kidney homeostatic and endocrine function. Uremic encephalopathy is the cerebral manifestation of uremia. It is expected that by the year 2030 upwards of 2 million patients with end-stage renal disease will be having ongoing dialysis treated in the United States,[22] and that Europe will experience a similar growth rate.[23] The prevalence of uremic encephalopathy will therefore follow.

Clinical Manifestations of Acute and Chronic Uremic Encephalopathy

The clinical description of uremic encephalopathy dates to the first century when Araetus, the Cappadocian, noted "...they are very pale, inert, sluggish, without appetite, without digestion...their eyes become dim, dull and rolling, hence many become epileptic; others are swollen, misty, dropsical; and other again are filled with melancholy and paralysis."[24] This definition correlates well with the modern, albeit less literary, description of anorexia, malnutrition, extracellular fluid expansion, encephalopathy and weakness, psychosis, insomnia, myoclonus, and focal and generalized seizures.[25]

Acute uremic encephalopathy is a florid neuropsychiatric illness whose clinical features, like other metabolic encephalopathies, range from subtle executive dysfunction to coma. Accordingly, early signs include reduced attention, impaired construction and writing, executive dysfunction, behavioral changes, and sleep disturbances, which can lead to an agitated delirium and coma. Hyperventilation may be present during periods of metabolic acidosis. Motor findings include generalized weakness, paratonia, mulitfocal myoclonus, action myoclonus, stimulus-sensitive myoclonus, tremor, and asterixis. Myoclonus is more prominent in uremia than in most other metabolic encephalopathies, and often responds to clonazepam. Asterixis is a periodic loss of muscle tone (ie, negative myoclonus), and can be seen as a flapping of the wrists with the arms outstretched and wrists hyperextended. Tetany from abnormal calcium homeostasis can also be seen. Seizures are typically generalized, and occur in the anuric or oligarch phase. Uremic coma, now uncommon, is typically accompanied by Kussmal breathing related to metabolic acidosis.

Chronic uremic encephalopathy is characterized by slowness of thought, headache, apathy, flattening of affect, inattention, and constructional impairment. Sleep disturbances and restless leg syndrome are also common. Diffuse motor findings of tremor, myoclonus, and asterixis may be present. Generalized convulsive seizures can occur in chronic uremic encephalopathy; however, this is typically seen at the very end stage of the disease, and may be accompanied by stupor or coma.[26] With improved treatment strategies, seizures have become less common.

The pathophysiology of uremic encephalopathy involves the accumulation of toxic compounds. No single substance is believed to be the sole cause of the clinical state of uremic encephalopathy. Putative toxins include guanidino compounds,[27] parathyroid hormone, urea, and middle molecules. Other toxins have been considered but none are substantiated.

ENCEPHALOPATHY RELATED TO TREATMENT OF UREMIA
Dialysis Disequilibrium

This encephalopathic state is caused by shifts of water and cerebral edema, and affects patients during or shortly after hemodialysis. Headache, nausea, vomiting, restlessness, myoclonus, disorientation, and somnolence are the classic features,[28] but in severe cases organic psychosis, generalized seizures, stupor, or coma may occur.[29]

Wernicke Encephalopathy

Wernicke encephalopathy is the triad of dementia, ophthalmoplegia, and ataxia, caused by thiamine deficiency. Patients with chronic renal failure are at risk for Wernicke encephalopathy if thiamine replacement is not given during dialysis. In addition, the cachexia, nausea, and vomiting that is present in some patients with chronic uremia may lead to dramatic reduction in oral thiamine intake (such as that seen in hyperemesis gravidarum). Ensuring proper replacement during dialysis and adequate nutritional status is necessary to prevent this debilitating condition.

Electroencephalographic Changes in Uremic Encephalopathy

The most common findings of EEG changes not influenced by dialysis therapy include: (1) poor regulation and slowing of the background rhythm—in this case the alpha rhythm is replaced or mixed with slower 5- to 7-Hz rhythm, and seen in almost all of the patients; (2) paroxysmal, high-voltage, slow (delta) synchronous bursts that are frontally predominant—this is seen in all patients with chronic renal failure and most of those with acute renal failure; (3) paradoxic response to eye opening with accentuation rather than suppression of the background rhythm; and (4) abnormal arousal response characterized by bursts of synchronous bilateral delta waves. Jacob and colleagues[30] and Hughes and Schreeder[31] described a predominantly frontal, low-amplitude theta (3–6 Hz) rhythm in patients with chronic renal failure. Epileptiform activity is less commonly seen. Triphasic waves have been reported in chronic renal failure. Although less common with aggressive dialysis, frontal predominant triphasic waves with a fronto-occipital gradient can be seen in severe azotemia,[32] or decompensated chronic renal failure (ie, sepsis, concomitant dialysis dementia), and is typically associated with reduced levels of consciousness that can range from somnolence to stupor and coma.[28]

POSTERIOR REVERSIBLE LEUKOENCEPHALOPATHY SYNDROME

In its initial description the posterior reversible leukoencephalopathy syndrome (PRLE or PRES), sometimes called reversible posterior leukoencephalopathy (RPL), affected those with hypertension associated with renal disease; preeclampsia, or immune suppressant therapy, and presented as a syndrome of headache, altered mental status (from confusion to stupor), and a variable combination of vomiting, seizures, and changes in visual perception **Box 1**.[33] summarizes the reported clinical features of PRLE. PRLE has now been associated with an ever growing number of medical conditions and exposures (**Box 2**). The lesions of PRLE are not always posterior: more than 80% of patients in one study had frontal involvement.[34] Furthermore, microhemorrhages and infarct are not infrequently seen.[35–37] Finally, cortical gray matter, in

---

Box 1
Common clinical features of PRLE

1. Headache
2. Nausea
3. Vomiting
4. Confusion
5. Lethargy
6. Somnolence
7. Stupor
8. Coma
9. Focal or generalized seizure
10. Visual perceptual changes
    a. blurred vision
    b. hemifield defect
    c. visual neglect
    d. hallucination
    e. cortical blindness
11. Focal weakness (less common)

Box 2
Conditions associated with PRLE

Hypertensive encephalopathy[33,43]

    Renal disease[44]

    Vasculitis

        Systemic lupus erythematosus[41,45]

        Polyarteritis nodosa[46]

        Wegener granulomatosis[47]

    Endocrinopathy

        Pheochromocytoma[48]

        Primary aldosteronism[49]

        Hypoglycemic coma[50]

    Porphyria[51]

    Scorpion venom[52]

    Cocaine, amphetamine use[53]

    Over-the-counter stimulants[54]

Eclampsia[33,55,56]

Thrombotic thrombocytopenic purpura[57]

Hemolytic uremic syndrome[58]

Hypercalcemia[59]

Immunosuppressive drugs

    Cyclosporin A[60,61]

    Tacrolimus[62]

    Vincristine[63]

    Cisplatin[64]

    Cytarabine[65]

    Interferon α[33]

    Combination chemotherapy[66,67]

Other drugs

    Antiretroviral therapy in human immunodeficiency virus–infected patients[68]

    Erythropoietin[69]

    Granulocyte-stimulating factor[70]

    Intravenous immunoglobulin[71,72]

Blood transfusion[73,74]

Contrast media exposure[75]

Ileocecal anastomosis breakdown[76]

Von Hippel-Lindau disease

Data from Lamy C, Oppenheim C, Meder JF, et al. Neuroimaging in posterior reversible encephalopathy syndrome. J Neuroimaging 2004;14:89–96.

Table 2
MRI distribution of vasogenic edema in PRLE in 109 cases: a Mayo experience

Location	Percent of Cases (%)
Parieto-occipital lobes	94
Frontal lobe	88
Temporal lobe	74
Cerebellum	61
Subcortical	99
Deep white matter	46
Basal ganglia	39
Brainstem	31
Cortical	12

Adapted from Fugate JE, Claassen DO, Cloft HJ, et al. Posterior reversible encephalopathy syndrome: associated clinical and radiologic findings. Mayo Clin Proc 2010;85:427–32; with permission.

addition to but often overlying affected white matter, can be involved.[36–39] An extensive review outlining the distribution of MRI clearly demonstrates a posterior predominance (**Table 2**); however, most areas can be affected. The lesions are at times irreversible,[35–37,40] a finding that underscores the observation that persistent deficits have been reported in up to 25% of cases. **Box 3**[34] summarizes the MRI characteristics of PRLE, which reflect the heterogeneity of the lesions. **Fig. 1** illustrates an example of combined vasogenic and cytotoxic edema that can be present in PRLE. In general, therapy is targeted at managing hypertension, withdrawal of the offending agent, and treating the underlying condition. It is interesting that in some cases of systemic lupus erythematosus (SLE), treatment with immunosuppressants is needed for the treatment of PRLE symptoms when return to normotension fails to reverse the clinical signs.[41] This approach gives important context to the role of immunosuppressants: they may be the cause of PRES, but in some case of systemic inflammatory disease they may be required for its treatment.[41,42]

Box 3
Common MRI characteristics in posterior reversible leukoencephalopathy

Parieto-occipital lesions of the subcortical white matter

Cortical lesions associated with subcortical lesions

Bilateral lesions, often symmetric lesions

Often does not follow arterial supply

Occasionally affects frontal and temporal regions

Hyperintense on T2 and fluid-attenuated inversion recovery sequences

Diffusion-weighted imaging lesions can be variably iso-, hypo-, or hyperintense

Apparent diffusion coefficient negativity indicates "irreversibility" and infarction

There can be mixed cytotoxic and vasogenic edema

Adapted from Lamy C, Oppenheim C, Meder JF, et al. Neuroimaging in posterior reversible encephalopathy syndrome. J Neuroimaging 2004;14:89–96; with permission.

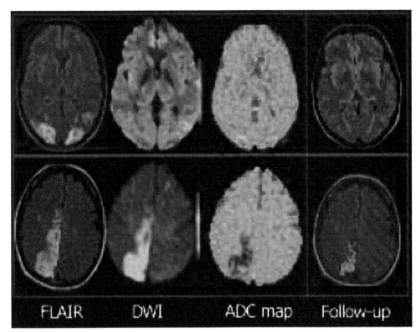

Fig. 1. Predictive value of apparent diffusion coefficient (ADC) in posterior reversible encephalopathy syndrome. (*Top row*) A 32-year-old woman with severe preeclampsia presenting with generalized seizures and cortical blindness. Magnetic resonance imaging (MRI) was performed 1 day after onset. Fluid-attenuated inversion recovery (FLAIR) showed cortical and subcortical hyperintensities with a posterior, bilateral, and symmetric distribution. Diffusion-weighted imaging (DWI) (b = 1000 s/mm^2) showed a slight hyposignal in the posterior areas, and ADC maps demonstrated increased ADC values in areas containing signal changes on FLAIR. This ADC-DWI pattern is consistent with the presence of vasogenic edema. The lesions are reversible, as confirmed by the 2-week follow-up FLAIR. (*Bottom row*) A 30-year-old woman with eclampsia. Three days after onset, she developed a motor deficit of the left lower limb. A striking hyperintense signal was seen posteriorly in the right hemisphere on FLAIR and DWI (b =1000 s/mm^2), with decreased ADC values. This pattern, similar to that of ischemic stroke, suggests the presence of cytotoxic edema. The 3-month follow-up FLAIR confirmed that most of the tissue was irreversibly damaged. (*From* Lamy C, Oppenheim C, Meder JF, et al. Neuroimaging in posterior reversible encephalopathy syndrome. J Neuroimaging 2004;14:89–96; with permission.)

The precise pathophysiology of PRLE is not entirely known; however, the combination of loss of cerebrovascular autoregulation and endothelial damage are thought to be two important factors that lead to vasogenic edema, with or without cytotoxic edema. In patients receiving calcineurin inhibitor immunosuppressive therapy or those with preeclampsia, PRLE may manifest at blood pressures that are not at the extreme ends of the autoregulatory curve. Thus, intrinsic endothelial damage may play a significant role in the development of PRLE. Cytotoxic drugs may exert effects directly on vascular endothelium, resulting in breakdown in the blood-brain barrier followed by vascular leakage and edema.[64] In the case of preeclamspsia, endothelial damage may be in response to circulating trophoblastic cytotoxic factors from the underperfused placenta.[77]

Therapy

For cases of PRLE related to accelerated hypertension, prompt lowering of blood pressure is indicated. Intravenous sodium nitroprusside and/or labetalol or sublingual nifedipine are most commonly used. A loading dose of phenytoin (15–20 mg/kg) or fosphenytoin (same dose in phenytoin equivalents) followed by a maintenance dose for a week is usually sufficient to prevent further seizures, as the disorder is usually self-limited in the uremic, hypertensive patient. In patients with underlying autoimmune disorders, however, treatment with immunosuppressants may be necessary in addition to correcting hypertension.[41,42]

PULMONARY ENCEPHALOPATHY

Pulmonary encephalopathy is an encephalopathic state caused by respiratory insufficiency often from mixed etiology and often complicated by systemic infection or congestive heart failure. Retention of carbon dioxide (CO_2) is the most common cause of pulmonary encephalopathy because its level most closely follows the central nervous system (CNS) disturbance,[78] although isolated hypoxia will also lead to impaired consciousness. Pulmonary encephalopathy is a potentially reversible condition, and correction of the CO_2 and O_2 levels usually results in prompt recovery.

Clinical Presentation

Headache, ataxia, reduced vigilance, inattention, confusion, drowsiness, stupor, and coma are common presenting features. Fundoscopic examination may reveal papilledema and absent spontaneous venous pulsations due to raised ICP. Motor signs include multifocal myoclonus and asterixis. Etiology includes hypercapnea; hypoxemic chronic obstructive pulmonary disease (COPD), carbon monoxide encephalopathy; acute mountain sickness, high-altitude cerebral edema, and nitrogen narcosis.

Etiology of Pulmonary Encephalopathy

Hypoxemic chronic obstructive pulmonary disease

Hypoxemic COPD can cause a chronic but reversible encephalopathic state. Patients with hypoxemic COPD who are treated with continuous oxygen supplementation show improved cognitive and motor learning skills in comparison with a similar group of patients who only have nighttime oxygen supplementation.[79] Neuropsychological studies on patients with hypoxemic COPD also demonstrate impaired verbal attainment, impaired deductive thinking, and inattention. These cognitive deficits were associated with anterior cerebral hypoperfusion on single-photon emission CT (SPECT) imaging. Patients with nonhypoxemic COPD failed to demonstrate similar SPECT findings.[80] Electrophysiologic testing in this population demonstrates prolonged event-related potentials (P300), and may therefore be a useful tool to determine early oxygen therapy for those patients engaged in employment that requires optimal neurocognitive processing.[81]

Hypercapnia

Hypercapnia is defined as arterial blood of CO_2 (PaCO_2) in excess of 60 mm Hg.

The classic article by Austen and colleagues[78] describes the syndrome of headache, altered mental status, and papilledema related to pulmonary insufficiency, and the neurologic manifestations of hypercapnia.

Symptomatic hypercapnia is usually the result of an acute metabolic, pulmonary, or cardiac decompensation in a person with chronic pulmonary disease. Other syndromes of hypoventilation that can result in hypercapnia are listed in **Table 3**. Symptoms are often worse in the morning because of reduced respiratory drive during

Table 3
Hypoventilation syndromes that may cause hypercapnia

Anatomic Site	Clinical Entity
Sensory	Loss of carotid sensitivity
Brainstem	Infarct; demyelination; tumor; sedative use; motor neuron disease; syringobulbia
Motor nerve	Guillain-Barré syndrome; critical illness polyneuropathy
Neuromuscular junction	Myasthenia gravis; Lambert-Eaton myasthenia; botulism
Muscle	Myopathy (congenital, inflammatory, critical illness)
Chest wall	Restrictive lung disease; Chest wall abnormalities; Obesity; Circumferential burns
Alveolus	Alveolar hypoventilation; Chronic obstructive pulmonary disease; Sleep apnea

sleep and periods of hypoxia. The presence of asterixis predicts encephalopathy.[82] Furthermore, the combination of encephalopathy, asterixis, and tremors with arterial hydrogen ion concentration above 54.9 μEq/L (pH 7.2) almost invariably precedes coma. In general, asterixis correlates with the degree of hypercapnia and acidemia. Myoclonus and general tremulousness of the upper limbs are commonly seen. Papilledema from raised ICP is variably present. Seizures are infrequent. The EEG findings in hypercapnia show generalized slowing.

Pathophysiology of hypercapnic encephalopathy
Although extensively studied, it is not clear how acute rises in CO_2 causes encephalopathy, and the pathophysiology is beyond the scope of this review and can be found elsewhere.[83] Hypercapnia may exert its effect on the CNS via cerebrospinal fluid (CSF) acidemia.[84] It is generally felt that the causes of impaired consciousness in hypercapnia are multifactorial, and include compensatory cerebral vasodilation and increased cerebral blood flow in response to CSF acidosis, with associated vascular congestion and increased CSF pressure. CSF acidosis per se may also impair neuronal excitability and neuronal metabolism.[85,86]

Carbon monoxide encephalopathy
Carbon monoxide (CO) can induce both acute and delayed encephalopathy. CO competes with O_2 for the binding sites on hemoglobin with more than 200 times the affinity, and impairs tissue oxygen delivery. Neurologic symptoms occur at 20% to 30% carboxy-hemoglobin (COHb) and include dizziness, confusion, nausea, vomiting, pounding headache, and memory impairment. With increased COHb ataxia, syncope, hallucinations, and depressed consciousness follow, with rapid death occurring at 80% COHb.[87] The pathophysiology of acute CO encephalopathy involves tissue hypoxia, which can cause endothelium and platelet activation from an N-methyl-D-aspartate (NMDA)-mediated generation of nitric oxide and peroxynitrite.[88] Survivors of acute symptomatic CO exposure may experience delayed CO encephalopathy 2 to 3 weeks after initial exposure. Delayed CO encephalopathy is characterized by recurrence of neurologic symptoms such as language dysfunction, parkinsonism, urinary incontinence, and memory loss.[89–91] MRI findings of delayed CO encephalopathy demonstrate bilateral, confluent T2 white matter lesions that have reduced apparent diffusion coefficient (ADC) values, suggesting the presence of delayed cytotoxic edema. The progressive brain damage related to delayed CO encephalopathy

may also be due to an immune-mediated neutrophil activation, lipid peroxidation, breakdown in cerebral vasculature,[92,93] and apoptosis.[94] Although hyperbaric oxygen therapy (HBO) is often given for acute or delayed CO encephalopathy, the benefit of HBO is highly controversial.[95]

HASHIMOTO ENCEPHALOPATHY

Lord Brain described a 40-year-old man with a previous autoimmune thyroiditis who had recurrent alternating hemiplegia, with visual disturbances and confusional states with abnormal EEG, elevated thyroid antibodies, and normal thyroid function, whose clinical and biochemical recovery occurred without intervention.[96] Brain and colleagues[96] stated "The association of the two disorders—the thyroiditis and the brain disease—suggests that antibody studies in other cases of unexplained encephalopathy might prove fruitful." Brain was the first to describe what, regrettably, would be termed Hashimoto encephalopathy.[97] His prediction was found to be accurate when patients with this condition were later shown to have elevated serum antithyroglobulin antibodies.[97] The role of antithyroglobulin antibodies and the CNS disease, however, remains both elusive and a source of ongoing controversy, as up to 30% of healthy individuals can have elevated antithyroglobulin antibodies.[98,99] Patients fulfilling the criteria for Hashimoto encephalopathy have been reported to have elevated CSF levels of antithyroglobulin antibodies, antithyroid peroxidase (antimicrosomal) antibodies, and circulating immune complexes: findings that were unique compared with controls.[100] Therefore such findings may represent an important diagnostic test for Hashimoto encephalopathy.

Reliable epidemiologic data on this condition are lacking. The best estimate on the prevalence of Hashimoto encephalopathy is 2.1 per 100,000.[101] Hashimoto encephalopathy is present in both the adult and pediatric populations.[102]

Clinical Presentation

There are two main presentations of Hashimoto encephalopathy: (1) a "vasculitic type" with multiple strokelike episodes, and (2) a diffuse progressive type with predominantly neuropsychiatric symptoms and dementia.[103] Both forms of Hashimoto encephalopathy can share common features such as myoclonus, seizures, tremor, and fluctuating levels of consciousness. Confusion and acute cognitive decline are the most common features. Impairment of consciousness has been reported in up to 30% of cases.[101] There are several case reports of isolated neurologic or psychiatric features that were felt to be a manifestation of Hashimoto encephalopathy, such as bipolar affective disorder,[104] major depressive episode,[105] schizophrenia-like disorder,[106,107] subacute cerebellar syndrome,[108] and amnesia. It is suggested that in a patient with an otherwise unexplained neurologic condition, the presence of CSF antithyroid antibodies is confirmatory of a diagnosis of Hashimoto encephalopathy.[101] The Ferracci criteria both address the protean nature of the clinical presentation of Hashimoto encephalopathy (**Box 4**), and also account for the potentially nonspecific nature of the presence of elevated serum antithyroid antibody levels. CSF antibody studies have not been routinely adopted by other workers, and tests for CSF antithyroglobulin antibodies are not universally available.

Laboratory Findings

CSF analysis in Hashimoto encephalopathy is bland. There may be a slight lymphocytic pleocytosis, but this is rare. CSF protein is usually elevated.[97] Patients are euthyroid,[97,100,101] or slightly hypothyroid[97,103] with CSF antithyroglobulin and

---

Box 4
Clinical features reported in patients with hashimoto encephalopathy

Cognitive impairment

Confusion

Somnolence

Impaired consciousness

Myoclonus

Focal or generalized seizure

Tremor

Myelopathy

Reversible strokelike episodes

Bipolar affective disorder

Major depressive disorder

Chorea

Nystagmus

Cerebellar syndrome

Reversible amnesia

Schizophrenia-like disorder

---

antithyroperoxidase antibodies, and circulating immune complexes should be elevated.[100,109] CSF IgG index is normal as is the CSF/serum albumin (Qalb)[101]; however, others report elevated CSF IgG levels that correlate with clinical severity in a single case.[110]

EEG Findings

Typical EEG abnormalities seen in this condition include generalized slowing,[111] focal slowing,[112] frontal intermittent rhythmic delta activity (FIRDA),[112] focal sharp waves,[101] triphasic waves[111,112] and epileptiform discharges.[111]

Neuroimaging

The MRI findings in Hashimoto encephalopathy are variable and nonspecific. In one review of the literature, half of the reported cases demonstrate normal cerebral MRI.[103] When present, MRI findings include subcortical white matter and cortical T2 changes, which are reversible on resolution of symptoms.[113] In the largest prospective study the most common finding was a normal MRI, while few had nonspecific white matter changes.[100] Conventional cerebral angiography has failed thus far to demonstrate abnormalities in Hashimoto encephalopathy.[97] Results from SPECT studies have been variable,[114,115] and therefore of questionable utility at present.

Pathophysiology

The encephalopathy does not result directly from thyroid disease. The proposed pathophysiologies of Hashimoto encephalopathy include autoimmune cerebral vasculitis,[116,117] global hypoperfusion,[114,115] brainstem vasculitis,[118] and primary demyelination.[119] No confirmed mechanism has been proved, given the rarity of disease and paucity of neuropathologic data. An immune-mediated process appears most compelling.[100,101,110,120-122]

Treatment

There is no consensus on the treatment of Hashimoto encephalopathy. Steroids are considered first-line therapy[123]; however Ferracci's group failed to demonstrate a relationship between corticosteroid use and clinical benefit. Further work clearly is required to determine the role of steroids and other immunosuppressants in Hashimoto encephalopathy.

ACUTE ADRENAL FAILURE

Adrenal failure is a medical emergency related to a deficiency of adrenal cortical hormones. Failure to identify this condition can lead to coma, cardiovascular collapse, and death. Primary adrenal cortical failure affects both cortisol and aldosterone secretion, whereas secondary adrenal failure affects only cortisol secretion. Cortisol secretion is under the direction of the hypothalamic-pituitary axis whereas aldosterone is regulated by the renal-adrenal axis.

Adrenocorticotropic hormone (ACTH), responsible for cortisol secretion by the adrenals, and its releasing hormone, corticotropin-releasing hormone (CRH), also have brain receptors. Aldosterone has a more limited action: an increase in sodium retention and potassium excretion by the kidney.

Epidemiology

Primary adrenal failure has a prevalence of 4 to 11 cases per 100,000 population.[124] Autoimmune adrenal damage accounts for most cases; some of these are associated with autoimmune polyendocrine syndromes (APSs). Other causes include infections (tuberculosis, fungal infections, cytomegalovirus, and human immunodeficiency virus), metastatic tumors, intra-adrenal hemorrhage (including meningococcemia), adrenoleukodystrophies, and adrenalectomy.

Secondary adrenal failure most commonly results from long-term corticosteroid usage with abrupt withdrawal or inadequate replacement at times of crisis, or less commonly from hypopituitarism of various causes.

Clinical Features

Impaired consciousness ranges from an acute confusional state, either quiet or agitated, to coma. Cognitive changes may sometimes relate to central effects of ACTH, CRF, or to a deficiency of cortisol on brain receptors. Hypotension, hypoglycemia, and the effects of cortisol on other endocrine glands or electrolyte disturbances (hyponatremia, hyperkalemia, hypercalcemia, and dehydration), as a consequence of relative cortisol deficiency, can also cause coma.

Treatment

Emergency therapy should be instituted as soon as the diagnosis of acute adrenal failure is considered. Hydrocortisone (100 mg) should be given intravenously every 6 hours. Hypotension, volume depletion, and hypoglycemia should be corrected. In cases of primary adrenal failure, the addition of a mineralocorticoid, such as fludrocortisone, is sometimes indicated. Investigation and treatment of underlying, reversible precipitants, such as infection, should be undertaken.

Maintenance replacement therapy should be undertaken once the patient is stable. Augmentation of corticosteroids at times of stress is advisable.

ENCEPHALOPATHY DUE TO ELECTROLYTE DISTURBANCES

Disruption of electrolyte balance is invariably secondary to other processes, whether iatrogenic or due to impairment of the organ function that regulates the particular electrolyte homeostasis. This section reviews the common encephalopathy syndrome related to common electrolytes disturbances **Table 4.** summarizes the neurologic features of electrolyte encephalopathy syndromes.

Sodium

Hyponatremia
Epidemiology Hyponatremia is defined as a serum sodium concentration less than 135 mmol/L. It has a 1% incidence and a prevalence of approximately 3% among inpatients within general hospitals.[125] Hyponatremia reflects alterations in the body's water balance, which thus influences plasma osmolality. Hyponatremia can either be of the hypoosmolar or isoosmolar variety. Hypoosmolar hyponatremia is more common, and this group can be further classified according to volume status: isovolemic, hypovolemic, and hypervolemic hyponatremia. Hypoosmolar hyponatremia is caused by a relative excess of solvent to solute.

The most common causes of hyponatremic encephalopathy are related to thiazide diuretic use, or the administration of hypotonic fluids in hospitals, that is, iatrogenic, especially in the postoperative period, and in conditions involving the presence of antidiuretic hormone (ADH) (ie, drugs and syndrome of inappropriate antidiuretic hormone secretion [SIADH]). The use of hypotonic fluid administration in the postoperative state is particularly risky due to SIADH from pain, nausea, and vomiting.[126,127] Symptomatic

Table 4		
Clinical features and laboratory definition of electrolyte encephalopathies		
	Laboratory Values	**Clinical Features**
Symptomatic Hyponatremia	<125 mmol/L	Acute: Headache, nausea, vomiting, seizures, weakness, behavioral changes, coma Chronic: usually asymptomatic (see text)
Hypernatremia	>160 mmol/L	Nausea, lethargy, seizure, coma
Hypocalcemia	<0.5 mmol/L ionized	Cognitive and behavioral changes, disorientation, confusion, cramps, agitated delirium, chorea
Hypercalcemia	>3 mmol/L	Cognitive impairment, personality changes, confusion, somnolence, stupor, coma
Hypophosphatemia	<0.5 mmol/L	GBS-like presentation, myopathy, irritability, confusion, multifocal myoclonus, seizures, coma
Hypomagnesemia	<0.5 mmol/L	Cramps, hyperreflexia, Chvostek sign, seizures, acute neuropsychiatric changes, impaired consciousness, bulbar dysfunction, athetosis, hemiparesis, aphasia
Hypermagnesemia	>2 mmol/L	Severe limb weakness, diaphragm weakness, respiratory compromise, parasympathetic blockade
Hypoglycemia	Variable (see text)	Nervousness, seizure, hemiplegia, coma, impaired cranial nerve function
Hyperglycemia	Variable (see text)	Confusion, lethargy, stupor, coma, hemichorea-hemiballism

acute hyponatremic encephalopathy has been reported following excessive water injection for pelvic ultrasound preparation.[128]

Clinical features Clinical features associated with hyponatremia can be divided into those symptoms caused by hyponatremia per se, and the clinical manifestations of improper treatment of hyponatremia (ie, the osmotic myelinolysis syndrome). Only the former is detailed in this article; however the reader is referred to Angel and colleagues[1] for detailed analysis of the osmotic myelinolysis syndrome.

Acute and chronic hyponatremia Severe hyponatremia per se can lead to severe and permanent brain damage.[126] Clinical symptoms typically occur following an acute drop in serum sodium. From the normonatremic state, symptoms commonly occur when serum levels drop below 125 mmol/L; however, severe symptoms have been reported at levels as high as 128 mmol/L. Symptoms of hyponatremic encephalopathy include headache, behavioral changes, and nausea and vomiting—symptoms similar to those seen in raised ICP. Focal neurologic signs such as monoparesis or hemiparesis, or ataxia have been reported, and may be related to preexisting structural lesions. MRI may show obliteration of the cortical sulci, restricted diffusion over the cortices and subcortical white matter, and pial enhancement.[128] EEG findings are typically nonspecific generalized slowing. Clinical symptoms are reversible with correction of the hyponatremia. Early symptoms may give way in a dramatic fashion to depressed levels of consciousness, seizures, respiratory arrest, coma, decerebrate posturing, and death.[126,129] In rare cases, the clinical symptoms of chronic hyponatremia may be similar to acute hyponatremia,[130] and prompt management of these patients is equally important. If the brain can adequately adapt to an acute hyponatremic stress, however, a relatively well tolerated state of chronic hyponatremia can be achieved, and the arbitrary designation of 48 hours from the onset of alterations in serum sodium concentration denotes chronic hyponatremia. When present, the symptoms attributable to chronic hyponatremia are more subtle and may include dizziness, confusion, and lethargy. Evidence of permanent brain damage from long-standing, chronic hyponatremia is lacking.[130] In addition, animal studies have failed to demonstrate histologic changes in long-standing, severe chronic hyponatremia.[131,132]

Pathophysiology of hyponatremic encephalopathy The encephalopathic features are attributable to the combined effects of hypoosmolar stresses and cerebral edema. In the presence of a hypoosmolar extracellular milieu, osmotic forces tend to drive water into the intracellular space. The brain, however, quickly responds by rapidly extruding first electrolytes (Na^+, K^+, and Cl^-), then organic osmolytes (glutamate, aspartate, glutamine, polyhydric alcohol, myoinositol, methylamine, taurine, and creatine) in a process known as regulatory volume decrease (RVD).[133,134] Together, movement of electrolytes and organic osmolytes work to reduce the shift of water into the intracellular space, and thus prevent cerebral edema.

If the hypoosmolar stress is severe and precipitous, the adaptive mechanisms may be overwhelmed and cerebral edema may follow. The symptoms and signs of headache, coma, decerebrate posturing, and respiratory failure may be satisfactorily explained by raised ICP, herniation, and coning. However, subtle impairment of consciousness, lethargy, inattention, and seizure may indicate alterations in cerebral function due to neuronal swelling per se.

Treatment of hyponatremic encephalopathy Recently a novel unified treatment for hyponatremic encephalopathy has been proposed, which involves a bolus of 2 mL/kg of 3% saline (maximum 100 mL), repeated until clinical improvement.[135] It is argued that this method rapidly corrects hyponatremia without risk of overtreatment, and is better controlled than continuous infusion. However, this approach has yet to be generally adopted.[129] A rational approach to treatment of hyponatremia is summarized in **Table 5**. The controversy surrounding the issue of treatment of hyponatremic encephalopathy arises from the sequelae of underly and overly aggressive correction of serum sodium. Correcting the serum sodium too slowly in patients with hyponatremic encephalopathy may prolong periods of cerebral edema and increase the risk of permanent brain damage.[131] Overly aggressive treatment, however, is a risk factor for osmotic demyelination syndrome (ODS). The literature is rife with conflicting reports on appropriate treatment strategies. Suggested approaches to initial treatment of various hyponatremic states are summarized in **Table 5**.

Chronic hyponatremic encephalopathy with permanent brain damage has been reported in a population of postmenopausal women.[130] This finding was important, as it showed that not all chronic hyponatremia is always well tolerated. Whether some of these patients had acute-on-chronic changes in their serum sodium is not known and remains an important caveat. Nevertheless, aggressive therapy in such patients is necessary to prevent permanent brain damage. It should be recognized that such chronically hyponatremic patients maybe encephalopathic not from the hyponatremia but from an associated, related disorder (eg, hypothyroidism, drug accumulation) or some intercurrent illness (eg, infection).

Alternative treatments for hyponatremic encephalopathy Urea is an effective treatment for symptomatic hyponatremia, inducing a sodium-retentive diuresis that reduces cerebral edema and raises serum sodium.[136] Another beneficial property of urea is its ability to raise intracellular osmolytes, which may be protective against ODS.[137] The rate of sodium change should remain 10 to 15 mEq/L per day. Vasopressin-2 antagonists have been introduced for treatment of hyponatremic

Table 5 Treatment of hyponatremia	
Acute symptomatic hyponatremia	Manage in ICU setting; Foley catheterization; infusion of 3% NaCl (0.514 mEq/mL) hypertonic saline to increase serum sodium at a rate of 1–2 mmol/L per hour; Target clinical improvement, not normonatremia, at which point 3% NaCl is stopped
Acute-on-chronic hyponatremia with encephalopathy	3% NaCl administered at a rate that results in a serum sodium change of 10–15 mEq/24 h. A rate of 10 mEq/24 h should not be exceeded in the presence of concomitant hypokalemia, liver disease, alcoholism, or malnutrition. Follow serum Na every 4 h. In the presence of brisk diuresis and rapid increase in serum sodium, desmopressin acetate and hypotonic saline should be administered over a 2-h period[129] to reduce serum sodium
Chronic symptomatic hyponatremia	NaCl 3%, at 1–2 mL/kg body weight/h for 4–5 h according to Arieff's group. Therapy should be stopped with symptom improvement
Chronic asymptomatic hyponatremia	These patients are considered clinically stable and rapid correction is not necessary

encephalopathy. Caution is advised when using these drugs because they can cause a brisk diuresis and rapid changes in serum sodium.[136,138] Vasopressin antagonists may be useful in patients with extracellular fluid overload (eg, cirrhosis, water intoxication, severe pulmonary edema).

Hypernatremic encephalopathy

Hypernatremia is defined as serum sodium greater than 145 mEq/L. Symptomatic hypernatremia is almost universal at serum levels greater than 160 mEq, above which 89% have hypernatremic encephalopathy.[139] The clinical picture of hypernatremic encephalopathy includes nausea, lethargy, seizures, and coma.[140] The two populations at highest risk for hypernatremic encephalopathy are the very young and very old. Gastrointestinal illness with vomiting and diarrhea coupled with a child's lack of access to water, or blunting of thirst in the elderly, increases this risk of developing hypernatremia.[141] Any situation whereby ADH secretion is impaired or the thirst response to ADH is impaired renders a patient at risk for hypernatremia (hypothalamic dysfunction from stroke, hemorrhage, tumor, and so forth). Excess salt intake can affect all ages, and this has been reported in the context of saltwater emetics[142–144] and pica syndrome.[145] Overly concentrated baby formula (incorrect preparation of powdered meal) can result in hypernatremia in babies. Hypernatremia may occur in response to subdural hemorrhages from nonaccidental head injury in the young.[146] Hypernatremic encephalopathy has also been reported to occur spontaneously in the postpartum state.[147] The mortality of hypernatremia can be as high as 20%, with severe brain damage in 33% of the pediatric population.[148]

Pathophysiology of hypernatremic encephalopathy In response to a hyperosmolar stress, water is driven out of neurons and glia. Reduction of whole brain volume occurs, due predominantly to oligodendroglia shrinkage.[149] Physical forces of volume loss can tear cortical bridging veins resulting in subdural hematoma, subarachnoid hemorrhage, intracranial hemorrhage,[150] and petechial hemorrhage.[109,151] Sinovenous thrombosis can also be seen. Case reports have shown several interesting imaging findings including isolated, transient cytotoxic edema of the thalamus,[152] diffuse cerebral edema,[153] and osmotic myelinolysis.[147,154]

Treatment of hypernatremic encephalopathy Reducing serum sodium at a rate of less than 0.5 mmol/L per hour is thus recommended.[155] Over-rapid correction of hypernatremia can lead to cerebral edema, seizures, and permanent brain damage.

Calcium

Extracellular calcium is held within a tight physiologic range by the interactions of parathyroid hormone (PTH), vitamin D, calcitonin, magnesium, phosphate, and calcium. A full description of calcium homeostasis is beyond the scope of this article. Calcium circulates in either a bound or ionized form. The ionized fraction exerts the biological action of calcium. The neurologic manifestations of abnormal calcium homeostasis depend on the severity and the rapidity of progression of the calcium imbalance. Calcium can have profound influences on neuronal processes, including alterations in membrane excitability and permeability, synaptic transmission, activation of second-messenger systems, organelle function, and glial-neuronal interactions (ie, the tripartite synapse).

Hypocalcemia

The common causes of hypocalcemia evoke their effects by inhibiting the PTH-vitamin D axis, by inducing redistribution of calcium, or by inhibiting the effects of calcium. **Table 6** summarizes common causes and mechanisms of hypocalcemia.

Table 6
Causes of hypocalcemia

Hypoparathyroidism	Postsurgical	↓PTH secretion
	Autoimmune disease	↓PTH secretion
	Infiltrative disease	↓PTH secretion
	Irradiation	↓PTH secretion
	Severe hypomagnesemia	Inhibition of PTH secretion
Pseudohypoparathyroidism	Albright syndrome	Insensitivity to PTH
Vitamin D deficiency	Insufficient intake	↓Formation of 25 or
	Hydroxy liver disease	1,25-Vitamin D
Redistribution of calcium	Acute pancreatitis	Sequestration of ionized calcium
	Rhabdomyolysis	In an acute situation (PTH not able to compensate)
	Tumor lysis syndrome	
	Phosphate infusion	
	Toxic shock syndrome	
	Critical illness	
	Alkalosis	
↑Osteoblastic activity	Hungry bone disease	Postparathyroidectomy
	Osteoblastic metastases cancer	Prostate or breast
Drugs		
Anticalcemic	Bisphosphonates	
	Plicamycin	
	Calcitonin	
	Gallium nitrate	
	Phosphate	
Antineoplastic	Asparaginase	
	Doxorubicin	
	ARA C	
	WR2721	
	Cisplatin	
Others	Ketoconazole	
	Pentamidine	
	Foscarnet	

Adapted from Young GB, DeRubeis R. Metabolic encephalopathies. In: Young GB, Ropper AH, Bolton CF, editors. Coma and impaired consciousness: a clinical perspective: McGraw-Hill; 1998. p. 307–92; with permission.

Laboratory findings Total serum calcium is made up of protein-bound, free ionized, and complex calcium. The range of normal total serum calcium is 2.12 to 2.62 mmol/L (8.5–10.5 mg/dL). Calcium concentration varies with serum albumin. For every 1g/L drop in albumin, there is a 0.02 mmol/L (0.8 mg/dL) decrease in calcium. Or:

Corrected [Ca] = measured [Ca] + {(40 − [albumin]) × 0.02}.

This is an estimate, and may vary during conditions whereby protein binding is affected, for example, sepsis, rhabdomyolysis, and cirrhosis. It is thus important to measure serum ionized calcium, as this is the physiologically relevant fraction of total serum calcium.

Symptomatic hypocalcemia is typically present when serum ionized calcium falls to less than 0.5 mmol/L (2 mg/dL; normal range1.02–1.27 mmol/L, or 4.1–5.1 mg/dL) or the total calcium drops below 1.8 to 1.875 mmol/L (7.0–7.5 mg/dL).

Clinical presentation Symptoms of hypocalcemic encephalopathy include cognitive and behavioral changes, disorientation, confusion, hypomania, an agitated delirium, and chorea.[156,157] In severe cases, obtundation and coma may result. Headache with papilledema can result from raised ICP.[158] Seizures may occur and may be focal, generalized, convulsive, or nonconvulsive. EEG findings are likewise variable with paroxysmal slowing, slowing of background rhythms, and focal and generalized spikes.[159,160] Generalized tonic-clonic seizures have been reported in association with kinesogenic paroxysmal dyskinesia in a patient with pseudohypoparathyroidsim.[161] A hypocalcemia-induced reversible encephalopathy and diffuse cerebral edema has likewise been reported in a patient with pseudohypoparathyroidism.[162] Neuromuscular irritability, presenting with hyperreflexia, Chvostek and Trousseau signs, and tetany are peripheral hallmarks of symptomatic hypocalcemia. Laryngeal stridor and spasm may compromise the airway.

Management of hypocalcemia Symptomatic hypocalcemia must be treated, and the presence of seizure or encephalopathy may necessitate intensive care monitoring and airway control. Specific treatment addressing the etiology of the hypocalcemia or other exacerbating factors is likewise important. For example, the concomitant treatment of hypomagnesemia will remove the hypomagnesemia-induced inhibition of PTH secretion.[163] Initial therapy for 10 to 20 mL of 10% intravenous calcium gluconate (contains 93 mg of elemental calcium) should be administered over 10 minutes, to avoid cardiac conduction abnormalities. Patients taking digoxin should be closely monitored during intravenous calcium replacement for digitalis toxicity.[164] Continuous infusion of 15 mg/kg will raise the serum calcium by 2 to 3 mg/dL. The aim of acute treatment is to reverse or improve the symptoms of hypocalcemia and not to target normocalcemia.[165] In the presence of hypophosphatemia, calcium supplementation should be delayed until serum phosphate is reduced to less than 1.5 mmol/L[164] to prevent soft-tissue calcium phosphate precipitations. Oral supplementation of 1 to 2.6 g daily may be sufficient in the presence of chronic stable hypocalcemia.

Hypercalcemia
Hypercalcemia is defined as total serum calcium levels greater than 2.63 mmol/L; however, symptomatic hypercalcemia typically occurs at a serum level of 3 mmol/L (12 mg/dL). Early neuropsychiatric symptoms tend to occur at serum levels above 3.0 mmol/L, and severe CNS dysfunction is seen at serum levels above 4 mmol/L (16 mg/dL).

Epidemiology Hypercalcemia is seen in about 5% of patients with cancer, and in 10% to 20% of patients with solid tumors.[166] The most common malignancies associated with hypercalcemia are multiple myeloma, and breast, lung, kidney, head, and neck cancers. Malignant neoplasms and hyperparathyroidism account for approximately 70% to 80% of cases of hypercalcemia.[167,168] Hypercalcemia has a prevalence of 0.5% of hospitalized patients.[169] A list of causes of hypercalcemia is presented in **Box 5**.

Clinical features Early neuropsychiatric symptoms include cognitive impairment, mental slowing, and personality changes. Posterior reversible leukoencephalopathy is not uncommon. Frank encephalopathy characterized by confusion, somnolence, stupor, and coma is typically reserved for those with severe hypercalcemia and usually with associated malignancy.[170]

Management Management of hypercalcemic encephalopathy involves determining and treating the underlying cause of hypercalcemia; aggressive administration of intravenous isotonic saline (these patients are almost uniformly in a state of severe

---

Box 5
Causes of hypercalcemia

1. Altered bone-extracellular fluid homeostasis

   a. Metastatic tumor

   b. Multiple myeloma

   c. Lymphoma

   d. Hyperthyroidism

   e. Immobilization

   f. Paget disease

2. Excessive parathyroid hormone or parathyroid hormone–related protein

   a. Primary hyperparathyroidism

   b. Lithium

   c. Familial hypocalciuric hypercalcemia

   d. Paraneoplastic secretion of parathyroid hormone, eg, breast, lung, renal cancer

3. Excessive vitamin D

   a. Hypervitaminosis

   b. Sarcoidosis

   c. Idiopathic hypercalcemia of childhood

4. Other

   a. Adrenal insufficiency

   b. Thiazide diuretics

   c. Milk-alkali syndrome

   d. Hypervitaminosis A

Adapted from Young GB, DeRubeis R. Metabolic encephalopathies. In: Young GB, Ropper AH, Bolton CF, editors. Coma and impaired consciousness: a clinical perspective. New York: McGraw-Hill; 1998. p. 307–92; with permission.

---

extracellular volume contraction and may require 1 to 3 L of isotonic saline)[166] and administration of drugs that modulate calcium homeostasis should be instituted. Dialysis may be required in the presence of severe renal or congestive heart failure. Bisphosphonates will inhibit osteoclastic activity and inhibit renal calcium reabsorption, and are the mainstay of treatment of recurrent hypercalcemia in malignancy.[166] A single dose of intravenous pamidronate, 90 mg over 2 to 24 hours, is an acceptable regimen and normalizes serum calcium within 2 days in 70% to 90% of patients.[171] Zolendronate, 4 mg or 8 mg single intravenous dose on a monthly basis, has shown very good results for refractory hypercalcemia.[172] Calcitonin, often used in conjunction with bisphosphonates, exerts its effects by inhibiting bone resorption and increasing renal excretion of calcium, and a regimen of 8 IU/kg every 6 hours for 5 days will achieve normocalcemia in a third of patients, and will last for 1 to 2 days.[166]

Magnesium

Hypomagnesemia

Hypomagnesemia is defined as a serum magnesium concentration less than 0.8 mmol/L (2.0 mg/dL). Neurologic complications related to hypomagnesemia, however, typically manifest at concentrations less than 0.5 mmol/L (1.2 mg/dL). Because more than 90% of total body magnesium resides in the intracellular compartment, serum magnesium levels fail to accurately reflect total body magnesium deficiency. Accordingly, a drop in serum magnesium may represent a profound total body magnesium deficit. Similarly, reduced total body magnesium may be present with normal serum concentrations. CSF magnesium tends to be higher than that of serum, due to its active secretion by the choroid plexus.

Hypomagnesemia affects 4% to 47% of hospitalized patients,[173–175] with those suffering from critical illness at highest risk. Populations most at risk for hypomagnesemia either lack adequate intake, or have excessive loss of magnesium through the kidney. Such conditions include protein-calorie malnutrition, malabsorption, diabetic ketoacidosis, sepsis, diuretic use, alcohol abuse, hyperaldosteronism, and hypocalcemia.[176] Drugs known to cause hypomagnesemia include loop diuretics, aminoglycosides, cisplatin,[177] cyclosporin A,[178] amphoteracin,[179] tacrolimius,[180] cetuximab,[181] and proton pump inhibitors.[182]

There are probably numerous ways in which reduced serum magnesium leads to altered CNS function and encephalopathy; however, the precise mechanism is not known.

The hypomagnesium-induced inhibition of PTH may induce hypocalcemia, therefore some of the clinical features of hypomagnesemia may in part be attributed to alterations in calcium homeostasis.

The clinical findings of hypomagnesemia are similar to hypocalcemia. Peripheral manifestations include muscle cramps, hyperreflexia, and Chvostek sign. CNS symptoms include seizures, acute neuropsychiatric changes, and impaired consciousness. Focal neurologic features include bulbar dysfunction (vertigo, dysphagia), athetosis, downbeat nystagmus, hemiparesis, and aphasia.[183–185] Although clinically worrisome, these features are potentially reversible. For severe hypomagnesemia (ie, with frank neurologic sequelae), parenteral magnesium sulfate (50% solution) should be given in divided doses, totaling 8 to 12 g of magnesium sulfate. Potassium replacement should be instituted when necessary, as hypokalemia is often coincident. Ongoing magnesium supplementation in parenteral nutrition is important, especially in the intensive care unit.

Hypermagnesemia

Hypermagnesemia is defined as serum magnesium levels greater than 1.05 mmol/L (2.4 mg/dL); however, clinical symptoms are usually manifest at serum concentrations above 2 to 3.5 mmol/L (5–8 mg/dL). Hypermagnesemia is considered to be a highly underrecognized condition.[175]

Symptomatic hypermagnesemia is rare in the absence of renal failure. Typically it occurs in the context of excessive administration of magnesium-containing compounds (laxatives, cathartics, antihypertensives) in patients with impaired renal excretion. Cases of severe hypermagnesemia from Epsom salts have been reported in healthy individuals.[186] Magnesium is known to inhibit neuromuscular transmission and cause parasympathetic blockade, resulting in a clinical picture of "pseudocoma."[187] How elevated serum magnesium leads to altered levels of consciousness is less clear, but contributing factors would include diaphragm weakness and hypercarbic encephalopathy. Calcium antagonizes the effects of magnesium, thus 10 mL of a 10% solution can be given repeatedly to reverse the neuromuscular blockade. Enhancement of renal excretion using loop diuretics is reasonable as well; however, some patients may require hemodialysis to remove excess magnesium.

Phosphate

Hypophosphatemia

Hypophosphatemia is defined as serum phosphate concentrations less than 2.5 mg/dL (0.83 mmol/L). Hypophosphatemic encephalopathy, however, is typically seen under conditions of severe hypophosphatemia, that is, serum concentrations less than 1.5 mg/dL (0.5 mmol/L).[188] The reported incidence of hypophosphatemia ranges from 0.2%[189] to 2.2%[190] among hospitalized patients. The incidence has been reported to be 30.4%[191] in alcoholics admitted to hospital, and in critically ill patients the prevalence has been reported as high as 80%.[192] Hypophosphatemia results from conditions that alter intestinal absorption, renal reabsorption, and distribution between extra intracellular stores, or a combination thereof. The "refeeding syndrome" is one of the main causes of acute symptomatic hypophosphatemia. The most common mechanism of hypophosphatemia is intracellular redistribution (**Box 6**), and this usually occurs in patients with multiple risk factors. For example, in the critically ill patient with sepsis mechanical ventilation, metabolic acidosis, volume expansion, and elevated catecholamines would all lower serum phosphate. Similarly in the chronic alcoholic, poor nutritional status and vitamin D deficiency would influence intracellular shifts and urinary excretion.[188,193]

Clinical manifestation of hypophosphatemia Neurologic manifestations occur only when hypophosphatemia is severe, and all levels of the nervous system can be affected. Hypophosphatemic encephalopathy can present as irritability, confusion,

---

Box 6
Causes of hypophosphatemia

Intracellular Redistribution

    Refeeding syndrome (chronic alcoholics, anorexia nervosa)

    Treatment of diabetic ketoacidosis

    Severe respiratory alkalosis (eg, sepsis, anxiety, alcohol withdrawal, hepatic coma)

    Glucose infusions

    Mechanical ventilation

Increased Urinary Excretion

    Hyperparathyroidism

    Vitamin D deficiency

    Renal tubular defects

    Volume expansion

    Metabolic acidosis

    Renal transplant

Decreased Intestinal Absorption

    Severe malnutrition

    Vitamin D deficiency

    Steatorrhea

    Vomiting, diarrhea

    Phosphate-binding antacids

multifocal myoclonus, seizures, and coma.[188,194–196] Muscle weakness from a Guillain-Barré–like syndrome and myopathy are well documented.[188] Severe weakness from profound myopathy has been reported to involve the diaphragm, causing encephalopathy at least in part due to respiratory insufficiency.[197–199] These features can be reversed with appropriate phosphate replacement (see later discussion). Central pontine myelinolysis has been reported in association with severe hypophosphatemia in the absence of overcorrection of hyponatremia.[200,201] Wernicke encephalopathy has been reported in association with severe hypophosphatemia, and this is of particular importance when standard therapy for Wernicke encephalopathy fails to improve the symptoms of what is almost universally considered a thiamine-deficient state.[202]

Treatment of hypophosphatemia Milk should be given by mouth or via gastric tube as a source of phosphate supplement. Intravenous administration of 9 mmol phosphorus in 77 mM NaCl over 12 hours provides 4 mg/kg body weight, and is also an appropriate therapy. Magnesium supplementation is indicated to prevent phosphate loss in the urine.[203]

Glucose

Hypoglycemia

The brain is dependent on glucose for its energy source. There is regional variability in both the brain's energy demand and the efficiency of glucose usage. Thus areas of higher cortical function (ie, neocortex) have higher metabolic demands and thus display increased glucose use and increased vulnerability to hypoglycemia, as opposed to the cerebellar cortex, which has both a reduced demand and a more efficient glucose transport system.[204,205]

Definition Hypoglycemia is defined as serum glucose concentration less than 2.5 mmol/L (40 mg/dL). Severe hypoglycemia is defined as the clinical state of hypoglycemia whereby the degree of impairment precludes self-treatment with food or medication, and assistance is required for management. In patients with diabetes who have consistently high basal serum glucose, the neuroglycopenic symptoms can occur at normal, or even slightly high levels. Likewise, patients with very tight glucose control often develop symptoms at lower serum glucose concentrations.[206]

Hypoglycemia is broadly classified into postprandial and fasting according to its etiology (**Box 7**). Most cases of severe hypoglycemia involve patients with either type 1 or type 2 diabetics on insulin therapy[207] or type 2 diabetics on sulfonylurea therapy.[208] In type 1 diabetes, severe hypoglycemia is common and potentially catastrophic, affecting approximately one-third of patients at least once per year. It is estimated that severe hypoglycemia is the cause of death in 2% to 4% of persons with type 1 diabetes.[209]

In the diabetic population, risk factors for severe hypoglycemia include: length of time from diagnosis of type 1 diabetes; previous episodes of severe hypoglycemia; loss of awareness of hypoglycemic symptoms (ie, impaired counterregulatory hormone function); reduced C-peptide levels (ie, well established insulin-requiring type 2 diabetes); and a history of low hemoglobin A_{1c}.[210]

Pathogenesis and pathology Neuroglycopenic symptoms are related to activation of the counterregulatory hormones, especially the catecholamine response. Severe symptomatic hypoglycemia occurs when counterregulatory mechanisms are overwhelmed, which can be due to an excessive insulin effect, diffuse hepatic dysfunction, or limited substrate for gluconeogensis.[206] Uncorrected severe hypoglycemia results

---

Box 7
Causes of hypoglycemia

Postprandial

Glucose-induced

Fructose-, galactose-, leucine-induced

Fasting Hypoglycemia

Hepatic disease

Excess endogenous insulin (insulinoma)

Exogenous insulin

Deficiency of growth hormone

Renal failure

Sepsis

Alcoholism

Drugs

Malnutrition

Heart failure

Tumors that secrete insulin-like growth factor (IGF-1)

Sarcoma

Mesothelioma

Hepatoma

Adapted from Young GB, DeRubeis R. Metabolic encephalopathies. In: Young GB, Ropper AH, Bolton CF, editors. Coma and impaired consciousness: a clinical perspective. New York: McGraw-Hill; 1998. p. 307–92; with permission.

---

in progressive impairment of consciousness, cerebral isoelectricity, and irreversible brain damage termed "selective necrosis."[211] Areas of the brain particularly suscep-tible to hypoglycemic brain damage include the medial subiculum, the crest of the dentate gyrus and dentate granule cells of the hippocampus, the superficial neocor-tical layers of the cerebral cortex, and the basal ganglia.[211–214]

EEG predicts reversible and irreversible cerebral dysfunction in hypoglycemia. Clin-ical somnolence correlates with the appearance of theta and coarse delta waves. Dominant delta waves correlate with stupor. With increased theta and delta activity, changes in cerebral monoamine (serotonin, noradrenaline, dopamine) occur.[215] Plasma membrane ion-channel functions become impaired,[216] and alterations in neuronal excitability contribute to the clinical picture of encephalopathy. With the onset of cerebral isoelectricity, the patient is invariably comatose. If uncorrected, selective neuronal necrosis and permanent brain damage will occur after 30 minutes of isoelectricity.[214] Diffusion-weighted sequences on MRI have revealed both symmetric and asymmetric focal cytotoxic edema in hypoglycemic coma that is potentially reversible if the patient is treated within a certain critical period.[50,217,218]

Imaging findings MR imaging in severe hypoglycemia has revealed signal changes involving cortical and subcortical structures, which may be reversible. Focal MRI abnormalities can be symmetric or asymmetric, and do not follow vascular boundaries (**Figs. 2** and **3**).

A

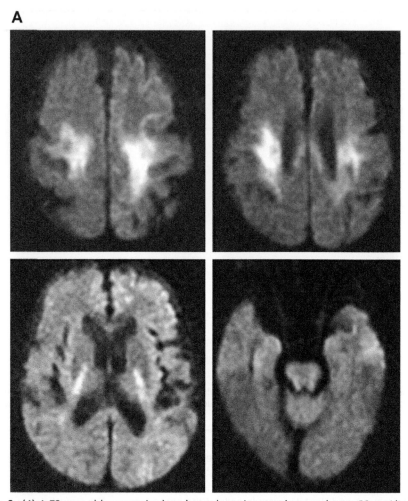

Fig. 2. (*A*) A 73-year-old woman in deep hypoglycemic coma (serum glucose 20 mg/dL; 0.5 mmol/L) with rolling eye movements, tetraparesis, and decerebrate rigidity to pain. Diffusion-weighted MRI shows hyperintense lesions within the bilateral internal capsule, corona radiata, and frontoparietal cortex. Note that bilateral hippocampi do not disclose any hyperintensity lesions. (*B*) Diffusion-weighted MRI 10 days after glucose infusion showing regression of the hyperintensity lesions. The patient had complete neurologic recovery. (*From* Aoki T, Sato T, Hesegawa K, et al. Reversible hyperintensity lesion on diffusion-weighted MRI in hypoglycemic coma. Neurology 2004;63:392–3; with permission.)

Table 7 compares the published case reports of diffusion-weighted imaging (DWI) and ADC findings in severe hypoglycemia. Of interest, clinically relevant permanent brain damage was present in all (3/3) cases in which DWI/ADC changes were present in the basal ganglia. This observation is in keeping with the T1-weighted and T2-weighted MR changes described in a small group of patients with irreversible hypoglycemic brain damage.[219] Thus DWI findings may offer important prognostic information. The lack of thalamic and cerebellar changes seen on MRI from severe hypoglycemia likely correlates with the thalamic and cerebellar "resistance" to

B

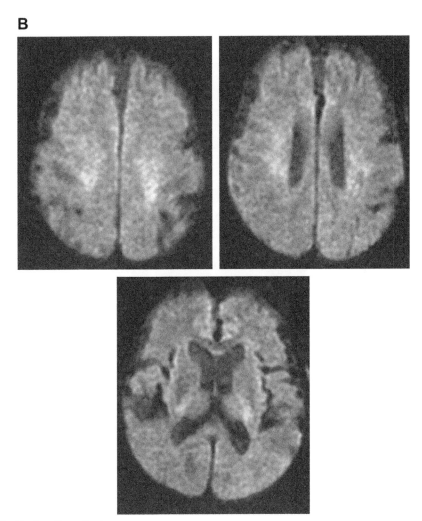

Fig. 2. (continued)

hypoglycemia. Such findings are in contrast to what is seen following hypoxic-ischemic insults.

Clinical presentation Serious CNS dysfunction is preceded by the well-known neuro-glycopenic symptoms of cold perspiration, tachycardia, lightheadedness, headache, and mild agitation. Initial dysfunction of higher cognitive processes can give way to more overt confusion, lethargy, and stupor. Seizures, often generalized, are common in severe hypoglycemia, and may contribute to further impairment of consciousness both from ictal and postictal-induced cerebral dysfunction, as well as cerebral edema, hypoxia, and excitotoxicity, especially in the presence of status epilepticus. Focal neurologic deficits in hypoglycemia can mimic stroke syndromes such as pure hemiplegia[218,220] and middle cerebral artery stroke.[221] Cranial nerve function can be abolished in profound hypoglycemia. Hypoglycemia is an important differential in a patient presenting with focal weakness, or impaired consciousness with brainstem deficits.[50]

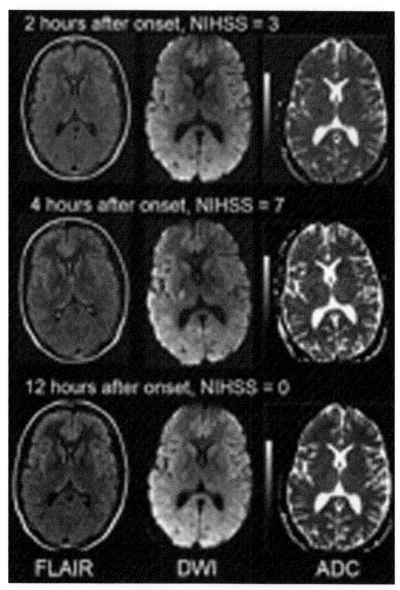

Fig. 3. A 24-year-old woman with sudden-onset left hemiparesis from hypoglycemia resulting from insulinoma (glucose level of 2.2 mmol/L; 85.8 mg/dL). Two hours after onset, the FLAIR image was normal whereas DWI showed a unilateral hypersignal in the right internal capsule with decreased ADC values (20% decreased). Four hours after onset, a slight signal increase was seen on FLAIR images with a clear-cut signal increase on DWI. Twelve hours after onset and treatment of hypoglycemia, the clinical symptoms had resolved and the MRI returned to normal. (*From* Cordonnier C, Oppenheim C, Lamy C, et al. Serial diffusion and perfusion-weighted MR in transient hypoglycemia. Neurology 2005;65:175; with permission.)

Table 7
Clinicoradiological correlation in hypoglycemic coma: summary of literature

Study	Symptoms	Hypoxia?	Imaging	Location	Reversible?	Outcome
255	Coma	No	T2 hyperintensities	Bilateral hippocampus	No	Seizure, amnesia
256	Stupor	Not reported	DWI+/ADC−	Bilateral basal ganglia; hippocampus; temporal cortex	Not repeated	Death
217	Hemiparesis	No	DWI+/ADC−	Bilateral corona radiata; splenium corpus callosum	Yes	Recovery
50	Coma, decerebrate	No	DWI+/ADC−	Bilateral corona radiata; internal capsule; frontoparietal cortex	Yes	Recovery
257	Encephalopathy; seizure	No	DWI+/ADC−	Bilateral (L>R) temporal/occipital lobes; frontoparietal cortex	No	Worsening seizure; death
258	Coma, decorticate	No	DWI+/ADC−	Bilateral occipital, hippocampi	Yes, after 14 days	Responds to commands
218	Hemiparesis	No	DWI+/ADC−	Right internal capsule	Yes	Recovery
259	Coma, decerebrate	Yes	ADC−/SPECT	Entire hemisphere; basal ganglia. Global hypoperfusion sparing basal ganglia	No (laminar necrosis along cortical rim, day 21)	Death
260	Coma	No	DWI+/ADC−	Left frontal; bilateral parieto-occipital; posterior temporal cortices; insular cortex; bilateral basal ganglia	No	Persistent coma
219	Coma; hemiplegia	No	DWI+	Pons	Yes	Recovery
261	Encephalopathy	No	DWI+	Entire cortex, sparing bilateral dorsal frontal cortex and occipital poles	Not reported	—
262 (case series 11 patients)	Encephalopathy; coma	No	DWI+/ADC−	Bilateral 10/11; Centrum semiovale 9/11; Corona radiata 7/11; int. capsule 6/11; corpus callosum 0/11; frontal lobe 7/11; parietal lob 4/11; temporal lobe 1/1; occipital lobe 2/11; insular cortex 1/11; basal ganglia 1/11; hippocampus 4/11	6/11 reversible 5/11 irreversible	7/11 recovery; 1/11 partial recovery; 2/11 death; 1/11 persistent deficits

Abbreviations: ADC−, reduced apparent diffusion coefficient; DWI +, bright signal on diffusion-weighted MRI; SPECT, single-photon emission computed tomography.
Adapted from Angel MJ, Chen R, Bryan YG. Metabolic encephalopathies. Handb Clin Neurol 2008;90:115–66; with permission.

Hypoglycemia-induced movement disorders including chorea and athetosis have been described.[222] At its most extreme, severe hypoglycemia can present as coma with decerebration or decortication. This advanced state may be reversible[50] and behooves serum glucose levels to be measured in such patients prior to other time-consuming investigations.

Treatment of hypoglycemia Severe hypoglycemia requires aggressive and sustained therapy and monitoring, particularly in sulfonylurea overdose. Bolus intravenous administration of 50 mL of 50% glucose solution followed by ongoing 5% intravenous glucose maintenance to target euglycemia is the standard therapy for acute management of severe hypoglycemia. Insulin overdose may require 30% glucose solution as intravenous maintenance. Serum glucose should be monitored every half hour, and maintenance intravenous glucose should continue until the patient is conscious and able to eat enough to replenish glycogen stores.

Investigations into liver dysfunction or the presence of an insulinoma is necessary when the cause of hypoglycemia is not abundantly clear. Idiopathic postprandial hypoglycemia is best treated with small, frequent meals.

Hyperglycemia

Acute, symptomatic hyperglycemia typically occurs in the context of diabetic ketoacidosis (DKA) or nonketotic hyperosmolar hyperglycemia (NKH)—two manifestations of decompensated diabetes. Encephalopathy is a common feature in NKH and less so in DKA. Both conditions are potentially life threatening and require diligent monitoring well beyond the point at which euglycemia is achieved.

Definition Hyperglycemia is defined as serum glucose greater than 7.8 mmol/L (140 mg/L). However, impairment of consciousness typically occurs when serum glucose values are greater than 16.7 mmol/L (300 mg/dL) in DKA, and greater than 33 mmol/L (600 mg/dL) in NKH.[223] The principal defect in these patients is either lack of insulin or insulin resistance, both of which prevent cellular uptake and use of circulating glucose. In general, hyperglycemia can be heterogeneous in etiology, with the common features of impaired "insulin effect" coupled with increased exogenous glucose, increased gluconeogenesis, or glycolysis.

Etiology and clinical features Although hyperglycemia with impaired consciousness usually occurs in the at-risk population during severe metabolic stress, such as infections, burns, inflammatory diseases, or steroid use, it can also occur spontaneously. **Box 8**[223] summarizes some common predisposing factors of nonketotic hyperglycemia.

Patients with NKH and DKA are severely volume contracted. Tissue turgor is reduced and mucus membranes are dry, with soft, sunken eyeballs. Kussmal breathing and breath of fruity odor is caused by metabolic acidosis, and expired acetone is characteristic of DKA. Neurologic manifestations of symptomatic hyperglycemia occur more frequently in NKH than in DKA. Impairment of consciousness follows a predictable course of confusion, lethargy, stupor, and coma.[223] In NKH, focal neurologic findings may be present including hemiplegia, aphasia, and focal motor seizures.[224–226] Hemichorea-hemiballism (HC-HB) is a movement disorder complication of NKH. These patients tend to be women,[227] and the neuroimaging correlates are reversible T1 hyperintensities and T2 hypointensities in the striatum.[227,228] Local metabolic changes from selective hypoperfusion and reduced oxygen delivery to the striatum have been implicated in HC-HB.[229] In one study the presence of acanthocytosis correlated with HC-HB.[230]

Box 8
Common conditions causing nonketotic hyperglycemia

1. Serious systemic illness

   a. Unobserved dehydration

   b. Metabolic change (infection, inflammation, burns, myocardial infarction, Cushing syndrome)

   c. Surgery or anesthesia

2. Reduction in carbohydrate tolerance with increased carbohydrate intake (eg, burns, drug therapy plus parenteral hyperalimentation)

3. Inhibition of fat mobilization in ketosis-susceptible patients (eg, propranolol therapy)

4. Inadequate insulin dosing

Adapted from Young GB, DeRubeis R. Metabolic encephalopathies. In: Young GB, Ropper AH, Bolton CF, editors. Coma and impaired consciousness: a clinical perspective. New York: McGraw-Hill; 1998. p. 307–92; with permission.

Epidemiology The incidence of DKA is 4.6 to 8.0 per 1000 person-years among patients with diabetes, and NKH incidence is less than 1.0 per 1000 person-years.[231] In one of the early prospective studies on NKH, the average age of patients was 62 years.[224] Clinical teaching usually categorizes NKH as a condition affecting the elderly, whereas DKA affects a relatively younger population; however, the explosion of childhood obesity and early-onset type 2 diabetes has had implications for the epidemiology of NKH.[232] The clinical outcome of death in the various case reports and case series ranges from 14% to 100%.[233–235]

Pathophysiology of impaired consciousness in hyperglycemia Arieff and Carroll[236] described a clear relationship between increased serum osmolality and progressive degree of impaired consciousness in hyperglycemic encephalopathy. Alterations in electrical activity of the reticular activating system (RAS) have been demonstrated following hyperosmolar stress.[237] Thus impairment of consciousness from severe hyperglycemia may localize to aberrations within the RAS in addition to diffuse and cellular dehydration. A rapid rate of osmolar change is particularly effective in depressing consciousness.[236] The metabolic acidosis per se does not cause altered levels of consciousness in DKA.[84] Alterations in specific neurotransmitter systems as the cause of impaired consciousness have yet to be described. It is likely that multiple transmitter systems are involved. Seizures in NKH have been proposed to be attributable to a decrease in GABA availability, because of glutamate shunting through the pentose phosphate shunt.[238]

Impairment of consciousness via cerebral edema can also occur following treatment of hyperglycemia; this can be seen in rapid correction of DKA, and only very rarely during treatment of NKH. Sudden alterations of consciousness after correction of hyperglycemia should prompt cranial imaging to assess signs of edema.

Treatment A detailed description of the management of NKH and DKA is beyond the scope of this article, and the reader is referred to a recent review of this topic.[239] The principles in the management of these disorders include (1) fluid replacement, (2) intravenous insulin therapy, (3) potassium replacement, (4) close monitoring of electrolytes and clinical state, and (5) treatment of the precipitating event.

Rapid extracellular fluid expansion is necessary, and—assuming adequate cardiopulmonary reserve—should be initiated by intravenous isotonic saline (0.9% NaCl) at

10 to 20 mL/kg (approximately 1–1.5 L in an average adult) in the first hour. Ongoing intravenous normal saline should be instituted at rate of 4 to 14 mL/kg/h until serum glucose is reaches12 to 14 mmol/L, at which point 5% dextrose in 0.45% NaCl intravenous fluids should be given to help prevent cerebral edema.[240,241] Intravenous insulin delivered by a pump at 0.1 U/kg/h should be started at the onset of fluid replacement. Insulin will reduce hyperglycemia by facilitating cellular uptake of glucose, and by inhibiting glycolysis and gluconeogenesis. Insulin will also arrest ketone production in DKA. Hypokalemia is usually present in severe hyperglycemia, and is worsened by insulin therapy because of the intracellular shift of potassium caused by insulin. If serum potassium is less than 3.3 mmol/L at the outset, insulin should be held, and 40 mEq of KCl should be added to the patient's intravenous fluids.[239] Potassium replacement of 20 mEq/L intravenous normal saline is typically used with potassium levels greater than 3.3 mmol/L and less than 5.0 mmol/L. Thus careful monitoring of electrolytes is necessary, and serum chemistries should be repeated every few hours until the patient is stable.

IDIOPATHIC RECURRENT STUPOR: ENDOZEPINE STUPOR

Endozepine stupor is a very uncommon syndrome characterized by recurrent spontaneous stupor with associated fast EEG (beta frequency) that is responsive to the $GABA_A$ antagonist, flumazenil. Recurrent idiopathic stupor is caused by the presence of endozepines, which are nonbenzodiazepine, nonprotein molecules that act as positive allosteric modulators of the $GABA_A$ receptor, and have the same action on the CNS as exogenous benzodiazepines.[242]

Epidemiology

The largest study indicates a male preponderance (16 male to 4 female), with involvement of both the young adult and elderly population (range of age 18–67 years).[243] There are no obvious risk factors or common premorbid conditions; however, 30% (6/20) had some form of respiratory disease (obstructive sleep apnea, 3; COPD, 3).[243]

Clinical Features

All patients have some impairment of consciousness, which can range from stupor to coma. Dysarthria and ataxia are also common features, and deep tendon reflexes are reduced.[243–245] Patients are usually amnestic of the episode, and of events hours to days preceding the attacks. The attacks can last 2 to 120 hours, and their frequency is also variable. For example, in the study by Lugaresi and colleagues[243] 9 of 20 patients had at some point more than 6 attacks per year. The attacks can occur at any time of the day and may be preceded by hours to days with fatigue, mental slowing, general malaise, and behavioral disturbances such as combativeness or docility.[245] Extensive investigations for other toxic or metabolic encephalopathies, or exogenous benzodiazepine ingestion, by definition, should not disclose an alternative diagnosis. Between attacks there is no published evidence for any neurologic sequelae.

EEG Findings

Interictally, the patients have normal EEG findings. During the attacks there is diffuse, low-amplitude, unreactive beta rhythm (13–16 Hz). Administration of intravenous flumazenil, 0.5 to 2 mg or more, reverses the abnormal EEG pattern to normal, reactive alpha rhythm, and correlates with clinical improvement.

Pathophysiology

As the name would suggest, the sine qua non of endozepine stupor is the presence of elevated serum endozepine that coincides with the appropriate clinical picture. It is believed that in the normal functioning nervous system endozepine release is physiologically regulated by neurons, and acts to modulate GABA-mediated neurotransmission.[246,247] In the syndrome of idiopathic recurrent stupor, high-performance liquid chromatography has shown that a subtype of endozepine molecule—endozepine-4—is massively elevated[244,248] during bouts of stupor. At present there is no known cause for the episodic increase in serum endozepine-4 in these patients.

ANTI-NMDA RECEPTOR ANTIBODY ENCEPHALITIS

This condition is a newly described, likely underrecognized, severe encephalopathy syndrome caused by the presence of antibodies directed against the brain NMDA receptor.[249] It is most commonly associated with ovarian teratomas in young non-Caucasian women[250]; however, the range of reported ages is from 20 months[251] to greater than 80 years,[252] and men are also affected, albeit less frequently. The largest case series (n = 100) reported 91% affected to be female, 59% of whom had ovarian tumors.[253] A case series in Europe using a more sensitive assay reported tumors in 9 of 34 patients, 11 of whom were male.[254] The nontumor antigenic stimulus may be an infectious/inflammatory event.[254]

The clinical picture is thus far fairly consistent: a neuropsychiatric prodrome lasting a median of 10 to 20 days that is characterized by behavioral changes, paranoia, anxiety, and psychotic symptoms gives way to seizure and protracted obtundation with or without nonconvulsive status epilepticus. On presentation to medical facilities, these patients are commonly triaged to an acute psychiatric care unit until seizure occurs followed by persistent loss of consciousness. The encephalopathy is somewhat unique, as it is associated with pronounced autonomic fluctuations including bradycardia or tachycardia, hypothermia, and hypoventilation.[249] A movement disorder characterized by facial and oral dyskinesia as well as limb posturing are well documented.[250]

CSF examination demonstrates that lymphocytic pleocytosis and protein may be elevated. Oligoclonal bands may be positive, as is the IgG index. Cranial MRI can be either normal or nonenhancing; T2-weighted abnormalities have been reported in the mesial temporal lobes. EEG findings vary from diffuse delta, rhythmic delta, to nonconvulsive status epilepticus.[250]

Treatment includes removal of the tumor and immunosuppression with intravenous IgG, high-dose steroids, or plasma exchange. Outcomes vary, but a significant proportion of patients (75%) can make excellent neurologic recovery, though often after protracted illness and rehabilitation.[250] This diagnosis should always be considered in the differential of viral encephalitis, and should be suspected in acute neuropsychiatric presentation in previously healthy persons.

REFERENCES

1. Angel MJ, Chen R, Bryan YG. Metabolic encephalopathies. Handb Clin Neurol 2008;90:115–66.
2. Maeda H, Sato M, Yoshikawa A, et al. Brain MR imaging in patients with hepatic cirrhosis: relationship between high intensity signal in basal ganglia on T1-weighted images and elemental concentrations in brain. Neuroradiology 1997;39:546–50.

3. Zeneroli ML, Cioni G, Crisi G, et al. Globus pallidus alterations and brain atrophy in liver cirrhosis patients with encephalopathy: an MR imaging study. Magn Reson Imaging 1991;9:295–302.

4. Wijdicks EF, Plevak DJ, Rakela J, et al. Clinical and radiologic features of cerebral edema in fulminant hepatic failure. Mayo Clin Proc 1995;70:119–24.

5. Demedts M, Pillen E, De Groote J, et al. Hepatic encephalopathy: comparative study of EEG abnormalities, neuropsychic disturbances and blood ammonia. Acta Neurol Belg 1973;73:281–8.

6. Van der Rijt CC, Schalm SW, De Groot GH, et al. Objective measurement of hepatic encephalopathy by means of automated EEG analysis. Electroencephalogr Clin Neurophysiol 1984;57:423–6.

7. Madl C, Grimm G, Ferenci P, et al. Serial recording of sensory evoked potentials: a noninvasive prognostic indicator in fulminant liver failure. Hepatology 1994;20: 1487–94.

8. Yang SS, Chu NS, Liaw YF. Somatosensory evoked potentials in hepatic encephalopathy. Gastroenterology 1985;89:625–30.

9. Davies MG, Rowan MJ, MacMathuna P, et al. The auditory P300 event-related potential: an objective marker of the encephalopathy of chronic liver disease. Hepatology 1990;12:688–94.

10. Senzolo M, Amodio P, D'Aloiso MC, et al. Neuropsychological and neurophysiological evaluation in cirrhotic patients with minimal hepatic encephalopathy undergoing liver transplantation. Transplant Proc 2005;37:1104–7.

11. Butterworth RF. Pathophysiology of hepatic encephalopathy: a new look at ammonia. Metab Brain Dis 2002;17:221–7.

12. Butterworth RF. The astrocytic ("peripheral-type") benzodiazepine receptor: role in the pathogenesis of portal-systemic encephalopathy. Neurochem Int 2000;36: 411–6.

13. Norenberg MD, Itzhak Y, Bender AS. The peripheral benzodiazepine receptor and neurosteroids in hepatic encephalopathy. Adv Exp Med Biol 1997;420: 95–111.

14. Swart GR, van den Berg JW, Wattimena JL, et al. Elevated protein requirements in cirrhosis of the liver investigated by whole body protein turnover studies. Clin Sci (Lond) 1988;75:101–7.

15. Kircheis G, Nilius R, Held C, et al. Therapeutic efficacy of L-ornithine-L-aspartate infusions in patients with cirrhosis and hepatic encephalopathy: results of a placebo-controlled, double-blind study. Hepatology 1997;25:1351–60.

16. Steinman TI, Becker BN, Frost AE, et al. Guidelines for the referral and management of patients eligible for solid organ transplantation. Transplantation 2001;71: 1189–204.

17. Rothstein JD, Olasmaa M. Endogenous GABAergic modulators in the pathogenesis of hepatic encephalopathy. Neurochem Res 1990;15:193–7.

18. Williams R, Bass N. Rifaximin, a nonabsorbed oral antibiotic, in the treatment of hepatic encephalopathy: antimicrobial activity, efficacy, and safety. Rev Gastroenterol Disord 2005;5(Suppl 1):10–8.

19. Bass NM, Mullen KD, Sanyal A, et al. Rifaximin treatment in hepatic encephalopathy. N Engl J Med 2010;362:1071–81.

20. Mantry PS, Munsaf S. Rifaximin for the treatment of hepatic encephalopathy. Transplant Proc 2010;42:4543–7.

21. Les I, Doval E, Garcia-Martinez R, et al. Effects of branched-chain amino acids supplementation in patients with cirrhosis and a previous episode of hepatic encephalopathy: a randomized study. Am J Gastroenterol 2011;106(6):1081–8.

22. Szczech LA, Lazar IL. Projecting the United States ESRD population: issues regarding treatment of patients with ESRD. Kidney Int Suppl 2004;90:S3–7.

23. Lameire N, Jager K, Van Biesen W, et al. Chronic kidney disease: a European perspective. Kidney Int Suppl 2005;(99):S30–8.

24. Adams F. The extant works of araetus, the cappadocian. London: The Sydenham Society; 1836.

25. Osler W. The principles and practice of medicine. 1st edition. London: Appleton; 1892.

26. Glaser GH. Brain dysfunction in uremia. Res Publ Assoc Res Nerv Ment Dis 1974;53:173–99.

27. De Deyn PP, Vanholder R, Eloot S, et al. Guanidino compounds as uremic (neuro) toxins. Semin Dial 2009;22:340–5.

28. Bolton CF, Young GB. Neurologic complication of renal disease. Boston: Butterworths; 1990.

29. Port FK, Johnson WJ, Klass DW. Prevention of dialysis disequilibrium syndrome by use of high sodium concentration in the dialysate. Kidney Int 1973;3:327–33.

30. Jacob JC, Gloor P, Elwan OH, et al. Electroencephalographic changes in chronic renal failure. Neurology 1965;15:419–29.

31. Hughes JR, Schreeder MT. EEG in dialysis encephalopathy. Neurology 1980; 30(11):1148–54.

32. Karnaze DS, Bickford RG. Triphasic waves: a reassessment of their significance. Electroencephalogr Clin Neurophysiol 1984;57:193–8.

33. Hinchey J, Chaves C, Appignani B, et al. A reversible posterior leukoencephalopathy syndrome. N Engl J Med 1996;334:494–500.

34. Covarrubias DJ, Luetmer PH, Campeau NG. Posterior reversible encephalopathy syndrome: prognostic utility of quantitative diffusion-weighted MR images. AJNR Am J Neuroradiol 2002;23:1038–48.

35. Ay H, Buonanno FS, Schaefer PW, et al. Posterior leukoencephalopathy without severe hypertension: utility of diffusion-weighted MRI. Neurology 1998;51:1369–76.

36. Kinoshita T, Moritani T, Shrier DA, et al. Diffusion-weighted MR imaging of posterior reversible leukoencephalopathy syndrome: a pictorial essay. Clin Imaging 2003;27:307–15.

37. Stott VL, Hurrell MA, Anderson TJ. Reversible posterior leukoencephalopathy syndrome: a misnomer reviewed. Intern Med J 2005;35:83–90.

38. Ahn KJ, You WJ, Jeong SL, et al. Atypical manifestations of reversible posterior leukoencephalopathy syndrome: findings on diffusion imaging and ADC mapping. Neuroradiology 2004;46:978–83.

39. Fugate JE, Claassen DO, Cloft HJ, et al. Posterior reversible encephalopathy syndrome: associated clinical and radiologic findings. Mayo Clin Proc 2010;85: 427–32.

40. Lamy C, Oppenheim C, Meder JF, et al. Neuroimaging in posterior reversible encephalopathy syndrome. J Neuroimaging 2004;14:89–96.

41. Fujieda Y, Kataoka H, Odani T, et al. Clinical features of reversible posterior leukoencephalopathy syndrome in patients with systemic lupus erythematosus. Mod Rheumatol 2011;21(3):276–81.

42. Kumar S, Rajam L. Posterior reversible encephalopathy syndrome (PRES/RPLS) during pulse steroid therapy in macrophage activation syndrome. Indian J Pediatr 2011;78(8):1002–4.

43. Schaefer PW, Buonanno FS, Gonzalez RG, et al. Diffusion-weighted imaging discriminates between cytotoxic and vasogenic edema in a patient with eclampsia. Stroke 1997;28:1082–5.

44. Weingarten K, Barbut D, Filippi C, et al. Acute hypertensive encephalopathy: findings on spin-echo and gradient-echo MR imaging. AJR Am J Roentgenol 1994;162:665–70.
45. Primavera A, Audenino D, Mavilio N, et al. Reversible posterior leucoencephalopathy syndrome in systemic lupus and vasculitis. Ann Rheum Dis 2001;60:534–7.
46. Vora J, Cooper J, Thomas JP. Polyarteritis nodosa presenting with hypertensive encephalopathy. Br J Clin Pract 1992;46:144–5.
47. Ohta T, Sakano T, Shiotsu M, et al. Reversible posterior leukoencephalopathy in a patient with Wegener granulomatosis. Pediatr Nephrol 2004;19:442–4.
48. de Seze J, Mastain B, Stojkovic T, et al. Unusual MR findings of the brain stem in arterial hypertension. AJNR Am J Neuroradiol 2000;21:391–4.
49. Kaplan NM. Primary aldosteronism with malignant hypertension. N Engl J Med 1963;269:1282–6.
50. Aoki T, Sato T, Hasegawa K, et al. Reversible hyperintensity lesion on diffusion-weighted MRI in hypoglycemic coma. Neurology 2004;63:392–3.
51. Kupferschmidt H, Bont A, Schnorf H, et al. Transient cortical blindness and bioccipital brain lesions in two patients with acute intermittent porphyria. Ann Intern Med 1995;123:598–600.
52. Sofer S, Gueron M. Vasodilators and hypertensive encephalopathy following scorpion envenomation in children. Chest 1990;97:118–20.
53. Grewal RP, Miller BL. Cocaine induced hypertensive encephalopathy. Acta Neurol (Napoli) 1991;13:279–81.
54. Lake CR, Gallant S, Masson E, et al. Adverse drug effects attributed to phenylpropanolamine: a review of 142 case reports. Am J Med 1990;89:195–208.
55. Digre KB, Varner MW, Osborn AG, et al. Cranial magnetic resonance imaging in severe preeclampsia vs eclampsia. Arch Neurol 1993;50:399–406.
56. Schwartz RB, Feske SK, Polak JF, et al. Preeclampsia-eclampsia: clinical and neuroradiographic correlates and insights into the pathogenesis of hypertensive encephalopathy. Radiology 2000;217:371–6.
57. Bakshi R, Shaikh ZA, Bates VE, et al. Thrombotic thrombocytopenic purpura: brain CT and MRI findings in 12 patients. Neurology 1999;52:1285–8.
58. Taylor MB, Jackson A, Weller JM. Dynamic susceptibility contrast enhanced MRI in reversible posterior leukoencephalopathy syndrome associated with haemolytic uraemic syndrome. Br J Radiol 2000;73:438–42.
59. Kaplan PW. Reversible hypercalcemic cerebral vasoconstriction with seizures and blindness: a paradigm for eclampsia? Clin Electroencephalogr 1998;29:120–3.
60. Schwartz RB, Bravo SM, Klufas RA, et al. Cyclosporine neurotoxicity and its relationship to hypertensive encephalopathy: CT and MR findings in 16 cases. AJR Am J Roentgenol 1995;165:627–31.
61. Truwit CL, Denaro CP, Lake JR, et al. MR imaging of reversible cyclosporin A-induced neurotoxicity. AJNR Am J Neuroradiol 1991;12:651–9.
62. Shutter LA, Green JP, Newman NJ, et al. Cortical blindness and white matter lesions in a patient receiving FK506 after liver transplantation. Neurology 1993;43:2417–8.
63. Hurwitz RL, Mahoney DH Jr, Armstrong DL, et al. Reversible encephalopathy and seizures as a result of conventional vincristine administration. Med Pediatr Oncol 1988;16:216–9.
64. Ito Y, Arahata Y, Goto Y, et al. Cisplatin neurotoxicity presenting as reversible posterior leukoencephalopathy syndrome. AJNR Am J Neuroradiol 1998;19:415–7.

65. Vaughn DJ, Jarvik JG, Hackney D, et al. High-dose cytarabine neurotoxicity: MR findings during the acute phase. AJNR Am J Neuroradiol 1993;14:1014–6.
66. Cooney MJ, Bradley WG, Symko SC, et al. Hypertensive encephalopathy: complication in children treated for myeloproliferative disorders—report of three cases. Radiology 2000;214:711–6.
67. Shin RK, Stern JW, Janss AJ, et al. Reversible posterior leukoencephalopathy during the treatment of acute lymphoblastic leukemia. Neurology 2001;56:388–91.
68. Giner V, Fernandez C, Esteban MJ, et al. Reversible posterior leukoencephalopathy secondary to indinavir-induced hypertensive crisis: a case report. Am J Hypertens 2002;15:465–7.
69. Delanty N, Vaughan C, Frucht S, et al. Erythropoietin-associated hypertensive posterior leukoencephalopathy. Neurology 1997;49:686–9.
70. Leniger T, Kastrup O, Diener HC. Reversible posterior leukencephalopathy syndrome induced by granulocyte stimulating factor filgrastim. J Neurol Neurosurg Psychiatry 2000;69:280–1.
71. Doss-Esper CE, Singhal AB, Smith MS, et al. Reversible posterior leukoencephalopathy, cerebral vasoconstriction, and strokes after intravenous immune globulin therapy in Guillain-Barre syndrome. J Neuroimaging 2005;15:188–92.
72. Mathy I, Gille M, Van Raemdonck F, et al. Neurologic complications of intravenous immunoglobulin (IVIg) therapy: an illustrative case of acute encephalopathy following IVIg therapy and a review of the literature. Acta Neurol Belg 1998;98:347–51.
73. Boughammoura A, Touze E, Oppenheim C, et al. Reversible angiopathy and encephalopathy after blood transfusion. J Neurol 2003;250:116–8.
74. Heo K, Park SA, Lee JY, et al. Post-transfusion posterior leukoencephalopathy with cytotoxic and vasogenic edema precipitated by vasospasm. Cerebrovasc Dis 2003;15:230–3.
75. Sticherling C, Berkefeld J, Auch-Schwelk W, et al. Transient bilateral cortical blindness after coronary angiography. Lancet 1998;351:570.
76. Zinn PO, Colen RR, Kasper EM, et al. Posterior leukoencephalopathy following repair of an ileocecal anastomosis breakdown: a case report and review of the literature. J Med Case Reports 2011;5:20.
77. Roberts JM, Redman CW. Pre-eclampsia: more than pregnancy-induced hypertension. Lancet 1993;341:1447–51.
78. Austen FK, Carmichael MW, Adams RD. Neurologic manifestations of chronic pulmonary insufficiency. N Engl J Med 1957;257:579–90.
79. Heaton RK, Grant I, McSweeny AJ, et al. Psychologic effects of continuous and nocturnal oxygen therapy in hypoxemic chronic obstructive pulmonary disease. Arch Intern Med 1983;143:1941–7.
80. Antonelli Incalzi R, Marra C, Giordano A, et al. Cognitive impairment in chronic obstructive pulmonary disease—a neuropsychological and SPECT study. J Neurol 2003;250:325–32.
81. Al Tahan AR, Zaidan R, Jones S, et al. Event-related evoked potentials in chronic respiratory encephalopathy. Int J Chron Obstruct Pulmon Dis 2010;5:21–7.
82. Kilburn KH. Neurologic manifestations of respiratory failure. Arch Intern Med 1965;116:409–15.
83. Ortiz Vasquez J. Neurologic manifestations of chronic respiratory disease. In: Vinken PJ, Bruyn GW, Klawans HL, editors. Handbook of clinical neurology. Amsterdam (The Netherlands): North Holland Publishing Co; 1979. p. 285–307.
84. Posner JB, Plum F. Spinal-fluid pH and neurologic symptoms in systemic acidosis. N Engl J Med 1967;277:605–13.

85. Borgstrom L, Norberg K, Siesjo BK. Glucose consumption in rat cerebral cortex in normoxia, hypoxia and hypercapnia. Acta Physiol Scand 1976;96: 569–74.

86. Siesjo BK, Borgstrom L, Johannsson H, et al. Cerebral oxygenation in arterial hypoxia. Adv Exp Med Biol 1976;75:335–42.

87. Von Berg R. Toxicology update: carbon monoxide. J Appl Toxicol 1999;19: 379–89.

88. Thom SR, Fisher D, Zhang J, et al. Neuronal nitric oxide synthase and N-methyl-D-aspartate neurons in experimental carbon monoxide poisoning. Toxicol Appl Pharmacol 2004b;194:280–95.

89. Choi IS. Delayed neurologic sequelae in carbon monoxide intoxication. Arch Neurol 1983;40:433–5.

90. Ginsberg MD, Myers RE, McDonagh BF. Experimental carbon monoxide encephalopathy in the primate. II. Clinical aspects, neuropathology, and physiologic correlation. Arch Neurol 1974;30:209–16.

91. Kim JH, Chang KH, Song IC, et al. Delayed encephalopathy of acute carbon monoxide intoxication: diffusivity of cerebral white matter lesions. AJNR Am J Neuroradiol 2003;24:1592–7.

92. Thom SR. Carbon monoxide-mediated brain lipid peroxidation in the rat. J Appl Physiol 1990;68:997–1003.

93. Thom SR, Bhopale VM, Fisher D, et al. Delayed neuropathology after carbon monoxide poisoning is immune-mediated. Proc Natl Acad Sci U S A 2004; 101:13660–5.

94. Rashidian J, Iyirhiaro G, Aleyasin H, et al. Multiple cyclin-dependent kinases signals are critical mediators of ischemia/hypoxic neuronal death in vitro and in vivo. Proc Natl Acad Sci U S A 2005;102:14080–5.

95. Scheinkestel CD, Jones K, Myles PS, et al. Where to now with carbon monoxide poisoning? Emerg Med Australas 2004;16:151–4.

96. Brain L, Jellinek EH, Ball K. Hashimoto's disease and encephalopathy. Lancet 1966;2:512–4.

97. Shaw PJ, Walls TJ, Newman PK, et al. Hashimoto's encephalopathy: a steroid-responsive disorder associated with high anti-thyroid antibody titers—report of 5 cases. Neurology 1991;41:228–33.

98. Hackett E, Beech M, Forbes IJ. Thyroglobulin antibodies in patients without clinical disease of the thyroid gland. Lancet 1960;2:402–4.

99. Mariotti S, Sansoni P, Barbesino G, et al. Thyroid and other organ-specific auto-antibodies in healthy centenarians. Lancet 1992;339:1506–8.

100. Ferracci F, Moretto G, Candeago RM, et al. Antithyroid antibodies in the CSF: their role in the pathogenesis of Hashimoto's encephalopathy. Neurology 2003;60:712–4.

101. Ferracci F, Bertiato G, Moretto G. Hashimoto's encephalopathy: epidemiologic data and pathogenetic considerations. J Neurol Sci 2004;217:165–8.

102. Vasconcellos E, Pina-Garza JE, Fakhoury T, et al. Pediatric manifestations of Hashimoto's encephalopathy. Pediatr Neurol 1999;20:394–8.

103. Chong JY, Rowland LP, Utiger RD. Hashimoto encephalopathy: syndrome or myth? Arch Neurol 2003;60:164–71.

104. Mussig K, Bartels M, Gallwitz B, et al. Hashimoto's encephalopathy presenting with bipolar affective disorder. Bipolar Disord 2005;7:292–7.

105. Laske C, Leyhe T, Buchkremer G, et al. Depression in Hashimoto's encephalopathy. Successful treatment of a severe depressive episode with a glucocorticoid as an add-on therapy. Nervenarzt 2005;76:617–22 [in German].

106. Arrojo M, Perez-Rodriguez MM, Mota M, et al. Psychiatric presentation of Hashimoto's encephalopathy. Psychosom Med 2007;69:200–1.
107. Lin YT, Liao SC. Hashimoto encephalopathy presenting as schizophrenia-like disorder. Cogn Behav Neurol 2009;22:197–201.
108. Passarella B, Negro C, Nozzoli C, et al. Cerebellar subacute syndrome due to corticosteroid-responsive encephalopathy associated with autoimmune thyroiditis (also called "Hashimoto's encephalopathy"). Clin Ter 2005;156:13–7.
109. Finberg L. Pathogenesis of lesions in the nervous system in hypernatremic states. I. Clinical observations of infants. Pediatrics 1959;23:40–5.
110. Gliebus G, Lippa CF. Cerebrospinal immunoglobulin level changes and clinical response to treatment of Hashimoto's encephalopathy. Am J Alzheimers Dis Other Demen 2009;24:373–6.
111. Schauble B, Castillo PR, Boeve BF, et al. EEG findings in steroid-responsive encephalopathy associated with autoimmune thyroiditis. Clin Neurophysiol 2003;114:32–7.
112. Henchey R, Cibula J, Helveston W, et al. Electroencephalographic findings in Hashimoto's encephalopathy. Neurology 1995;45:977–81.
113. Pozo-Rosich P, Villoslada P, Canton A, et al. Reversible white matter alterations in encephalopathy associated with autoimmune thyroid disease. J Neurol 2002;249:1063–5.
114. Forchetti CM, Katsamakis G, Garron DC. Autoimmune thyroiditis and a rapidly progressive dementia: global hypoperfusion on SPECT scanning suggests a possible mechanism. Neurology 1997;49:623–6.
115. Zettinig G, Asenbaum S, Fueger BJ, et al. Increased prevalence of subclinical brain perfusion abnormalities in patients with autoimmune thyroiditis: evidence of Hashimoto's encephalitis? Clin Endocrinol (Oxf) 2003;59:637–43.
116. Shein M, Apter A, Dickerman Z, et al. Encephalopathy in compensated Hashimoto thyroiditis: a clinical expression of autoimmune cerebral vasculitis. Brain Dev 1986;8:60–4.
117. Thrush DC, Boddie HG. Episodic encephalopathy associated with thyroid disorders. J Neurol Neurosurg Psychiatry 1974;37:696–700.
118. Nolte KW, Unbehaun A, Sieker H, et al. Hashimoto encephalopathy: a brainstem vasculitis? Neurology 2000;54:769–70.
119. Mahad DJ, Staugaitis S, Ruggieri P, et al. Steroid-responsive encephalopathy associated with autoimmune thyroiditis and primary CNS demyelination. J Neurol Sci 2005;228:3–5.
120. Fujii A, Yoneda M, Ito T, et al. Autoantibodies against the amino terminal of alpha-enolase are a useful diagnostic marker of Hashimoto's encephalopathy. J Neuroimmunol 2005;162:130–6.
121. Jacob S, Rajabally YA. Hashimoto's encephalopathy: steroid resistance and response to intravenous immunoglobulins. J Neurol Neurosurg Psychiatry 2005;76:455–6.
122. Ochi H, Horiuchi I, Araki N, et al. Proteomic analysis of human brain identifies alpha-enolase as a novel autoantigen in Hashimoto's encephalopathy. FEBS Lett 2002;528:197–202.
123. Castillo P, Woodruff B, Caselli R, et al. Steroid-responsive encephalopathy associated with autoimmune thyroiditis. Arch Neurol 2006;63:197–202.
124. Oelkers W. Adrenal insufficiency. N Engl J Med 1996;335:1206–12.
125. Anderson RJ. Hospital-associated hyponatremia. Kidney Int 1986;29:1237–47.
126. Arieff AI. Hyponatremia, convulsions, respiratory arrest, and permanent brain damage after elective surgery in healthy women. N Engl J Med 1986;314:1529–35.

127. Fraser CL, Arieff AI. Epidemiology, pathophysiology, and management of hyponatremic encephalopathy. Am J Med 1997;102:67–77.

128. Yalcin-Cakmakli G, Karli OK, Shorbagi A, et al. Hyponatremic encephalopathy after excessive water ingestion prior to pelvic ultrasound: neuroimaging findings. Intern Med 2010;49:1807–11.

129. Soupart A, Decaux G. Therapeutic recommendations for management of severe hyponatremia: current concepts on pathogenesis and prevention of neurologic complications. Clin Nephrol 1996;46:149–69.

130. Ayus JC, Arieff AI. Chronic hyponatremic encephalopathy in postmenopausal women: association of therapies with morbidity and mortality. JAMA 1999;281:2299–304.

131. Arieff AI. Hyponatremia associated with permanent brain damage. Adv Intern Med 1987;32:325–44.

132. Verbalis JG, Martinez AJ. Neurological and neuropathological sequelae of correction of chronic hyponatremia. Kidney Int 1991;39:1274–82.

133. Ordaz B, Tuz K, Ochoa LD, et al. Osmolytes and mechanisms involved in regulatory volume decrease under conditions of sudden or gradual osmolarity decrease. Neurochem Res 2004;29:65–72.

134. Pasantes-Morales H. Volume regulation in brain cells: cellular and molecular mechanisms. Metab Brain Dis 1996;11:187–204.

135. Moritz ML, Ayus JC. 100 cc 3% sodium chloride bolus: a novel treatment for hyponatremic encephalopathy. Metab Brain Dis 2010;25:91–6.

136. Decaux G, Soupart A. Treatment of symptomatic hyponatremia. Am J Med Sci 2003;326:25–30.

137. Silver SM, Schroeder BM, Sterns RH, et al. Myoinositol administration improves survival and reduces myelinolysis after rapid correction of chronic hyponatremia in rats. J Neuropathol Exp Neurol 2006;65:37–44.

138. Gross P, Palm C. The treatment of hyponatraemia using vasopressin antagonists. Exp Physiol 2000;85(Spec No):253S–7S.

139. Snyder NA, Feigal DW, Arieff AI. Hypernatremia in elderly patients. A heterogeneous, morbid, and iatrogenic entity. Ann Intern Med 1987;107:309–19.

140. Arieff AI, Guisado R. Effects on the central nervous system of hypernatremic and hyponatremic states. Kidney Int 1976;10:104–16.

141. Finberg L. Hypernatremic (hypertonic) dehydration in infants. N Engl J Med 1973;289:196–8.

142. Casavant MJ, Fitch JA. Fatal hypernatremia from saltwater used as an emetic. J Toxicol Clin Toxicol 2003;41:861–3.

143. Kupiec TC, Goldenring JM, Raj V. A nonfatal case of sodium toxicity. J Anal Toxicol 2004;28:526–8.

144. Turk EE, Schulz F, Koops E, et al. Fatal hypernatremia after using salt as an emetic–report of three autopsy cases. Leg Med (Tokyo) 2005;7:47–50.

145. Ofran Y, Lavi D, Opher D, et al. Fatal voluntary salt intake resulting in the highest ever documented sodium plasma level in adults (255 mmol L^{-1}): a disorder linked to female gender and psychiatric disorders. J Intern Med 2004;256:525–8.

146. Handy TC, Hanzlick R, Shields LB, et al. Hypernatremia and subdural hematoma in the pediatric age group: is there a causal relationship? J Forensic Sci 1999;44:1114–8.

147. Naik KR, Saroja AO. Seasonal postpartum hypernatremic encephalopathy with osmotic extrapontine myelinolysis and rhabdomyolysis. J Neurol Sci 2010;291:5–11.

148. Morris-Jones PH, Houston IB, Evans RC. Prognosis of the neurological complications of acute hypernatraemia. Lancet 1967;2:1385–9.
149. Luse SA, Harris B. Brain ultrastructure in hydration and dehydration. Arch Neurol 1961;4:139–52.
150. Simmons MA, Adcock EW III, Bard H, et al. Hypernatremia and intracranial hemorrhage in neonates. N Engl J Med 1974;291:6–10.
151. Luttrell CN, Finberg L. Hemorrhagic encephalopathy induced by hypernatremia. I. Clinical, laboratory, and pathological observations. AMA Arch Neurol Psychiatry 1959;81:424–32.
152. Hartfield DS, Loewy JA, Yager JY. Transient thalamic changes on MRI in a child with hypernatremia. Pediatr Neurol 1999;20:60–2.
153. Mocharla R, Schexnayder SM, Glasier CM. Fatal cerebral edema and intracranial hemorrhage associated with hypernatremic dehydration. Pediatr Radiol 1997;27:785–7.
154. Alorainy IA, O'Gorman AM, Decell MK. Cerebral bleeding, infarcts, and presumed extrapontine myelinolysis in hypernatraemic dehydration. Neuroradiology 1999;41:144–6.
155. Kahn A, Blum D, Casimir G, et al. Controlled fall in natremia in hypertonic dehydration: possible avoidance of rehydration seizures. Eur J Pediatr 1981;135:293–6.
156. Hossain M. Neurological and psychiatric manifestations in idiopathic hypoparathyroidism: response to treatment. J Neurol Neurosurg Psychiatry 1970;33:153–6.
157. Simpson JA. The neurological manifestation of idiopathic hypoparathyroidism. Brain 1952;75:76–90.
158. Glaser GH, Levy LL. Seizures and idiopathic hypoparathyroidism: a clinical-electrophysiologic study. Epilepsia 1959;1:454–65.
159. Rose GA, Vas CJ. Neurological complications and electroencephalographic changes in hypoparathyroidism. Acta Neurol Scand 1966;42:537–50.
160. Huang CW, Chen YC, Tsai JJ. Paroxysmal dyskinesia with secondary generalization of tonic-clonic seizures in pseudohypoparathyroidism. Epilepsia 2005;46:164–5.
161. Oechsner M, Pfeiffer G, Timmermann K, et al. Acute reversible encephalopathy with brain edema and serial seizures in pseudohypoparathyroidism. Nervenarzt 1996;67:875–9 [in German].
162. Graber ML. Magnesium deficiency: pathophysiologic and clinical overview. Am J Kidney Dis 1995;25:973.
163. Weiss-Guillet EM, Takala J, Jakob SM. Diagnosis and management of electrolyte emergencies. Best Pract Res Clin Endocrinol Metab 2003;17:623–51.
164. Tohme JF, Bilezikian JP. Hypocalcemic emergencies. Endocrinol Metab Clin North Am 1993;22:363–75.
165. Spinazze S, Schrijvers D. Metabolic emergencies. Crit Rev Oncol Hematol 2006;58:79–89.
166. Casez J, Pfammatter R, Nguyen Q, et al. Diagnostic approach to hypercalcemia: relevance of parathyroid hormone and parathyroid hormone-related protein measurements. Eur J Intern Med 2001;12:344–9.
167. Lafferty FW. Differential diagnosis of hypercalcemia. J Bone Miner Res 1991;6(Suppl 2):S51–9.
168. Fisken RA, Heath DA, Somers S, et al. Hypercalcaemia in hospital patients. Clinical and diagnostic aspects. Lancet 1981;1:202–7.

169. Wang CA, Guyton SW. Hyperparathyroid crisis: clinical and pathologic studies of 14 patients. Ann Surg 1979;190:782–90.
170. Nussbaum SR, Younger J, Vandepol CJ, et al. Single-dose intravenous therapy with pamidronate for the treatment of hypercalcemia of malignancy: comparison of 30-, 60-, and 90-mg dosages. Am J Med 1993;95:297–304.
171. Major P, Lortholary A, Hon J, et al. Zoledronic acid is superior to pamidronate in the treatment of hypercalcemia of malignancy: a pooled analysis of two random-ized, controlled clinical trials. J Clin Oncol 2001;19:558–67.
172. Croker JW, Walmsley RN. Routine plasma magnesium estimation: a useful test? Med J Aust 1986;145(71):74–6.
173. Ryzen E, Wagers PW, Singer FR, et al. Magnesium deficiency in a medical ICU population. Crit Care Med 1985;13:19–21.
174. Whang R, Ryder KW. Frequency of hypomagnesemia and hypermagnesemia. Requested vs routine. JAMA 1990;263:3063–4.
175. Olerich MA, Rude RK. Should we supplement magnesium in critically ill patients? New Horiz 1994;2:186–92.
176. Schilsky RL, Anderson T. Hypomagnesemia and renal magnesium wasting in patients receiving cisplatin. Ann Intern Med 1979;90:929–31.
177. Hauben M. Cyclosporine neurotoxicity. Pharmacotherapy 1996;16:576–83.
178. Barton CH, Pahl M, Vaziri ND, et al. Renal magnesium wasting associated with amphotericin B therapy. Am J Med 1984;77:471–4.
179. Nijenhuis T, Hoenderop JG, Bindels RJ. Downregulation of Ca(2+) and Mg(2+) transport proteins in the kidney explains tacrolimus (FK506)-induced hypercal-ciuria and hypomagnesemia. J Am Soc Nephrol 2004;15:549–57.
180. Schrag D, Chung KY, Flombaum C, et al. Cetuximab therapy and symptomatic hypomagnesemia. J Natl Cancer Inst 2005;97:1221–4.
181. Hoorn EJ, van der HJ, de Man RA, et al. A case series of proton pump inhibitor-induced hypomagnesemia. Am J Kidney Dis 2010;56:112–6.
182. Hall RC, Joffe JR. Hypomagnesemia. Physical and psychiatric symptoms. JAMA 1973;224:1749–51.
183. Hamed IA, Lindeman RD. Dysphagia and vertical nystagmus in magnesium deficiency. Ann Intern Med 1978;89:222–3.
184. Leicher CR, Mezoff AG, Hyams JS. Focal cerebral deficits in severe hypomag-nesemia. Pediatr Neurol 1991;7:380–1.
185. Birrer RB, Shallash AJ, Totten V. Hypermagnesemia-induced fatality following Epsom salt gargles (1). J Emerg Med 2002;22:185–8.
186. Rizzo MA, Fisher M, Lock JP. Hypermagnesemic pseudocoma. Arch Intern Med 1993;153:1130–2.
187. Knochel JP. The pathophysiology and clinical characteristics of severe hypo-phosphatemia. Arch Intern Med 1977;137:203–20.
188. King AL, Sica DA, Miller G, et al. Severe hypophosphatemia in a general hospital population. South Med J 1987;80:831–5.
189. Betro MG, Pain RW. Hypophosphataemia and hyperphosphataemia in a hospital population. Br Med J 1972;1:273–6.
190. Ryback RS, Eckardt MJ, Pautler CP. Clinical relationships between serum phos-phorus and other blood chemistry values in alcoholics. Arch Intern Med 1980;140:673–7.
191. Barak V, Schwartz A, Kalickman I, et al. Prevalence of hypophosphatemia in sepsis and infection: the role of cytokines. Am J Med 1998;104:40–7.
192. Territo MC, Tanaka KR. Hypophosphatemia in chronic alcoholism. Arch Intern Med 1974;134:445–7.

193. Jansen A, Velkeniers B. Neurological involvement in a case of hypophosphatemia. Eur J Intern Med 2003;14:326–8.
194. Lee JL, Sibbald WJ, Holliday RL, et al. Hypophosphatemia associated with coma. Can Med Assoc J 1978;119:143–5.
195. Prins JG, Schrijver H, Staghouwer JH. Hyperalimentation, hypophosphataemia, and coma. Lancet 1973;1:1253–4.
196. Aubier M, Murciano D, Lecocguic Y, et al. Effect of hypophosphatemia on diaphragmatic contractility in patients with acute respiratory failure. N Engl J Med 1985;313:420–4.
197. Knochel JP. The clinical status of hypophosphatemia: an update. N Engl J Med 1985;313:447–9.
198. Newman JH, Neff TA, Ziporin P. Acute respiratory failure associated with hypophosphatemia. N Engl J Med 1977;296:1101–3.
199. Falcone N, Compagnoni A, Meschini C, et al. Central pontine myelinolysis induced by hypophosphatemia following Wernicke's encephalopathy. Neurol Sci 2004;24:407–10.
200. Michell AW, Burn DJ, Reading PJ. Central pontine myelinolysis temporally related to hypophosphataemia. J Neurol Neurosurg Psychiatry 2003;74:820.
201. Vanneste J, Hage J. Acute severe hypophosphataemia mimicking Wernicke's encephalopathy. Lancet 1986;1:44.
202. Vannatta JB, Whang R, Papper S. Efficacy of intravenous phosphorus therapy in the severely hypophosphatemic patient. Arch Intern Med 1981;141:885–7.
203. Agardh CD, Kalimo H, Olsson Y, et al. Hypoglycemic brain injury: metabolic and structural findings in rat cerebellar cortex during profound insulin-induced hypoglycemia and in the recovery period following glucose administration. J Cereb Blood Flow Metab 1981;1:71–84.
204. LaManna JC, Harik SI. Regional comparisons of brain glucose influx. Brain Res 1985;326:299–305.
205. Carroll MF, Burge MR, Schade DS. Severe hypoglycemia in adults. Rev Endocr Metab Disord 2003;4:149–57.
206. DCCT Hypoglycemia in the Diabetes Control and Complications Trial. The Diabetes Control and Complications Trial Research Group. Diabetes 1997;46:271–86.
207. Shorr RI, Ray WA, Daugherty JR, et al. Incidence and risk factors for serious hypoglycemia in older persons using insulin or sulfonylureas. Arch Intern Med 1997;157:1681–6.
208. Laing SP, Swerdlow AJ, Slater SD, et al. The British Diabetic Association Cohort Study, II: cause-specific mortality in patients with insulin-treated diabetes mellitus. Diabet Med 1999;16:466–71.
209. Frier BM. Morbidity of hypoglycemia in type 1 diabetes. Diabetes Res Clin Pract 2004;65(Suppl 1):S47–52.
210. Auer RN, Wieloch T, Olsson Y, et al. The distribution of hypoglycemic brain damage. Acta Neuropathol (Berl) 1984;64:177–91.
211. Auer RN, Kalimo H, Olsson Y, et al. The temporal evolution of hypoglycemic brain damage. I. Light- and electron-microscopic findings in the rat cerebral cortex. Acta Neuropathol (Berl) 1985;67:13–24.
212. Auer RN, Kalimo H, Olsson Y, et al. The temporal evolution of hypoglycemic brain damage. II. Light- and electron-microscopic findings in the hippocampal gyrus and subiculum of the rat. Acta Neuropathol (Berl) 1985;67:25–36.
213. Auer RN, Olsson Y, Siesjo BK. Hypoglycemic brain injury in the rat. Correlation of density of brain damage with the EEG isoelectric time: a quantitative study. Diabetes 1984;33:1090–8.

214. Agardh CD, Carlsson A, Linqvist M, et al. The effect of pronounced hypoglycemia on monoamine metabolism in rat brain. Diabetes 1979;28:804–9.

215. Agardh CD, Chapman AG, Pelligrino D, et al. Influence of severe hypoglycemia on mitochondrial and plasma membrane function in rat brain. J Neurochem 1982;38:662–8.

216. Bottcher J, Kunze A, Kurrat C, et al. Localized reversible reduction of apparent diffusion coefficient in transient hypoglycemia-induced hemiparesis. Stroke 2005;36:e20–2.

217. Cordonnier C, Oppenheim C, Lamy C, et al. Serial diffusion and perfusion-weighted MR in transient hypoglycemia. Neurology 2005;65:175.

218. Fujioka M, Okuchi K, Hiramatsu KI, et al. Specific changes in human brain after hypoglycemic injury. Stroke 1997;28:584–7.

219. Shirayama H, Ohshiro Y, Kinjo Y, et al. Acute brain injury in hypoglycaemia-induced hemiplegia. Diabet Med 2004;21:623–4.

220. Kossoff EH, Ichord RN, Bergin AM. Recurrent hypoglycemic hemiparesis and aphasia in an adolescent patient. Pediatr Neurol 2001;24:385–6.

221. Newman RP, Kinkel WR. Paroxysmal choreoathetosis due to hypoglycemia. Arch Neurol 1984;41:341–2.

222. Arieff AI, Carroll HJ. Nonketotic hyperosmolar coma with hyperglycemia: clinical features, pathophysiology, renal function, acid-base balance, plasma-cerebrospinal fluid equilibria and the effects of therapy in 37 cases. Medicine (Baltimore) 1972;51:73–94.

223. Duncan MB, Jabbari B, Rosenberg ML. Gaze-evoked visual seizures in nonketotic hyperglycemia. Epilepsia 1991;32:221–4.

224. Hennis A, Corbin D, Fraser H. Focal seizures and non-ketotic hyperglycaemia. J Neurol Neurosurg Psychiatry 1992;55:195–7.

225. Venna N, Sabin T. Tonic focal seizures in nonketotic hyperglycemia of diabetes mellitus. Arch Neurol 1981;38(8):512–4.

226. Oh SH, Lee KY, Im JH, et al. Chorea associated with non-ketotic hyperglycemia and hyperintensity basal ganglia lesion on T1-weighted brain MRI study: a meta-analysis of 53 cases including four present cases. J Neurol Sci 2002; 200:57–62.

227. Lin JJ, Lin GY, Shih C, et al. Presentation of striatal hyperintensity on T1-weighted MRI in patients with hemiballism-hemichorea caused by non-ketotic hyperglycemia: report of seven new cases and a review of literature. J Neurol 2001;248:750–5.

228. Chang MH, Li JY, Lee SR, et al. Non-ketotic hyperglycaemic chorea: a SPECT study. J Neurol Neurosurg Psychiatry 1996;60:428–30.

229. Pisani A, Diomedi M, Rum A, et al. Acanthocytosis as a predisposing factor for non-ketotic hyperglycaemia induced chorea-ballism. J Neurol Neurosurg Psychiatry 2005;76:1717–9.

230. Vivian EM. Type 2 diabetes in children and adolescents–the next epidemic? Curr Med Res Opin 2006;22:297–306.

231. Fishbein HA, Palumbo PJ. Acute metabolic complications in diabetes. In: Diabetes in America. National Diabetes Data Group, National Institutes of Health; 1995. p. 283.

232. Carchman RM, Dechert-Zeger M, Calikoglu AS, et al. A new challenge in pediatric obesity: pediatric hyperglycemic hyperosmolar syndrome. Pediatr Crit Care Med 2005;6:20–4.

233. Fourtner SH, Weinzimer SA, Levitt Katz LE. Hyperglycemic hyperosmolar non-ketotic syndrome in children with type 2 diabetes*. Pediatr Diabetes 2005;6:129–35.

234. Morales AE, Rosenbloom AL. Death caused by hyperglycemic hyperosmolar state at the onset of type 2 diabetes. J Pediatr 2004;144:270–3.
235. Arieff AI, Carroll HJ. Cerebral edema and depression of sensorium in nonketotic hyperosmolar coma. Diabetes 1974;23:525–31.
236. Tachibana Y, Yasuhara A. Hyperosmolar syndrome and diffuse CNS dysfunction with clinical implications. Funct Neurol 1986;1:140–55.
237. Tiamkao S, Pratipanawatr T, Tiamkao S, et al. Seizures in nonketotic hyperglycaemia. Seizure 2003;12:409–10.
238. Chiasson JL, Aris-Jilwan N, Belanger R, et al. Diagnosis and treatment of diabetic ketoacidosis and the hyperglycemic hyperosmolar state. CMAJ 2003; 168:859–66.
239. Arieff AI, Kleeman CR. Studies on mechanisms of cerebral edema in diabetic comas. Effects of hyperglycemia and rapid lowering of plasma glucose in normal rabbits. J Clin Invest 1973;52:571–83.
240. Arieff AI, Kleeman CR. Cerebral edema in diabetic comas. II. Effects of hyperosmolality, hyperglycemia and insulin in diabetic rabbits. J Clin Endocrinol Metab 1974;38:1057–67.
241. Rothstein JD, Garland W, Puia G, et al. Purification and characterization of naturally occurring benzodiazepine receptor ligands in rat and human brain. J Neurochem 1992;58:2102–15.
242. Lugaresi E, Montagna P, Tinuper P, et al. Endozepine stupor. Recurring stupor linked to endozepine-4 accumulation. Brain 1998;121(Pt 1):127–33.
243. Chen R, Rothstein JD, Frey KA, et al. Idiopathic recurring stupor: a new syndrome? Neurology 1995;45(Suppl 4). Ref Type: Abstract.
244. Tinuper P, Montagna P, Cortelli P, et al. Idiopathic recurring stupor: a case with possible involvement of the gamma-aminobutyric acid (GABA)ergic system. Ann Neurol 1992;31:503–6.
245. Cortelli P, Avallone R, Baraldi M, et al. Endozepines in recurrent stupor. Sleep Med Rev 2005;9:477–87.
246. Rothstein JD, Garland W, Puia G, et al. The role of endogenous benzodiazepine receptor ligands in physiology and pathology. In: Barnard EA, Costa E, editors. Transmitter amino acid receptors: structures, transduction and models for drug development. New York: Thieme Medical Publishers; 1991. p. 325–39.
247. Rothstein JD, Guidotti A, Tinuper P, et al. Endogenous benzodiazepine receptor ligands in idiopathic recurring stupor. Lancet 1992;340:1002–4.
248. Sansing LH, Tuzun E, Ko MW, et al. A patient with encephalitis associated with NMDA receptor antibodies. Nat Clin Pract Neurol 2007;3:291–6.
249. Dalmau J, Lancaster E, Martinez-Hernandez E, et al. Clinical experience and laboratory investigations in patients with anti-NMDAR encephalitis. Lancet Neurol 2011;10:63–74.
250. Wong-Kisiel LC, Ji T, Renaud DL, et al. Response to immunotherapy in a 20-month-old boy with anti-NMDA receptor encephalitis. Neurology 2010;74:1550–1.
251. Day GS, High SM, Cot B, et al. Anti-NMDA-receptor encephalitis: case report and literature review of an under-recognized condition. J Gen Intern Med 2011;26(7):811–6.
252. Dalmau J, Gleichman AJ, Hughes EG, et al. Anti-NMDA-receptor encephalitis: case series and analysis of the effects of antibodies. Lancet Neurology 2008; 12:1091–8.
253. Irani SR, Bera K, Waters P, et al. N-methyl-D-aspartate antibody encephalitis: temporal progression of clinical and paraclinical observations in a predominantly non-paraneoplastic disorder of both sexes. Brain 2010;133:1655–67.

254. Soupart A, Penninckx R, Crenier L, et al. Prevention of brain demyelination in rats after excessive correction of chronic hyponatremia by serum sodium lowering. Kidney Int 1994;45:193–200.
255. Finelli PF. Diffusion-weighted MR in hypoglycemic coma. Neurology 2001; 57:933.
256. Chan R, Erbay S, Oljeski S, et al. Case report: hypoglycemia and diffusion-weighted imaging. J Comput Assist Tomogr 2003;27:420–3.
257. Maekawa S, Aibiki M, Kikuchi K, et al. Time related changes in reversible MRI findings after prolonged hypoglycemia. Clin Neurol Neurosurg 2005;108(5): 511–3.
258. Yoneda Y, Yamamoto S. Cerebral cortical laminar necrosis on diffusion-weighted MRI in hypoglycaemic encephalopathy. Diabet Med 2005;22:1098–100.
259. Jung SL, Kim BS, Lee KS, et al. Magnetic resonance imaging and diffusion-weighted imaging changes after hypoglycemic coma. J Neuroimaging 2005; 15:193–6.
260. Cho SJ, Minn YK, Kwon KH. Severe hypoglycemia and vulnerability of the brain. Arch Neurol 2006;63:138.
261. Kang EG, Jeon SJ, Choi SS, et al. Diffusion MR imaging of hypoglycemic encephalopathy. AJNR Am J Neuroradiol 2010;31:559–64.
262. Katzman R, Pappius HM. Brain electrolytes and fluid metabolism. Philadelphia (PA): Williams & Wilkins; 1973. p. 419.

Trauma and Impaired Consciousness

Sandrine de Ribaupierre, MD

KEYWORDS

- Traumatic brain injury • Concussion • Diffuse axonal injury
- Vegetative state • Consciousness • Coma

Consciousness has been defined by many investigators as the combination of wakefulness, consisting of arousal or the capacity for consciousness, and awareness, consisting of the content of consciousness itself.[1–4]

Arousal is based on mechanisms of the ascending reticular activating system in the brainstem, whereas the content of consciousness depends on the integrity of the limbic structures (hypothalamus, amygdala, hippocampus, cingulum, septal area, and basal forebrain), as well as the thalamus and basal ganglia.[5] The reticular formation has three ascending pathways. The first projects to the cortex via the thalamus (mostly the intralaminar nuclei) and is inhibitory.[6] The second projects to the basal forebrain and limbic system through the hypothalamus.[7] The third projects broadly through the neocortex through norepinephrine neurons of the locus ceruleus[8–10] and serotonin neurons of the midbrain raphe.[11]

In addition, recent studies on consciousness and vegetative states have shown the presence of a "default mode network" that is active when someone is at rest but modified when the person is in a decreased level of consciousness.[12] This network has been identified with functional MRI (fMRI) and is composed of the precuneus, the temporoparietal junction, and the medial prefrontal cortex.[13]

Therefore, the integrity of both systems, as well as a working connection between the two, is essential for an individual to experience normal consciousness. In turn, this relies on the functionality of the cells in those areas (mostly the neurons), and on the availability of various neurotransmitters. Other physiologic effects on the neurons mean that the composition of the extracellular space is also important in determining function.

Whereas the ascending reticular activating system has a large part of its function determined by acetylcholine and glutamate receptors, the hypothalamus has histaminergic receptors, the raphe nuclei depend more on serotonin, and the transmitters are noradrenergic for the locus coeruleus and cholinergic for the basal forebrain.[8–11]

The author has nothing to disclose.

Division of Neurosurgery, Department of Clinical Neurological Sciences, University of Western Ontario, Victoria Hospital, 800 Commissioners Road East, London, ON N6A 5W9, Canada

E-mail address: Sandrine.deRibaupierre@lhsc.on.ca

After trauma, whereas a local injury will result in a focal deficit, a more diffuse cortical injury, either with wide bilateral cortical lesions or something acting on the brainstem-activating centers, is required for a perturbation of consciousness.[14,15]

There are different levels of impaired consciousness. Whereas some are transient, like the loss of consciousness in a concussion, some are more permanent, as seen in neuronal death. They can also be classified into acute and chronic phases, or described as increasingly more impaired states such as confusional state, delirium, obtundation, stupor, vegetative state, akinetic mutism, coma, and brain death (**Box 1**). Some investigators add locked-in syndrome, but this is controversial because such patients are fully conscious but lack a way of communicating. A new definition, written by a multidisciplinary working group addressing the "minimally conscious state," allows for some variability of the state of the patient. In that state, the patient might follow simple commands or show some other purposeful attitude although he or she otherwise seems to be in a vegetative state.[16] The term vegetative state was first used by Jennett and Plum[17] to describe a set of patients who were unresponsive but not in a coma. In 1994, a task force redefined the term to a "wakeful unconscious state."[18,19] In some countries, such as United Kingdom, it is further categorized into two groups: persistent vegetative state, when the patient is in that condition for more than 4 weeks, and permanent vegetative state, when the patient has been in that state for more than 12 months after a traumatic brain injury (TBI).

Lately the understanding of unresponsive patients has greatly improved with the study by Owen and Coleman.[21] Their experiments using fMRI in patients previously

---

Box 1
States of impaired consciousness

Confusion

Deficit in attention, with disorientation to time, person, and/or place. The alertness is usually normal.

Obtundation

Mild reduction in alertness, slower responses to stimulation.

Stupor

Can be aroused by vigorous stimuli, decreased reaction to external stimuli.

Akinetic mutism

No spontaneous motor activity, patient seems alert however. Seen in bilateral cingulate-septal area, or thalamus or hypothalamus lesions.[20]

Minimally conscious state

Might follow some simple commands inconsistently; variable neurologic status. Decreased reaction to external stimuli. Closer to a vegetative state than to an awake state.

Vegetative state

The "wakeful unconscious state." Some eye opening, no response to commands, some sleep-awake cycle. Preserved autonomic functions. Might have some preserved cognitive function but unable to interact with environment.

Coma

Cannot be aroused, no response to external stimuli. No voluntary movements.

Brain death

No cortical, subcortical, or brainstem function remaining.

deemed to be vegetative have shown that some of them have more preserved cognitive functions than previously thought.

TRAUMA

TBI can be caused by a direct blow to the head, or as the result of an acceleration-deceleration force transmitted to the head causing a distortion of the brain. Penetrating injuries (firearms) is the last category with a more complex mechanism (focal and blast injury). There are different levels of severity that can be further classified as focal or more diffuse injuries.

Primary brain injury is directly linked to the affect of the trauma, whereby the mechanical forces will affect different parts of the brain depending on their nature. A compression force will lead to a focal neuronal or vascular injury, whereas acceleration-deceleration or rotational forces will lead to shearing of axons and diffuse axonal injury (DAI).

Secondary brain injury is linked to both the systemic and the brain reactions to the trauma. Well known and illustrated are the effects of hypoxia and hypotension when there is a systemic injury necessitating resuscitation[22–25]; however, there is also a local cascade of events within the brain itself that is responsible for some secondary injuries.

This secondary cascade of events is not completely understood yet. Among other factors, there is a release of neurotransmitters, an inflammatory response, but also an ischemic-reperfusion problem as seen in stroke.[26]

Most patients will develop secondary brain injury and demonstrate signs and symptoms such as cerebral edema and raised intracranial pressure (ICP).[27–30]

Pathophysiology

The pathophysiology of impaired consciousness is first described. There is no strict rule as to which pathologic events occur in each category of trauma but, more likely, there is a continuum of progressive severity. Therefore, a proposed cascade of events is described and then summarized for each specific category. With increased severity of the trauma and increased progression through the cascade, there is a transition from transient to permanent deficit, as well as from functional to structural lesions.

Directly after the trauma there is a cascade of events, including deregulation of cellular metabolism and cerebral blood flow, disruption of the extracellular and intracellular ions, and the release of neurotransmitters.

Axonal stretching and shearing leads to an acute release of *neurotransmitters* that are mostly excitatory (glutamate). Stimulation of the neurons by neurotransmitters creates a subsequent efflux of potassium. This extracellular potassium triggers neuronal depolarization, increasing the efflux of potassium ions (K^+) and influx of sodium ions (Na^+), as well as the release of more neurotransmitters. To return to baseline, there is a need for extra work from the Na^+-K^+ pump[31–33] to pump the sodium out and the potassium in. The increased ATP requirements of the pumps lead to a global increase in glucose metabolism.[31] However, because of the recent trauma, the brain is also in a state of diminished blood flow and impaired autoregulation[34,35] and the resulting increased demand leads to an energy crisis.

The increased energy need also leads to accelerated glycolysis, producing more lactate.[36] Again, in the context of diminished blood flow, there will be an increase of regional lactate levels that will then lead to further neuronal dysfunction because of the acidosis, membrane damage, altered blood brain barrier permeability, and cerebral edema. Following the initial hypermetabolism, there is a decrease in brain metabolism.

Changes in electrolytes

As discussed above, the shearing of neurons produces an efflux of K^+, which then leads to an increase in excitability of the neurons and further efflux of K^+. A high K^+ concentration will then impede neuronal activity and is thought to be part of the phenomenon of concussion.[37]

Experiments that modeled concussion by a blow to the vertex of the heads of mice and rats showed that the impact was followed by an increase of about 4 Mmol/L of cortical and brainstem K^+. This lead to an episode of apnea, bradycardia, and low-voltage electroencephalogram (EEG) that spontaneously recovered within a few minutes. In the group that succumbed to the injury, the extracellular K^+ increased continuously after the impact until greater than 50 Mmol/L.[37]

The release of neurotransmitters, especially excitatory amino acids, activates N-methyl-D-aspartate receptors,[38,39] enabling intravasation of calcium ions (Ca^{2+}). Calcium accumulation is seen within hours and persists for 2 to 4 days.[40] With an increase axonal Ca^{2+} concentration, there is a risk for microtubules to break down, leading to more accumulation of organelles at the site of the axonal damage, and finally to secondary axotomy.[41–43] However, an increase in intracellular Ca^{2+} concentration does not always lead to axonal death.[40]

That cascade of events also leads to a decrease of intracellular magnesium ions (Mg^{2+}), which can remain depressed for up to 4 days. This may be responsible for neuronal dysfunction because of impaired glycolytic and oxidative generation of ATP, which is magnesium-dependent.[44–47]

Cerebrovascular reactivity

To keep a constant cerebral blood volume and flow, the brain has different mechanisms. One is the cerebrovascular reactivity, which is the capacity of the walls of the cerebral arteries to react to changes of transmural pressure, and dilate when the CPP is low. When the reactivity is intact, if the systemic pressure is high, there is a vasoconstriction leading to a reduction of cerebral blood volume and, therefore, a decrease in ICP. However, if the reactivity is impaired, such as seen in some brain injuries, then the ICP will directly follow the systemic blood pressure, and increase when the systemic blood pressure increases. As studied by Zweifel and colleagues,[48] the cerebrovascular pressure reactivity index seems to correlate with outcome after trauma.

Cerebral perfusion pressure autoregulation

Autoregulation is another mechanism by which the brain can maintain a constant cerebral blood flow even during variation of the systemic blood pressure. To meet the brain's oxygen requirements, the blood flow is relatively constant. It varies depending on the nature of the tissue, but is around 50 mL/100 g globally [30–45 mL/100 g for white, 75 mL/100 g for gray matter].[49] A significant decrease will lead to permanent damage if the flow is less than 10 to 15 mL/100 mg.[50] In a normal subject, this autoregulation phenomenon can maintain the cerebral blood flow constant when the mean arterial blood pressure is between 50 and 150 mm Hg.[51]

After severe trauma, 49% to 87% of patients have impaired autoregulation[3,52,53] and, therefore, cannot regulate their cerebral blood flow. This deficit can lead to either ischemia or hyperemia, and secondary brain lesions after the trauma.[51,52,54] The loss of autoregulation will lead to the congestion of the vascular compartment. The lack of autoregulation is not uniform across the brain, and increases with more severe injuries.[55]

TYPES OF TRAUMA
Concussion

Concussion can be caused by a direct blow or an indirect force to the head, leading to the rapid onset of transient neurologic impairment. It is diagnosed based on a series of symptoms, not all of them needing to be present, such as loss of consciousness immediately after the impact, headaches, nausea and vomiting, confusion, disorientation, attention deficit, dizziness, and unsteadiness.[31] The loss of consciousness is not considered a necessary prerequisite for the diagnosis of concussion.[56] Because the symptoms seen after a concussion are transient, they must be based on a temporary neuronal disturbance instead of neuronal damage or death.[31] Clinically, the unresponsive patient has reactive pupils, ocular reflexes, is eupneic, and more or less flaccid. He or she can experience a period of confusion after the initial loss of consciousness, which is a nonspecific symptom. After recovery, the patient can experience acute postconcussive symptoms that can last from a few hours to a few days, including headaches, visual disturbances, nausea, vomiting, and amnesia.[57] More subtle symptoms (chronic headaches, sensibility to noise or light, memory and attention deficits, irritability) can last for months.[58–60]

Concussion is frequent, because 8% to 19% of sport-related injuries involve a loss of consciousness.[61] Most patients (65%) are between the ages of 5 and18 years. By definition, they have a negative CT scan and anatomic MRI. There are different grading systems to describe concussion depending on the duration of the loss of consciousness and the posttraumatic amnesia (eg, those of the American Academy of Neurology and Colorado Medical Society).[1,62–71] These are based on consensus of experts and are not evidenced-based. Nonetheless, the real and cumulative effect on the brain of concussion has lead an increasing number of sport league to adopt the guidelines.

Because of the prevalence of the injury in athletes, concussion and neuropsychology are increasingly studied clinically and with the use of other imaging technologies. There is typically some pressure within team-based sporting organizations (amateur or professional) for the player to return to play.[72] However, cases of death after a second small impact have lead to more cautious guidelines.[72–74] After an initial trauma, the brain is prone to malignant edema after another small impact. This is usually seen in children and adolescents, but can also be seen in adults.[75–78]

A pediatric study on mild and moderate TBI has shown changes in fractional anisotropy (see below) relatively soon after the injury—from a few days up to 6 to 12 months postinjury[79] in patients who had a normal or near normal anatomic MRI.[79,80]

Pathophysiology

A variety of theories has been published on concussion. In conjunction with and addition to the events described above, here is a brief summary of the different theories.[81,82] One of the first described is the *vascular hypothesis*, now a defunct theory.[83] It was believed that the impact would cause the brain to compress some vessels leading to an arrest of the cerebral blood flow and, therefore, the symptoms were occurring because of an episode of cerebral ischemia. Researchers have also portrayed a *convulsive hypothesis*, in which the impact would result in a diffuse depolarization (mechanically induced) leading to a synchronized discharge as seen in general epilepsy.[82] The *reticular hypothesis* is based on the activity of the reticular activating system in the brainstem, which would be temporarily disturbed by the impact.[84] Similarly, the *pontine cholinergic system hypothesis* implies that only the inhibitory cholinergic system within the dorsal pontine tegmentum would be affected by the impact.[85] The last common hypothesis is the *centripetal hypothesis*, which suggests that the impact leads to a functional disconnection of neurons in a centripetal fashion and, therefore, a small impact would affect only the cortico-subcortical areas, whereas a greater impact would also affect the central structures. Whereas a smaller impact would be transient, a greater one would lead to irreversible damage. The latter theory is in agreement with a continuum of severity in the lesions and depicts the concussion as a mild DAI.[86]

DAI

Patients diagnosed with DAI have an immediate loss of consciousness and remain at a low GCS for a variable amount of time, from a few hours to a few months, or may never regain awareness. The impact of the trauma is such that the axons have been stretched or disrupted by the sudden acceleration-deceleration or rotational forces.[87,88] Typically DAI is found in frontal and temporal regions, as well as in the corpus callosum and the upper brainstem.[89]

In 1974, Ommaya and Gennarelli[81] postulated that TBI followed a centripetal model: the periphery of the brain is more prone to damage and, therefore, already damaged with a mild injury, whereas deeper structures need more force to be damaged. It was found that the depth of the parenchymal lesions seen on MRI were directly related to the duration of impaired consciousness and that deeper lesions (corpus callosum or brainstem) also correlated with a greater degree of impaired consciousness.[2] These findings are consistent with the grading system of DAI, introduced by Adams and colleagues[89] in 1989, depending whether they affect the hemisphere (Grade I), the corpus callosum (Grade II), or the brainstem (Grade III).

There is evidence that in DAI, as in concussion, neurons encounter secondary injuries after the initial impact, because of biochemical cascades that are more marked in their activation than in less severe injuries.[90,91] Neuronal damage is followed by the appearance of secondary lesions that are not seen on the first images owing to loss of white matter over time. Positron emission tomography (PET) studies using [18F] fluorodeoxyglucose and flumazenil in DAI patients also showed focal damage mostly in the medial frontal gyrus, the cingulate gyrus, and the thalamus.[92]

Focal Lesions

In the more focal brain lesions, such subdural and epidural hematomas and contusions (**Figs. 1–3**), the decreased level of consciousness is due to the mass effect exerted by the lesion directly on the diencephalon, mesencephalon, or brainstem, and/or by the increased ICP due to the volume of the lesion leading to herniation (discussed elsewhere in this issue). There are three types of supratentorial herniation that might cause impaired consciousness: cingulate (subfalcial; see **Fig. 1**), central, or uncal. Herniations (**Box 2**) might then contribute to an obstructive hydrocephalus or a compressive vascular problem (ischemia from arterial compression or venous engorgement). With an infratentorial mass effect, there is direct compression of the brainstem and the clinical examination will demonstrate the level of the injury: mitotic pupils and absent caloric reflex in the case of a pons compression, wheras a compression of the midbrain will produce midposition fixed pupils.

INVESTIGATIONS
Imaging

Advances in technology have made the recognition and diagnosis of some pathology easier. For example, DAIs were not seen on CT scan and, therefore, patients were diagnosed on the bases of history, clinical symptoms, and the absence of lesions

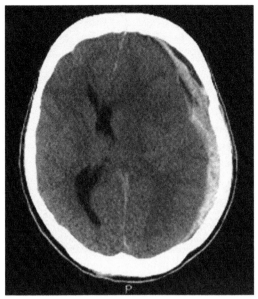

Fig. 1. Axial CT scan showing a left acute subdural shift with a significant mass effect on the ventricle and a midline shift with a subfalcine herniation. The patient presented with an impaired level of consciousness (GCS of 4) after a motor vehicle accident.

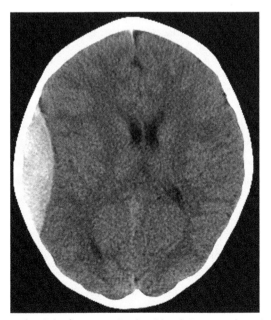

Fig. 2. Axial CT scan of a right fronto-parietal epidural. Because there is only a focal mass effect from the clot, there is no decreased level of consciousness in this patient.

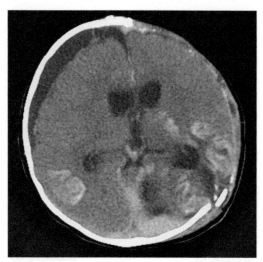

Fig. 3. Axial CT scan of a pediatric patient who required a left hemicraniectomy after a trauma. The CT scan shows bilateral contusions and the ICP was refractory to all the medical treatments. There was significant left-sided edema with a midline shift preoperatively which was corrected by allowing the brain to have more room by removing the bone on the left.

on CT scan. Therefore, the final diagnosis was usually made at autopsy. With MRI technologies (T1 and T2 sequences), axonal tears with subsequent edema were discovered. Newer sequences such as FLAIR (fluid-attenuated inversion recovery) made the lesions more apparent[93] but, with the study of water diffusion through diffusion tensor imaging, more precise images of tracts could be obtained.

Whereas the CT scan is still the imaging modality of choice in the acute setting of a trauma, when the patient is unconscious, other imaging techniques are emerging. A CT scan results in irradiation and has a relatively poor resolution for small lesions. Although essential to rule out a large hemorrhagic lesion needing an adequate treatment, a CT scan does not detect DAIs. There are Canadian guidelines for indications for a CT scan after a head injury.[94]

Box 2
Herniation syndromes

Cingulate or subfalcine

> Compression of the ACA and internal cerebral veins. Obstruction of the Monro foramen interfering with cerebrospinal fluid circulation.

Central transtentorial

> Downward displacement of the diencephalon and midbrain. Compression of the PCA and the great cerebral veins leading to increased hydrostatic pressure. Compression of the aqueduct of Sylvius interfering with cerebrospinal fluid circulation.

Uncal

> Direct pressure on the midbrain, pushing the contralateral side against the tentorium, compressing the third nerve and the PCA.

Abbreviations: ACA, anterior cerebral artery; PCA, posterior cerebral artery.

Standard MRI sequences (T1-weighted, T2-weighted, and FLAIR images) can reveal small contusions as well as some of the DAIs. They allow for better discrimination of the structural lesions than a CT scan. Although not usually indicated when the neurologic status is normal after a concussion, some MRI studies have shown subacute and chronic changes with brain atrophy in more severe injuries (decrease in white matter and ventricular enlargement).[95,96]

The study of fiber tracts with diffusion tensor MRI, which takes advantage of the anisotropic motion of water within the axons, has enabled the identification of white matter tract disruption and, therefore, the detection of smaller areas of DAI. Maps of fractional anisotropy are disturbed when the sheaths of myelin are disrupted or when there is edema around the axons. Studies of mild TBIs have shown abnormalities in the genu of the corpus callosum (reduction in fractional anisotropy).[79,97,98] Although this finding is currently mostly used as a research tool,[61,88,99] it is progressively being used clinically in TBIs.[88,100,101] It might even be useful in follow-up for consciousness recovery after TBI and support the possible use of diffusion tensor imaging as a biomarker for early classification of patients.[102]

Proton magnetic resonance spectroscopy is a noninvasive way of looking at brain metabolites. Differences in ratio of metabolites as well the presence of some metabolites are the signature for neuronal or other cell injuries. Disruption of neurons will also lead to changes in metabolite regulation (eg, impaired mitochondrial energy production will reduce N-acetyl-aspartate (NAA), a neuronal marker, and membrane degradation might increase choline [Cho]). The presence of lactate indicates some degree of anaerobic metabolism. After trauma, a decrease in NAA to creatine (Cr) ratio, which is the signature for neuronal damage, has been shown in the corpus callosum,[103,104] in the brainstem, in basal ganglia,[105] and in and near contused areas.[106–108] In concussion, changes in the NAA to Cr ratio have been shown,[109,110] but those changes are transient, coming back to baseline within a few days[109,111] to months,[109,110,112] although it remains disturbed in more severe trauma. The Cho to Cr ratio, which is seen in membrane disruption, increases after TBI and remains high up to 6 months after the injury,[110,112,113] even in some concussion patients. This could be reflective of glial proliferation or inflammation in the perilesional region. Lactate to creatine (Lac to Cr) ratio was elevated during the first week after TBI.[56,113,114] Absolute peak value for glutamate to glutamine (Glx) and Cho were found to be significantly elevated in the occipital and parietal white matter early after injury in patients with poor long-term (6–12-month) outcomes in one study.[115] That study showed that Glx and Cho values predicted long-term outcome with 94% accuracy and, when combined with the motor GCS, score provided the highest predictive accuracy (97%), whereas somatosensory-evoked potentials (SSEPs) were not as accurate. Previous research suggests that magnetic resonance spectroscopy might be helpful in showing the true extent of axonal damage, especially when combined with MRI (T2*, FLAIR, and diffusion) images.[116]

The fMRI has been used to study a variety of brain injuries of varying severity. In concussion in athletes, studies have found different patterns of activity in patients versus controls[117–119] in tasks involving working memory.[119] For example, in patients with a severe TBI, those with a better recovery showed a near-normal activation pattern when completing a Tower of London task (prefrontal and parietal activation), whereas the patients with a worse recovery had an inconsistent pattern of activation and poor behavioral performance.[120] Nevertheless, fMRI is used mostly as a research tool.

Single-photon emission computed tomography (SPECT) has been used in trauma to look at cerebral blood flow and has shown abnormalities in the medial temporal lobe.[121] However, this involves exposure to radioisotopes. Furthermore, SPECT is qualitative, not quantitative, and compares regions of the brain to each other. It is not sensitive to a global disturbance.[122]

PET is used to observe the metabolism of the brain, usually using fluorodeoxyglucose. Some studies have shown that there are differences in patients who have had a concussion compared with controls with a reduced mesial temporal metabolism,[121] as well as more globally in the frontal and temporal cortex.[123,124] Some studies have also shown a decrease in the global glucose metabolism for up to 4 weeks after injury, without correlation with the GCS. PET is currently used only as a research tool and not clinically.

EEG and Evoked and Event-Related Potentials

Spontaneous brain activity can be measured with EEG and has been shown to be perturbed in TBI, correlating with severity and outcome.[125] Although EEG is usually not used in acute brain injuries, it has been studied in animal models and has shown a significant decrease in amplitude.[126,127] Bispectral index, which is been used in the operating room to record the depth of general anesthesia, has been used in a study and showed some correlation with outcome.[128] One of the main applications is in the detection of seizures in patients with TBI. Most seizures are nonconvulsive and can only be detected by continuous EEG monitoring (ideally for 48 hours after the patient is admitted to the ICU).[129] There is mounting evidence that such seizures occur in more than 20% of TBI patients in the ICU[130] and can contribute to brain damage.[131]

Measures of EEG variability have been explored by Vespa and colleagues[130] and appear to have prognostic value: low alpha variability is associated with thalamic damage and poor outcomes.

Reduction of spontaneous and evoked cortical electrical activity has been identified in an ischemic model[132–135] as well as in TBI.[136–138] Reduction of cortical activity after trauma has been described as "spreading depression." It is a transient phenomenon, however, seen in conjunction with changes in interstitial ion concentration, blood flow, and metabolism.[139] Although animal models have shown that provoked spreading depression in normal brain does not automatically lead to cell death,[139] it might still be involved in secondary injury mechanism.[138]

Evoked potentials have been used clinically to try to predict the outcome by testing some pathways in the brainstem. Although they are, by definition, less global than EEG, they are also less perturbed by the anesthetic drugs given to the patient.[140] The absence of SSEPs from the primary sensory cortex has a strong association with poor outcome.[141] Because the brainstem is an essential part of the nervous system, measures of dysfunction of the brainstem auditory pathways (brainstem auditory-evoked potentials) in the mesencephalon and pons are relatively helpful in prognosticating outcome.[142–146]

Event-related potentials rely on the brain to discriminate sounds or words and require more complex processing than SSEPs or auditory-evoked potentials. Their presence may indicate a more favorable outcome. Mismatch negativity can even be performed on clinically unresponsive patients in the acute phase.[147]

MANAGEMENT

After a concussion, patients should be careful not to have a second impact injury (**Box 3**). When playing sports, they should restrain from practicing until completely asymptomatic, then gradually return to play, depending on their symptoms (or lack of symptoms).[72] Nonathletes can gradually start their activity again when they are asymptomatic. Individuals with long-lasting symptoms could benefit from neuropsychological testing.[148]

Box 3
Management of unresponsive patient in a trauma situation

Airway or **Breathing**: oxygenation, make sure the airways are clear

Circulation: monitor and keep the blood pressure within normal range if possible; cervical-spine precautions if necessary

Glucose: check or administer; if unknown circumstances, keep in mind that the patient may have fallen following hypoglycemia

ICP: if signs it is raised (pupil asymmetry), lower by administrating mannitol or 3% saline

Stop seizures

Restore electrolytes and acid-base balance

Adjust body temperature

Thiamine, because the patient might have fallen due to alcohol influence and have a chronic condition

Specific antidotes if the cause of the trauma is unclear and the patient might be under some drug influence

---

Patients with more severe injury are scanned to assess the necessity of a neurosurgical intervention. When the GCS is lower than eight and the imaging is abnormal, a pressure monitoring probe is usually inserted.[149] The ICP can, therefore, be monitored and treated if necessary.[150,151] Lesions creating mass effect will need to be evacuated surgically. Hemispheric edema with raised ICP refractory to medical treatment (hypertonic saline, mannitol, etc) might require a hemicraniectomy.[152,153]

Abnormal cerebral autoregulation can also be monitored using continuous Trans-Cranial Doppler ultrasonography, or Pressure Reactivity index monitoring.[51] The Pressure Reactivity index is the slope of the regression line relating mean arterial blood pressure and ICP[154] Near Infrared Spectroscopy (NIRS) is progressively being investigated and used to monitor the cerebral blood flow or brain oxygenation. It is based on the different absorption characteristics of oxyhemoglobin and desoxyhemoglobin.[155–159] These new techniques to monitor patients are currently still research-oriented, but they could become clinical tools in the near future.

SUMMARY

Traumatic brain injury can affect consciousness by different mechanisms, depending on the type of trauma. Since there is an increasing severity in the repercussion of trauma: concussion, focal lesions and diffuse axonal injuries, they will affect the level of consciousness differently. With the increasing number of investigation tools developed, the mechanism per which the decrease level of consciousness occurs in trauma is better understood. Correlations, in different studies, between levels of metabolites, brain networks in functional MRI, EEG and Event-Related Potentials, and Fractional Anisotropy, for example, and outcome, might lead, in a near future, to the developments of new techniques and tools to enable physicians to provide more accurate prognosis.

REFERENCES

1. Kelly JP. Loss of consciousness: pathophysiology and implications in grading and safe return to play. J Athl Train 2001;36(3):249–52.

2. Levin HS, Williams D, Crofford MJ, et al. Relationship of depth of brain lesions to consciousness and outcome after closed head injury. J Neurosurg 1988;69(6): 861–6.
3. Plum F, Brennan RW. Dissociation of autoregulation and chemical regulation in cerebral circulation following seizures. Trans Am Neurol Assoc 1970;95:27–30.
4. Teasdale G, Jennett B. Assessment of coma and impaired consciousness. A practical scale. Lancet 1974;2(7872):81–4.
5. Plum F, Posner JB. The diagnosis of stupor and coma. New York: Oxford University Press; 1982.
6. Yingling CD, Skinner JE. Regulation of unit activity in nucleus reticularis thalami by the mesencephalic reticular formation and the frontal granular cortex. Electroencephalogr Clin Neurophysiol 1975;39(6):635–42.
7. Saper CB, Swanson LW, Cowan WM. The efferent connections of the anterior hypothalamic area of the rat, cat and monkey. J Comp Neurol 1978;182(4):575–99.
8. Jones BE, Harper ST, Halaris AE. Effects of locus coeruleus lesions upon cerebral monoamine content, sleep-wakefulness states and the response to amphetamine in the cat. Brain Res 1977;124(3):473–96.
9. Jones BE, Moore RY. Ascending projections of the locus coeruleus in the rat. II. Autoradiographic study. Brain Res 1977;127(1):25–53.
10. Levitt P, Moore RY. Noradrenaline neuron innervation of the neocortex in the rat. Brain Res 1978;139(2):219–31.
11. Moore RY, Halaris AE, Jones BE. Serotonin neurons of the midbrain raphe: ascending projections. J Comp Neurol 1978;180(3):417–38.
12. Cruse D, Owen A. Consciousness revealed: new insights into the vegetative and minimally conscious states. Curr Opin Neurol 2010;23(6):656–60.
13. Gusnard DA, Raichle ME. Searching for a baseline: functional imaging and the resting human brain. Nat Rev Neurosci 2001;2(10):685–94.
14. Crompton MR, Teare RD, Bowern DA. Prolonged coma after head injury. Lancet 1966;2(7470):938–40.
15. Jellinger K, Seitelberger F. Protracted post-traumatic encephalopathy. Pathology, pathogenesis and clinical implications. J Neurol Sci 1970;10(1):51–94.
16. Giacino JT, Ashwal S, Childs N, et al. The minimally conscious state: definition and diagnostic criteria. Neurology 2002;58(3):349–53.
17. Jennett B, Plum F. Persistent vegetative state after brain damage. A syndrome in search of a name. Lancet 1972;1(7753):734–7.
18. Medical aspects of the persistent vegetative state (2). The Multi-Society Task Force on PVS. N Engl J Med 1994;330(22):1572–9.
19. Medical aspects of the persistent vegetative state (1). The Multi-Society Task Force on PVS. N Engl J Med 1994;330(21):1499–508.
20. Buge A, Escourolle R, Rancurel G, et al. Akinetic mutism and bicingular softening. 3 anatomo-clinical cases. Rev Neurol (Paris) 1975;131(2):121–31 [in French].
21. Owen A, Coleman MR. Functional MRI in disorders of consciousness: advantages and limitations. Curr Opin Neurol 2007;20(17992081):632–7.
22. Bayir H, Clark RS, Kochanek PM. Promising strategies to minimize secondary brain injury after head trauma. Crit Care Med 2003;31(Suppl 1):S112–7.
23. Bayir H, Kochanek PM, Clark RS. Traumatic brain injury in infants and children: mechanisms of secondary damage and treatment in the intensive care unit. Crit Care Clin 2003;19(3):529–49.
24. Chesnut RM, Marshall LF, Klauber MR, et al. The role of secondary brain injury in determining outcome from severe head injury. J Trauma 1993;34(2):216–22.

25. Rosomoff HL, Kochanek PM, Clark R, et al. Resuscitation from severe brain trauma. Crit Care Med 1996;24(Suppl 2):S48–56.

26. Schmidt OI, Infanger M, Heyde C, et al. The role of neuroinflammation in traumatic brain injury. Eur J Trauma 2004;30:135–49.

27. Eisenberg HM, Gary HE Jr, Aldrich EF, et al. Initial CT findings in 753 patients with severe head injury. A report from the NIH Traumatic Coma Data Bank. J Neurosurg 1990;73(5):688–98.

28. Golding EM. Sequelae following traumatic brain injury. The cerebrovascular perspective. Brain Res Brain Res Rev 2002;38(3):377–88.

29. Leker RR, Shohami E. Cerebral ischemia and trauma-different etiologies yet similar mechanisms: neuroprotective opportunities. Brain Res Brain Res Rev 2002;39(1):55–73.

30. Wahl M, Schilling L, Unterberg A, et al. Mediators of vascular and parenchymal mechanisms in secondary brain damage. Acta Neurochir Suppl (Wien) 1993;57:64–72.

31. Giza CC, Hovda DA. The neurometabolic cascade of concussion. J Athl Train 2001;36(3):228–35.

32. Hubschmann OR, Kornhauser D. Effects of intraparenchymal hemorrhage on extracellular cortical potassium in experimental head trauma. J Neurosurg 1983;59(2):289–93.

33. Rosenthal M, LaManna J, Yamada S, et al. Oxidative metabolism, extracellular potassium and sustained potential shifts in cat spinal cord in situ. Brain Res 1979;162(1):113–27.

34. Yamakami I, McIntosh TK. Effects of traumatic brain injury on regional cerebral blood flow in rats as measured with radiolabeled microspheres. J Cereb Blood Flow Metab 1989;9(1):117–24.

35. Yuan XQ, Prough DS, Smith TL, et al. The effects of traumatic brain injury on regional cerebral blood flow in rats. J Neurotrauma 1988;5(4):289–301.

36. Biros MH, Dimlich RV. Brain lactate during partial global ischemia and reperfusion: effect of pretreatment with dichloroacetate in a rat model. Am J Emerg Med 1987;5(4):271–7.

37. Takahashi H, Manaka S, Sano K. Changes in extracellular potassium concentration in cortex and brain stem during the acute phase of experimental closed head injury. J Neurosurg 1981;55(5):708–17.

38. Katayama Y, Becker DP, Tamura T, et al. Massive increases in extracellular potassium and the indiscriminate release of glutamate following concussive brain injury. J Neurosurg 1990;73(6):889–900.

39. Katayama Y, Becker DP, Tamura T, et al. Early cellular swelling in experimental traumatic brain injury: a phenomenon mediated by excitatory amino acids. Acta Neurochir Suppl (Wien) 1990;51:271–3.

40. Fineman I, Hovda DA, Smith M, et al. Concussive brain injury is associated with a prolonged accumulation of calcium: a 45Ca autoradiographic study. Brain Res 1993;624(1/2):94–102.

41. Blumbergs PC, Scott G, Manavis J, et al. Staining of amyloid precursor protein to study axonal damage in mild head injury. Lancet 1994;344(8929):1055–6.

42. Maxwell WL, Graham DI. Loss of axonal microtubules and neurofilaments after stretch-injury to guinea pig optic nerve fibers. J Neurotrauma 1997;14(9):603–14.

43. Pettus EH, Povlishock JT. Characterization of a distinct set of intra-axonal ultrastructural changes associated with traumatically induced alteration in axolemmal permeability. Brain Res 1996;722(1/2):1–11.

44. Gorman LK, Fu K, Hovda DA, et al. Effects of traumatic brain injury on the cholinergic system in the rat. J Neurotrauma 1996;13(8):457–63.

45. Vink R, McIntosh TK, Demediuk P, et al. Decrease in total and free magnesium concentration following traumatic brain injury in rats. Biochem Biophys Res Commun 1987;149(2):594–9.

46. Vink R, Head VA, Rogers PJ, et al. Mitochondrial metabolism following traumatic brain injury in rats. J Neurotrauma 1990;7(1):21–7.

47. Vink R, McIntosh TK. Pharmacological and physiological effects of magnesium on experimental traumatic brain injury. Magnes Res 1990;3(3):163–9.

48. Zweifel C, Lavinio A, Steiner LA, et al. Continuous monitoring of cerebrovascular pressure reactivity in patients with head injury. Neurosurg Focus 2008; 25(18828700):E2.

49. Attwell D, Laughlin SB. An energy budget for signaling in the grey matter of the brain. J Cereb Blood Flow Metab 2001;21(10):1133–45.

50. Astrup J, Siesjo BK, Symon L. Thresholds in cerebral ischemia—the ischemic penumbra. Stroke 1981;12(6):723–5.

51. Rangel-Castilla L, Gasco J, Nauta HJ, et al. Cerebral pressure autoregulation in traumatic brain injury. Neurosurg Focus 2008;25(18828705):E7.

52. Bouma GJ, Muizelaar JP. Cerebral blood flow, cerebral blood volume, and cerebrovascular reactivity after severe head injury. J Neurotrauma 1992;9(Suppl 1): S333–48.

53. Hlatky R, Valadka AB, Robertson CS. Intracranial pressure response to induced hypertension: role of dynamic pressure autoregulation. Neurosurgery 2005; 57(5):917–23 [discussion: 917–23].

54. Bouma GJ, Muizelaar JP, Bandoh K, et al. Blood pressure and intracranial pressure-volume dynamics in severe head injury: relationship with cerebral blood flow. J Neurosurg 1992;77(1):15–9.

55. Marion DW, Darby J, Yonas H. Acute regional cerebral blood flow changes caused by severe head injuries. J Neurosurg 1991;74(3):407–14.

56. Signoretti S, Vagnozzi R, Tavazzi B, et al. Biochemical and neurochemical sequelae following mild traumatic brain injury: summary of experimental data and clinical implications. Neurosurg Focus 2010;29(5):E1.

57. Makdissi M, Darby D, Maruff P, et al. Natural history of concussion in sport: markers of severity and implications for management. Am J Sports Med 2010; 38(3):464–71.

58. Belanger H, Spiegel E, Vanderploeg R. Neuropsychological performance following a history of multiple self-reported concussions: a meta-analysis. J Int Neuropsychol Soc 2010;16(2):262.

59. Brenner LA, Ivins BJ, Schwab K, et al. Traumatic brain injury, posttraumatic stress disorder, and postconcussive symptom reporting among troops returning from Iraq. J Head Trauma Rehabil 2010;25(5):307–12.

60. Sroufe N, Fuller D, West B, et al. Postconcussive symptoms and neurocognitive function after mild traumatic brain injury in children. Pediatrics 2010;125(6): e1331–9.

61. Davis G, Iverson G, Guskiewicz K, et al. Contributions of neuroimaging, balance testing, electrophysiology and blood markers to the assessment of sport-related concussion. Br J Sports Med 2009;43(Suppl 1):i36–45.

62. Centers for Disease Control and Prevention (CDC). Sports-related recurrent brain injuries—United States. MMWR Morb Mortal Wkly Rep 1997;46(10):224–7.

63. Bazarian JJ, Veenema T, Brayer AF, et al. Knowledge of concussion guidelines among practitioners caring for children. Clin Pediatr (Phila) 2001;40(4):207–12.

64. Fick DS. Management of concussion in collision sports. Guidelines for the side-lines. Postgrad Med 1995;97(2):53–6, 59–60.
65. Gebke KB. Mild traumatic brain injury. Curr Sports Med Rep 2002;1(1):23–7.
66. Johnston KM, McCrory P, Mohtadi NG, et al. Evidence-based review of sport-related concussion: clinical science. Clin J Sport Med 2001;11(3):150–9.
67. Kelly JP, Rosenberg JH. The development of guidelines for the management of concussion in sports. J Head Trauma Rehabil 1998;13(2):53–65.
68. Leclerc S, Lassonde M, Delaney JS, et al. Recommendations for grading of concussion in athletes. Sports Med 2001;31(8):629–36.
69. Lovell MR, Collins MW, Iverson GL, et al. Grade 1 or "ding" concussions in high school athletes. Am J Sports Med 2004;32(1):47–54.
70. Reddy CC, Collins MW. Sports concussion: management and predictors of outcome. Curr Sports Med Rep 2009;8(1):10–5.
71. Spinos P, Sakellaropoulos G, Georgiopoulos M, et al. Postconcussion syndrome after mild traumatic brain injury in Western Greece. J Trauma 2010;69(4):789–94.
72. Putukian M, Aubry M, McCrory P. Return to play after sports concussion in elite and non-elite athletes? Br J Sports Med 2009;43(Suppl 1):i28–31.
73. Echlin P, Tator C, Cusimano M, et al. Return to play after an initial or recurrent concussion in a prospective study of physician-observed junior ice hockey concussions: implications for return to play after a concussion. Neurosurg Focus 2010;29(5):E5.
74. McCrory P, Meeuwisse W, Johnston K, et al. Consensus statement on concus-sion in sport: the 3rd International Conference on Concussion in Sport held in Zurich, November 2008. Br J Sports Med 2009;43(Suppl 1):i76–84.
75. Laurer HL, Bareyre FM, Lee VM, et al. Mild head injury increasing the brain's vulnerability to a second concussive impact. J Neurosurg 2001;95(5):859–70.
76. McCrory PR, Berkovic SF. Second impact syndrome. Neurology 1998;50(3):677–83.
77. McQuillen JB, McQuillen EN, Morrow P. Trauma, sport, and malignant cerebral edema. Am J Forensic Med Pathol 1988;9(1):12–5.
78. Saunders RL, Harbaugh RE. The second impact in catastrophic contact-sports head trauma. JAMA 1984;252(4):538–9.
79. Wozniak JR, Krach L, Ward E, et al. Neurocognitive and neuroimaging corre-lates of pediatric traumatic brain injury: a diffusion tensor imaging (DTI) study. Arch Clin Neuropsychol 2007;22(5):555–68.
80. Wilde EA, McCauley SR, Hunter JV, et al. Diffusion tensor imaging of acute mild traumatic brain injury in adolescents. Neurology 2008;70(12):948–55.
81. Ommaya AK, Gennarelli TA. Cerebral concussion and traumatic unconscious-ness. Correlation of experimental and clinical observations of blunt head injuries. Brain 1974;97(4):633–54.
82. Shaw NA. The neurophysiology of concussion. Prog Neurobiol 2002;67(4):281–344.
83. Nilsson B, Ponten U. Exerimental head injury in the rat. Part 2: regional brain energy metabolism in concussive trauma. J Neurosurg 1977;47(2):252–61.
84. Hayes RL, Stonnington HH, Lyeth BG, et al. Metabolic and neurophysiologic sequelae of brain injury: a cholinergic hypothesis. Cent Nerv Syst Trauma 1986;3(2):163–73.
85. Saija A, Hayes RL, Lyeth BG, et al. The effect of concussive head injury on central cholinergic neurons. Brain Res 1988;452(1/2):303–11.
86. Stein SC, Spettell C. The head injury severity scale (HISS): a practical classifi-cation of closed-head injury. Brain Inj 1995;9(5):437–44.

87. Risling M, Plantman S, Angeria M, et al. Mechanisms of blast induced brain injuries, experimental studies in rats. Neuroimage 2010;54(Suppl 1): S89–97.

88. Xu J, Rasmussen IA, Lagopoulos J, et al. Diffuse axonal injury in severe traumatic brain injury visualized using high-resolution diffusion tensor imaging. J Neurotrauma 2007;24(17518531):753–65.

89. Adams JH, Doyle D, Ford I, et al. Diffuse axonal injury in head injury: definition, diagnosis and grading. Histopathology 1989;15(1):49–59.

90. Bigler ED. Quantitative magnetic resonance imaging in traumatic brain injury. J Head Trauma Rehabil 2001;16(2):117–34.

91. Buki A, Povlishock JT. All roads lead to disconnection?–Traumatic axonal injury revisited. Acta Neurochir (Wien) 2006;148(2):181–93 [discussion: 193–4].

92. Kawai N, Maeda Y, Kudomi N, et al. Focal neuronal damage in patients with neuropsychological impairment after diffuse traumatic brain injury: evaluation using 11C-flumazenil positron emission tomography with statistical image analysis. J Neurotrauma 2010;27(12):2131–8.

93. Parizel PM, Ozsarlak O, Van Goethem JW, et al. Imaging findings in diffuse axonal injury after closed head trauma. Eur Radiol 1998;8(6):960–5.

94. Stiell IG, Wells GA, Vandemheen K, et al. The Canadian CT head rule for patients with minor head injury. Lancet 2001;357(9266):1391–6.

95. Azouvi P. Neuroimaging correlates of cognitive and functional outcome after traumatic brain injury. Curr Opin Neurol 2000;13(11148667):665–9.

96. Ding K, Marquez de la Plata C, Wang JY, et al. Cerebral atrophy after traumatic white matter injury: correlation with acute neuroimaging and outcome. J Neurotrauma 2008;25(19072588):1433–40.

97. Niogi SN, Mukherjee P, Ghajar J, et al. Extent of microstructural white matter injury in postconcussive syndrome correlates with impaired cognitive reaction time: a 3T diffusion tensor imaging study of mild traumatic brain injury. AJNR Am J Neuroradiol 2008;29(5):967–73.

98. Niogi SN, Mukherjee P, Ghajar J, et al. Structural dissociation of attentional control and memory in adults with and without mild traumatic brain injury. Brain 2008;131(Pt 12):3209–21.

99. Benson BW, Hamilton GM, Meeuwisse WH, et al. Is protective equipment useful in preventing concussion? A systematic review of the literature. Br J Sports Med 2009;43(Suppl 1):i56–67.

100. Gupta RK, Saksena S, Agarwal A, et al. Diffusion tensor imaging in late posttraumatic epilepsy. Epilepsia 2005;46(9):1465–71.

101. Salmond CH, Menon DK, Chatfield DA, et al. Diffusion tensor imaging in chronic head injury survivors: correlations with learning and memory indices. Neuroimage 2006;29(1):117–24.

102. Perlbarg V, Puybasset L, Tollard E, et al. Relation between brain lesion location and clinical outcome in patients with severe traumatic brain injury: a diffusion tensor imaging study using voxel-based approaches. Hum Brain Mapp 2009; 30(12):3924–33.

103. Cecil KM, Hills EC, Sandel ME, et al. Proton magnetic resonance spectroscopy for detection of axonal injury in the splenium of the corpus callosum of brain-injured patients. J Neurosurg 1998;88(5):795–801.

104. Sinson G, Bagley LJ, Cecil KM, et al. Magnetization transfer imaging and proton MR spectroscopy in the evaluation of axonal injury: correlation with clinical outcome after traumatic brain injury. AJNR Am J Neuroradiol 2001;22(1): 143–51.

105. Ariza M, Junque C, Mataro M, et al. Neuropsychological correlates of basal ganglia and medial temporal lobe NAA/Cho reductions in traumatic brain injury. Arch Neurol 2004;61(4):541–4.

106. Nakabayashi M, Suzaki S, Tomita H. Neural injury and recovery near cortical contusions: a clinical magnetic resonance spectroscopy study. J Neurosurg 2007;106(17367057):370–7.

107. Son BC, Park CK, Choi BG, et al. Metabolic changes in pericontusional oedematous areas in mild head injury evaluated by 1H MRS. Acta Neurochir Suppl 2000;76:13–6.

108. Sutton LN, Wang Z, Duhaime AC, et al. Tissue lactate in pediatric head trauma: a clinical study using 1H NMR spectroscopy. Pediatr Neurosurg 1995;22(2): 81–7.

109. Garnett MR, Blamire AM, Corkill RG, et al. Early proton magnetic resonance spectroscopy in normal-appearing brain correlates with outcome in patients following traumatic brain injury. Brain 2000;123(Pt 10):2046–54.

110. Garnett MR, Blamire AM, Rajagopalan B, et al. Evidence for cellular damage in normal-appearing white matter correlates with injury severity in patients following traumatic brain injury: a magnetic resonance spectroscopy study. Brain 2000;123(Pt 7):1403–9.

111. Gasparovic C, Arfai N, Smid N, et al. Decrease and recovery of N-acetylaspartate/ creatine in rat brain remote from focal injury. J Neurotrauma 2001;18(3):241–6.

112. Brooks WM, Stidley CA, Petropoulos H, et al. Metabolic and cognitive response to human traumatic brain injury: a quantitative proton magnetic resonance study. J Neurotrauma 2000;17(8):629–40.

113. Babikian T, Marion SD, Copeland S, et al. Metabolic levels in the corpus callosum and their structural and behavioral correlates after moderate to severe pediatric TBI. J Neurotrauma 2010;27(3):473–81.

114. Lescot T, Fulla-Oller L, Po C, et al. Temporal and regional changes after focal traumatic brain injury. J Neurotrauma 2010;27(19705964):85–94.

115. Shutter L, Tong KA, Holshouser BA. Proton MRS in acute traumatic brain injury: role for glutamate/glutamine and choline for outcome prediction. J Neurotrauma 2004;21(15684761):1693–705.

116. Carpentier A, Galanaud D, Puybasset L, et al. Early morphologic and spectroscopic magnetic resonance in severe traumatic brain injuries can detect "invisible brain stem damage" and predict "vegetative states." J Neurotrauma 2006; 23(5):674–85.

117. Chen JK, Johnston KM, Frey S, et al. Functional abnormalities in symptomatic concussed athletes: an fMRI study. Neuroimage 2004;22(1):68–82.

118. Jantzen KJ, Anderson B, Steinberg FL, et al. A prospective functional MR imaging study of mild traumatic brain injury in college football players. AJNR Am J Neuroradiol 2004;25(5):738–45.

119. Lovell MR, Pardini JE, Welling J, et al. Functional brain abnormalities are related to clinical recovery and time to return-to-play in athletes. Neurosurgery 2007; 61(2):352–9 [discussion: 359–60].

120. Cazalis F, Feydy A, Valabregue R, et al. fMRI study of problem-solving after severe traumatic brain injury. Brain Inj 2006;20(10):1019–28.

121. Umile EM, Sandel ME, Alavi A, et al. Dynamic imaging in mild traumatic brain injury: support for the theory of medial temporal vulnerability. Arch Phys Med Rehabil 2002;83(11):1506–13.

122. Agrawal D, Gowda NK, Bal CS, et al. Is medial temporal injury responsible for pediatric postconcussion syndrome? A prospective controlled study with

single-photon emission computerized tomography. J Neurosurg 2005;102(Suppl 2):167–71.

123. Kato T, Nakayama N, Yasokawa Y, et al. Statistical image analysis of cerebral glucose metabolism in patients with cognitive impairment following diffuse traumatic brain injury. J Neurotrauma 2007;24(6):919–26.

124. Zhang J, Mitsis EM, Chu K, et al. Statistical parametric mapping and cluster counting analysis of [18F] FDG-PET imaging in traumatic brain injury. J Neurotrauma 2010;27(1):35–49.

125. Dow RS, Ulett G, Raaf J. Electroencephalographic studies immediately following head injury. Am J Psychiatry 1944;101:174–83.

126. Dixon CE, Lyeth BG, Povlishock JT, et al. A fluid percussion model of experimental brain injury in the rat. J Neurosurg 1987;67(1):110–9.

127. McIntosh TK, Noble L, Andrews B, et al. Traumatic brain injury in the rat: characterization of a midline fluid-percussion model. Cent Nerv Syst Trauma 1987; 4(2):119–34.

128. Fabregas N, Gambus PL, Valero R, et al. Can bispectral index monitoring predict recovery of consciousness in patients with severe brain injury? Anesthesiology 2004;101(1):43–51.

129. Claassen J, Mayer SA, Kowalski RG, et al. Detection of electrographic seizures with continuous EEG monitoring in critically ill patients. Neurology 2004;62(10): 1743–8.

130. Vespa PM, Nuwer MR, Nenov V, et al. Increased incidence and impact of nonconvulsive and convulsive seizures after traumatic brain injury as detected by continuous electroencephalographic monitoring. J Neurosurg 1999;91(5): 750–60.

131. Vespa PM, McArthur DL, Xu Y, et al. Nonconvulsive seizures after traumatic brain injury are associated with hippocampal atrophy. Neurology 2010;75(9): 792–8.

132. Horiguchi T, Kis B, Rajapakse N, et al. Cortical spreading depression (CSD)-induced tolerance to transient focal cerebral ischemia in halothane anesthetized rats is affected by anesthetic level but not ATP-sensitive potassium channels. Brain Res 2005;1062(1/2):127–33.

133. Horiguchi T, Snipes JA, Kis B, et al. The role of nitric oxide in the development of cortical spreading depression-induced tolerance to transient focal cerebral ischemia in rats. Brain Res 2005;1039(1/2):84–9.

134. Kawahara N, Ruetzler CA, Klatzo I. Protective effect of spreading depression against neuronal damage following cardiac arrest cerebral ischaemia. Neurol Res 1995;17(1):9–16.

135. Kobayashi S, Harris VA, Welsh FA. Spreading depression induces tolerance of cortical neurons to ischemia in rat brain. J Cereb Blood Flow Metab 1995;15(5): 721–7.

136. Hebb MO, McArthur DL, Alger J, et al. Impaired percent alpha variability on continuous electroencephalography is associated with thalamic injury and predicts poor long-term outcome after human traumatic brain injury. J Neurotrauma 2007;24:579–90.

137. Mayevsky A, Doron A, Manor T, et al. Cortical spreading depression recorded from the human brain using a multiparametric monitoring system. Brain Res 1996;740(1/2):268–74.

138. Strong AJ, Fabricius M, Boutelle MG, et al. Spreading and synchronous depressions of cortical activity in acutely injured human brain. Stroke 2002;33(12): 2738–43.

139. Nedergaard M, Hansen AJ. Spreading depression is not associated with neuronal injury in the normal brain. Brain Res 1988;449(1/2):395–8.
140. Drummond JC, Todd MM, Schubert A, et al. Effect of the acute administration of high dose pentobarbital on human brain stem auditory and median nerve somatosensory evoked responses. Neurosurgery 1987;20(6):830–5.
141. Amantini A, Grippo A, Fossi S, et al. Prediction of 'awakening' and outcome in prolonged acute coma from severe traumatic brain injury: evidence for validity of short latency SEPs. Clin Neurophysiol 2005;116(1):229–35.
142. Carter BG, Butt W. Are somatosensory evoked potentials the best predictor of outcome after severe brain injury? A systematic review. Intensive Care Med 2005;31(6):765–75.
143. Carter BG, Butt W. A prospective study of outcome predictors after severe brain injury in children. Intensive Care Med 2005;31(6):840–5.
144. Garcia-Larrea L, Fischer C, Artru F. [Effect of anesthetics on sensory evoked potentials]. Neurophysiol Clin 1993;23(2/3):141–62 [in French].
145. Rothstein TL. The role of evoked potentials in anoxic-ischemic coma and severe brain trauma. J Clin Neurophysiol 2000;17(5):486–97.
146. Sherman AL, Tirschwell DL, Micklesen PJ, et al. Somatosensory potentials, CSF creatine kinase BB activity, and awakening after cardiac arrest. Neurology 2000;54(4):889–94.
147. Zarza-Lucianez D, Arce-Arce S, Bhathal H, et al. [Mismatch negativity and conscience level in severe traumatic brain injury]. Rev Neurol 2007;44(8):465–8 [in Spanish].
148. Ingebrigtsen T, Romner B, Kock-Jensen C. Scandinavian guidelines for initial management of minimal, mild, and moderate head injuries. The Scandinavian Neurotrauma Committee. J Trauma 2000;48(4):760–6.
149. Padayachy LC, Figaji AA, Bullock MR. Intracranial pressure monitoring for traumatic brain injury in the modern era. Childs Nerv Syst 2010;26(19937249):441–52.
150. Chesnut RM, Marshall LF. Management of head injury. Treatment of abnormal intracranial pressure. Neurosurg Clin N Am 1991;2(2):267–84.
151. Francony G, Fauvage B, Falcon D, et al. Equimolar doses of mannitol and hypertonic saline in the treatment of increased intracranial pressure. Crit Care Med 2008;36(18209674):795–800.
152. Aarabi B, Hesdorffer DC, Ahn ES, et al. Outcome following decompressive craniectomy for malignant swelling due to severe head injury. J Neurosurg 2006;104(4):469–79.
153. Rutigliano D, Egnor MR, Priebe CJ, et al. Decompressive craniectomy in pediatric patients with traumatic brain injury with intractable elevated intracranial pressure. J Pediatr Surg 2006;41(1):83–7 [discussion: 83–7].
154. Steiner LA, Czosnyka M, Piechnik SK, et al. Continuous monitoring of cerebrovascular pressure reactivity allows determination of optimal cerebral perfusion pressure in patients with traumatic brain injury. Crit Care Med 2002;30(4):733–8.
155. Adelson PD, Nemoto E, Colak A, et al. The use of near infrared spectroscopy (NIRS) in children after traumatic brain injury: a preliminary report. Acta Neurochir Suppl 1998;71:250–4.
156. Crespi F. Near-infrared spectroscopy (NIRS): a non-invasive in vivo methodology for analysis of brain vascular and metabolic activities in real time in rodents. Curr Vasc Pharmacol 2007;5(4):305–21.

157. Kampfl A, Pfausler B, Denchev D, et al. Near infrared spectroscopy (NIRS) in patients with severe brain injury and elevated intracranial pressure. A pilot study. Acta Neurochir Suppl 1997;70:112–4.
158. Rohlwink UK, Figaji AA. Methods of monitoring brain oxygenation. Childs Nerv Syst 2010;26(19937250):453–64.
159. van Rossem K, Garcia-Martinez S, De Mulder G, et al. Brain oxygenation after experimental closed head injury. A NIRS study. Adv Exp Med Biol 1999;471: 209–15.

Syncope

Paul Angaran, MD, FRCPC, George J. Klein, MD, FRCPC,
Raymond Yee, MD, FRCPC, Allan C. Skanes, MD, FRCPC,
Lorne J. Gula, MD, FRCPC, Peter Leong-Sit, MD, FRCPC,
Andrew D. Krahn, MD, FRCPC*

KEYWORDS

• Syncope • Neurocardiogenic syncope • Diagnosis • Vasovagal

Syncope is defined as a sudden and transient loss of consciousness associated with a loss of postural tone, with spontaneous recovery. Although this definition was originally restricted to a loss of consciousness caused by diminished cardiac output, it is now predominately used without an implication of origin. It is common, with an overall incidence of a first occurrence of 6.2 per 1000 person-years.[1] It accounts for 3% to 5% of emergency room visits and 1% to 6% of hospital medical admissions.[2–4] It is associated with considerable health care costs, estimated at $1.7 to $2.4 billion annually.[5,6] Mortality is generally low but is related to the underlying cause.[1,5] Age at presentation is typically bimodal, with the first peak in adolescence and early adulthood (predominantly neurocardiogenic) and the second peak in the sixth and seventh decade, reflecting arrhythmias from structural heart disease and also being neurocardiogenic.

Syncope is often diagnostically challenging because of its various causes and periodic and unpredictable occurrence. Cardiac syncope is important to distinguish from other neurologic disorders of consciousness, such as seizures and transient ischemic attacks. This article focuses primarily on cardiac causes of syncope, particularly arrhythmias, and neurocardiogenic syncope.

ETIOLOGY

In general, cardiac syncope reflects a loss of adequate cerebral perfusion to maintain consciousness, caused by a decrease in blood pressure. It is often related to cardiovascular disease but can also be from underlying neurologic processes. The most

Dr Krahn is a Career Investigator of the Heart and Stroke Foundation of Ontario. The study was supported by the Heart and Stroke Foundation of Ontario (T6730).

Drs Klein, Yee, and Krahn are consultants to Medtronic. Dr Krahn receives research funding from St Jude Medical and Boston Scientific. Drs Yee, Krahn, and Klein receive research funding from Medtronic.

Division of Cardiology, University of Western Ontario, London, 339 Windermere Road, London, ON N6A 5A5, Canada

* Corresponding author. Arrhythmia Service, London Health Sciences Centre, 339 Windermere Road, London, ON N6A 5A5, Canada.

E-mail address: akrahn@uwo.ca

common cause of syncope in the general population is vasovagal or neurocardiogenic syncope.[1] The cardiovascular causes of syncope (**Fig. 1**; **Table 1**) can be generally divided into reflex syncope (vasovagal, situational, orthostatic, and carotid sinus hypersensitivity) and cardiac causes (arrhythmias, hemodynamic).

Diagnosing the underlying cause of syncope is often challenging. In a large series of patients presenting either to a primary care setting or an emergency department, the origin of syncope was found in only approximately 60% of patients.[7] Cardiovascular causes accounted for 90% of the diagnosed cases, with the most common cause being vasomotor and reactive syncope (50%). Neurocardiogenic syncope and orthostatic hypotension accounted for 28% and 17% of diagnosed cases. Arrhythmias were the cause in 34% of patients, with a high incidence of ventricular tachycardia (19%). The true incidence of ventricular tachycardia was likely overestimated, because the basis for classification in most of these patients was nonsustained ventricular tachycardia on monitoring, in contrast with confirmation of ventricular tachycardia during a clinical episode. On the other end of the spectrum, bradyarrhythmias were probably underestimated because of their intermittent nature and the lack of prolonged monitoring tools to detect them. In a large cohort of patients from the Framingham Heart Study, the most frequently identified causes of syncope were vasovagal (21.2%), cardiac (9.5%), orthostatic (9.4%), medication (6.8%), seizure (4.9%), stroke or transient ischemic attack (4.1%), other causes (7.5%), and unknown (37%).[1] These studies highlight that the underlying cause of syncope is most often cardiovascular, with vasomotor and arrhythmic causes predominating.

PATHOPHYSIOLOGY

Although the underlying pathophysiology can vary widely, syncope is a direct result of inadequate cerebral perfusion. The spectrum of presyncope to syncope will depend

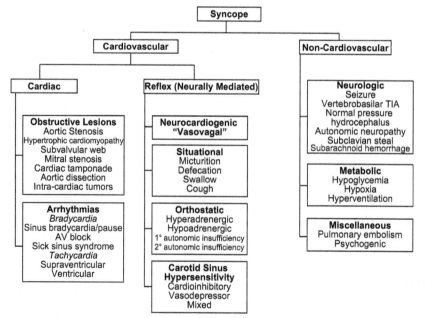

Fig. 1. Flow diagram illustrating the differential diagnosis of syncope. Most episodes of loss of consciousness are cardiovascular in origin, largely related to vasovagal syncope.

Table 1
Classification of syncope

Cardiovascular	Noncardiovascular
Cardiac	**Neurologic**
Arrhythmias	
Bradycardia	Seizure
Sinus bradycardia/pause	Vertebrobasilar transient ischemic attack
Atrioventricular block	Normal pressure hydrocephalus
Sick sinus syndrome	Autonomic neuropathy
Tachycardia	Subclavian steal
Supraventricular	Subarachnoid hemorrhage
Ventricular	
Obstructive Cardiac Lesions	*Metabolic*
Aortic stenosis	Hypoglycemia
Hypertrophic cardiomyopathy	Hypoxia
Subvalvular web	Hyperventilation
Mitral stenosis	
Cardiac tamponade	
Aortic dissection	
Intracardiac tumors	
Reflex (Neurally Mediated)	
Neurocardiogenic Vasovagal	*Miscellaneous*
Postural tachycardia syndrome	Pulmonary embolism
	Psychogenic
Situational	
Micturition	
Defecation	
Swallow	
Cough	
Orthostatic	
Hyperadrenergic	
Hypoadrenergic	
Primary or secondary autonomic insufficiency	
Carotid Sinus Hypersensitivity	
Cardioinhibitory	
Vasodepressor	
Mixed	

Data from Manolis AS, Linzer M, Salem D, et al. Syncope: current diagnostic evaluation and management. Ann Intern Med 1990;112(11):850–63.

on the duration and degree of reduction of cerebral blood compromise. Under normal physiologic circumstances, when standing upright, venous distension and blood pooling compromise venous return to the heart and its ability to perfuse the brain. Compensation occurs through a set of complex reflexes, especially baroreflexes, that maintain venous return and cardiac output through peripheral vasoconstriction and autonomically mediated increase in the heart rate.

Reflex or Neurally Mediated Syncope

Reflex or neurally mediated syncope constitutes a group of disorders characterized by an abrupt and transient autonomic dysfunction leading to hypotension or bradycardia.[8] Neurocardiogenic syncope is the most common, with an estimated lifetime prevalence of 30% to 40%.[9–11] Other disorders in this category include situational syncope and carotid sinus hypersensitivity. Situational syncope is in effect neurocardiogenic syncope associated with a specific trigger. Although many triggers exist, common ones include micturition, deglutition, defecation, blood phobia, venipuncture, and trumpet player's syncope. Carotid sinus hypersensitivity is an exaggerated or inappropriate baroreflex from carotid sinus stimulation, resulting in presyncope or syncope.[12] This reflex is composed of two components; a vasodepressor component that leads to vasodilation and hypotension, and a cardioinhibitory component that leads to bradycardia. Postural tachycardia syndrome is another variant of autonomically mediated presyncope and syncope. It is characterized by an exaggerated increase in heart rate during standing, with minimal blood pressure change.[13] Patients are more likely to experience presyncope than syncope, and may also report fatigue, exercise intolerance, and gastrointestinal symptoms. The origin has not been elucidated, but reduced cardiac size and intravascular volume, baroreceptor sensitivity, and deconditioning have been implicated.[14–17]

The underlying pathophysiology of neurocardiogenic syncope remains controversial.[18] Under normal physiologic circumstances, gravity causes venous pooling of blood on standing, with a subsequent decrease in venous return. Arterial baroreceptors located primarily in the aortic arch and carotid artery sense the reduction in cardiac output and send afferent signals to the medulla, leading to an increase in sympathetic tone. Left ventricular mechanoreceptors, responsive to pressure and stretch, modulate this response through parasympathetic tone. This feedback system autoregulates blood pressure within a remarkably narrow range during changes in posture. The popular hypothesis for neurocardiogenic syncope suggests a predisposition to excessive peripheral venous pooling, leading to a sudden reduction in cardiac venous return.[19] This reduction in left ventricular volume triggers a reflex increase in sympathetic-mediated contractility. This hypercontractile cardiac state activates left ventricular mechanoreceptors (c-fibers), causing a paradoxic withdrawal of sympathetic activity and increase in parasympathetic activity, leading to hypotension, bradycardia, and syncope. Some evidence also suggests central sympathetic regulation dysfunction, with reduced sympathetic nerve activity just before syncope in patients undergoing tilt table testing.[20]

Orthostatic Hypotension

Orthostatic hypotension is a related cause of syncope, and entails dysfunction of reflex compensation for hypotension when upright. Mechanisms include primary and secondary autonomic failure, and volume depletion (**Fig. 2**). The first account of primary chronic autonomic failure associated with other neurologic abnormalities, now termed *multiple systems atrophy*, was first described by Shy and Drager[21] in 1960. This syndrome is characterized by autonomic dysfunction and orthostatic hypotension. Autonomic failure can be divided into primary and secondary causes. Secondary causes are numerous and include diabetic neuropathy, Parkinson's disease, and paraneoplastic autonomic failure. Orthostatic hypotension is more common with advancing age.[22] An often-overlooked cause is drug-induced hypotension from diuretics, vasodilators, and antihypertensive medications. In one series involving 100 patients with moderate to severe orthostatic hypotension referred to a tertiary center, 27% had primary autonomic failure, 35% had secondary autonomic failure, and 38% had hypotension with no evidence of autonomic dysfunction.[23]

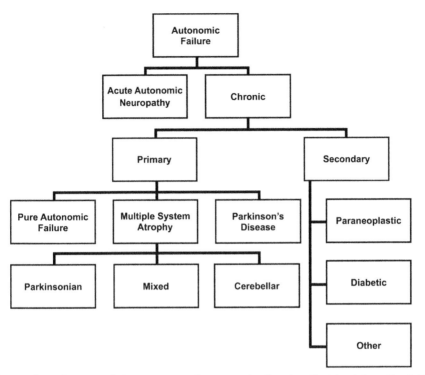

Fig. 2. Flow diagram of the spectrum of autonomic disorders that lead to orthostatic intolerance.

Arrhythmias

Syncope can be caused by either bradyarrhythmias or tachyarrhythmias. Bradyarrhythmias tend to be the more common cause, especially in elderly people, when symptom-rhythm correlation can be obtained. Although extreme bradycardia or tachycardia can result in hemodynamic compromise, the more important factor is the rate of heart rate change, as opposed to the absolute heart rate, which explains why symptoms are most pronounced at arrhythmia onset. The efficiency with which the peripheral vasculature can adapt to sudden changes in cardiac output caused by the arrhythmia influences the severity of symptoms.

INVESTIGATIONS

Because of the variety of underlying disease processes that lead to syncope, the key first step is differentiating benign from malignant causes of syncope. The fundamental issue is whether life-threatening ventricular arrhythmias may be responsible for the clinical presentation. These typically occur in the context of structural heart disease, such as ischemic or nonischemic cardiomyopathy. Less common but equally important are rare inherited causes of arrhythmias, such a long QT syndrome, diagnosed through resting adrenaline-induced or treadmill-provoked QT prolongation on the electrocardiogram (ECG). Propensity to ventricular arrhythmias related to underlying structural heart disease can be diagnosed through history and confirmatory imaging with a transthoracic echocardiogram, whereas syncope in patients with an inherited "channelopathy" is often associated with unusual triggers, such as exercise or auditory stimulation, variably associated with familial syncope and sudden death (**Fig. 3**).

Incorrect diagnoses can lead to unnecessary life-altering consequences, such as loss of personal freedoms from the inability to drive a vehicle to loss of employment. The diagnostic gold standard for cardiovascular syncope includes physiologic and electrocardiographic monitoring during a spontaneous syncopal episode, but unfortunately this is difficult to achieve.[24] Clinical history and physical examination remain the most important diagnostic tools; if the diagnosis is not apparent, cardiovascular syncope may not be detected in approximately 50% of cases because of its infrequent and unpredictable nature.[25]

The ideal approach to investigate syncope has not been established. One approach categorizes investigations into three different levels.[26] In the first level, a detailed history and physical examination, resting ECG, and discretionary short-term ECG monitoring and echocardiography are performed as initial investigations. If unrewarding, a second level involves provocative testing, with a goal of reproducing the physiologic state that led to the syncopal event. Head-up tilt table testing, an electrophysiology study, and sleep-deprived electroencephalogram may be useful tests if initial investigations did not yield a diagnosis. The third level of testing involves

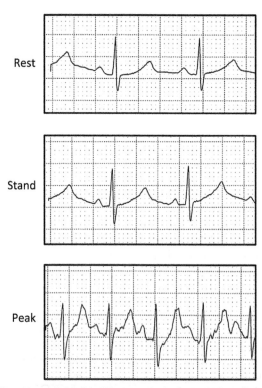

Fig. 3. ECG lead II in a 14-year-old girl with syncope during exercise. The resting QTc is at the upper limit of normal but fails to shorten with the minimal heart rate acceleration of standing, and throughout exercise. The abnormal circumstances of syncope and the provoked QT abnormalities lead to the diagnosis of long QT syndrome.

longer-term electrocardiographic monitoring, so that if a patient experiences another spontaneous syncopal event, the heart rhythm can be correlated to the event. This technique requires a recurrence of syncope, which may be associated with a risk of injury or even death. Current long-term monitoring strategies include Holter monitoring (24–48 hours), external loop recorders (2–8 weeks), and implantable loop recorders (36 months).

History and Physical Examination

The history and physical examination remains the cornerstone for diagnosing the cause of syncope, with several studies showing a diagnostic yield of approximately 50%.[25,27] Patients use various terms to describe their episodes, including dizziness, lightheadedness, fainting, and blackouts. Many will experience a prodrome, often more protracted with vasovagal episodes, typically abrupt with loss of consciousness caused by arrhythmia or seizure. The speed of recovery is also useful, being classically rapid for syncope caused by transient arrhythmia and more drawn out with fatigue and lightheadedness with vasovagal syncope or postictal confusion after a seizure. Common key clinical findings associated with the main causes of loss of consciousness are listed in **Table 2**.

An important first step is differentiating cardiac syncope from seizures. Seizures are typically associated with epileptiform movements, along with a distinct prodrome, abrupt onset, tongue biting, bowel and bladder incontinence, and a prolonged postictal phase during which the patient is confused. In contrast, patients with cardiogenic syncope will not have seizure activity unless the hypotension is more severe and longer lasting, although minor twitching is commonly observed, attributed to transient cerebral hypoperfusion.[28] A simple evidence-based point scoring system of historical features has been developed that reliably distinguishes seizures from cardiac syncope (**Table 3**).[29] Obtaining a history from a witness is well worth the effort, especially when the patient is a poor historian.

Neurocardiogenic syncope can be provoked by prolonged standing or intense emotional stress, fear, or pain, and sometimes after exercising in a warm environment. The prodrome (weakness, lightheadedness, diaphoresis, nausea, and visual blurring) can last several minutes before the syncopal event. Most episodes occur when patients are in the standing or sitting position, and rarely when they are supine. Episodes can often be averted if the patient recognizes the prodrome and immediately sits or lies down. Loss of consciousness is brief, usually lasting less than a minute, with recovery within minutes. Patients commonly experience fatigue, lightheadedness, or poor energy for minutes to hours after the event. Episodes may also occur in clusters.[8,29]

Stokes-Adams attacks are classically described as a sudden loss of consciousness with no warning symptoms, and are associated with rapid recovery. These attacks were originally described in patients with bradycardia secondary to atrioventricular block.[30,31] Patients regain consciousness quickly, usually within seconds to minutes, and may experience injury if standing. An arrhythmic cause should be suspected with a typical Stokes-Adams type of history.

Palpitations associated with presyncope or preceding a syncopal event may suggest arrhythmia or may be nonspecific. Irregular palpitations suggest the presence of atrial fibrillation and, in conjunction with sinus node disease, can lead to a long conversion pause on resumption of sinus rhythm (tachybrady or sick sinus syndrome). Ventricular arrhythmias may also cause palpitations but, in general, rapid ventricular tachycardia often causes syncope without awareness of rapid heart beat. In a series of 516 consecutive patients with unexplained syncope, a diagnostic point scoring system was developed, called the European Guidelines in Syncope Study score, to help identify patients

Table 2
Clinical findings differentiating causes of syncope and seizure

History	Arrhythmic	Neurocardiogenic	Seizure
Precipitant	Often none	Prolonged standing, fear, emotional stress, pain	Sleep deprivation, repetitive stimuli (strobe lights)
Prodrome	Palpitations	Warm Diaphoresis Nausea Visual blurring	Aura
Onset	Sudden	Usually gradual	Sudden
Duration	Seconds to minutes	Usually <60 s	Variable, can be longer than several minutes
Seizure activity	Unlikely	Rare	Always
Time to complete recovery	Seconds to minutes	Minutes	Minutes to hours
Presyncope	Sometimes	Often	Rare
Relationship of episodes to posture	None, although may be worse upright	Usually upright	None
Palpitations	Sometimes	Sometimes	None
Physical Examination			
Postural blood pressure changes	No	Often	No
Physical signs of obstructive cardiac origin	No	No	No
Structural heart disease	Often	No	No
Neurologic deficit	No	No	Often
Maneuvers			
Valsalva	No effect	No effect	No effect
Carotid sinus massage	May see bradycardia	May see bradycardia	No effect

with a cardiac cause of syncope.[32] Historical features consistent with a cardiac cause of syncope included palpitations preceding syncope, a history of heart disease or abnormal ECG, syncope during effort or while supine, and the absence of autonomic prodrome or predisposing/precipitating factors. In another study, a simple point score of historical features was able to differentiate vasovagal syncope from other causes of syncope with 89% sensitivity and 91% specificity.[33] Rarely, patients can also present with trauma secondary to a syncopal event. Possible scenarios include unexplained motor vehicle collision and soft tissue injuries or fractures from a fall.

Although most of the diagnostic yield is from the history, physical examination can be useful. Postural vital signs should be obtained, and a significant change may indicate orthostatic hypotension. The cardiovascular examination should focus on identifying obstructive lesions, such as aortic stenosis or hypertrophic obstructive

Table 3
Questions differentiating syncope from seizure

Historical Question	Diagnostic Score for Positive Response
At times do you wake with a cut tongue after your spells?	2
At times do you have a sense of déjà vu or jamais vu before your spells?	1
At times is emotional stress associated with losing consciousness?	1
Has anyone ever noted your head turning during a spell?	1
Has anyone ever noted that you are unresponsive, have unusual posturing, or have jerking limbs during your spells or have no memory of your spells afterwards?	1 for any positive response
Has anyone ever noted that you are confused after a spell?	1
Have you ever had lightheaded spells?	−2
At times do you sweat before spells?	−2
Is prolonged sitting or standing associated with your spells?	−2

Seizures if diagnostic score ≥1, syncope if diagnostic score <1.
Adapted from Sheldon R, Rose S, Ritchie D, et al. Historical criteria that distinguish syncope from seizures. J Am Coll Cardiol 2002;40(1):142–8; with permission.

cardiomyopathy. Structural heart disease, such as coronary artery disease and cardiomyopathies, may predispose patients to ventricular arrhythmias and sudden death. A neurologic examination may, of course, also implicate seizure, stroke, or subarachnoid hemorrhage.

Carotid sinus massage (CSM) can be performed as an adjunct to the physical examination if carotid sinus hypersensitivity (CSH) is suspected. CSH can cause sinus bradycardia, sinus arrest, or atrioventricular block leading to presyncope or syncope. CSM is contraindicated in the presence of suspected or known carotid artery disease, and auscultation of the carotids before the procedure is required at minimum. CSM should be performed with continuous ECG, and ideally blood pressure monitoring. To perform CSM, the carotid pulse should be palpated at the level of the carotid sinus, just inferior to the mandible at the level of the thyroid cartilage. Firm steady pressure, rather than pulsatile pressure, should be applied for 5 to 10 seconds.[34] If a positive result is not obtained, CSM can be repeated on the other side or in the upright position, which can increase the sensitivity of the test.[35] Neurologic complications occur with a frequency of 0.28%.[36] Normally, CSM will cause slowing of the sinus rate, and sometimes AV block, with a sinus pause no longer than 3 seconds. The test is considered positive if symptoms are reproduced in combination with asystole longer than 3 seconds (cardioinhibitory response) or a decrease of 50 mm Hg or more in systolic blood pressure (vasodepressor response). The presence of an abnormal response suggests but does not prove that this caused the clinical syncope.

Electrocardiogram

Although its diagnostic yield is only 5%, an ECG should be performed in all patients presenting with syncope.[37] ECG abnormalities (**Table 4**) may show evidence of structural heart disease (eg, myocardial infarction, hypertrophic cardiomyopathy), arrhythmias, and conduction disturbances. Certain ECG findings can be considered diagnostic of arrhythmia-related syncope, such as profound sinus bradycardia (<40 bpm) or sinus pauses greater than 3 seconds, Mobitz II second- or third-degree

Table 4
Electrocardiogram abnormalities in syncope

Conduction Abnormalities	Arrhythmias	Arrhythmogenic Syndromes	Other
Between atrium and ventricle	*Bradyarrhythmias/ pauses*	QT prolongation (congenital or acquired)	Q waves; previous myocardial infarct
First-degree heart block	Sinus bradycardia (<50 beats per minute)	Brugada syndrome	Left ventricular hypertrophy
Second-degree heart block	Sinus pauses (>3 s)	Arrhythmogenic right ventricular cardiomyopathy	
- Mobitz type I	Junctional bradycardia	Catecholaminergic polymorphic ventricular tachycardia	
- Mobitz type II	Ventricular escape rhythm (associated with third-degree heart block)	Pre-excitation syndrome	
Third-degree heart block			
Intraventricular			
Right or left bundle branch block	*Tachyarrhythmias*		
Bifascicular block	Supraventricular		
Alternating bundle branch block	Ventricular		
	Tachy-brady or sick sinus syndrome		

atrioventricular block, alternating bundle branch block, rapid supraventricular tachycardia or ventricular tachycardia, or pacemaker malfunction with pauses.[37]

Cardiac Imaging

Routine cardiac imaging with echocardiography or radionuclide ventriculography has low diagnostic yield (1%–3%).[38,39] However, imaging is much more useful for determining prognosis because structural heart disease, such as previous myocardial infarction and cardiomyopathies, increases the probability of sudden cardiac death. It is typically performed as a risk-stratifying tool to help triage patients who require inpatient or ambulatory investigation.

Exercise Stress Testing

Exercise testing may be helpful in patients with exertional symptoms or those at risk for coronary artery disease, but generally has low diagnostic yield (<1%). It can also be helpful in diagnosing several inherited arrhythmia syndromes, such as long QT syndrome, if clinical suspicion exists.

Laboratory Investigations

Routine blood work, along with cardiac biomarkers for screening for myocardial infarction, has a very low diagnostic yield and should not be routinely performed unless indicated by the clinical history and examination.

Head-up Tilt Testing

Head-up tilt table testing is a provocative test that attempts to reproduce the hemodynamic conditions and symptoms that occur in neurocardiogenic syncope.[13] It provides an orthostatic stress that subsequently leads to peripheral venous pooling. Tilt table testing is typically performed in an electrophysiology laboratory or dedicated room using a motorized table with a foot rest and safety restraints, which allows for rapid elevation and lowering between 0° and 90° (**Fig. 4**). The room should be some-what quiet. Continuous ECG and noninvasive blood pressure monitoring occurs throughout the test. A peripheral intravenous catheter is inserted for administration of fluids and isoproterenol or nitroglycerin. The patient is then monitored in the supine position for 5 to 15 minutes to obtain a baseline steady state. Tilt testing should not be performed if baseline orthostatic changes occur.

Various tilt protocols have been described with varying angles of tilt, duration of tilt, and use of pharmacologic provocation.[37,40–42] In a typical tilt test, the patient is tilted to an angle of 60° to 70° for 20 to 45 minutes during the passive phase. If the passive phase is negative, the active phase is performed after the patient is returned to the supine position. Pharmacologic provocation with isoproterenol or nitroglycerin is given and the patient is retilted and monitored for an additional 15 to 20 minutes. The test is considered positive if the patient loses consciousness or the ability to maintain posture, with a significant decrease in heart rate or blood pressure.

The most common pharmacologic agents used in tilt table testing are isoproterenol and nitroglycerin. Isoproterenol is a β_2-agonist with positive chronotropic and inotropic effects that decreases peripheral vascular resistance, leading to peripheral venous blood pooling. It is given in doses of 1 to 3 μg/min to increase the hypercontractile state

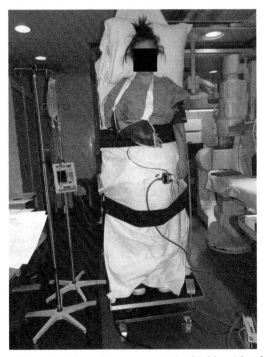

Fig. 4. Tilt table test. The patient is resting on a motorized table with a foot rest and safety restraints, which allows for elevation to 80° (pictured here) and rapid lowering in the event of syncope. Continuous electrocardiogram and noninvasive blood pressure monitoring occurs throughout the test, with a peripheral intravenous catheter inserted for administration of fluids and isoproterenol or nitroglycerin. The patient is monitored in the supine position at baseline, and then elevated to 60° to 80° for 15 to 45 minutes, which typically includes a pharmacologic adjunct if syncope does not occur in the first 15 minutes of orthostatic stress.

that leads to abrupt sympathetic withdrawal. Nitroglycerin is a vasodilator that causes peripheral blood pooling, thereby increasing orthostatic stress while patients are upright. It is often given sublingually, in a dose of 400 μg, but can also be administered as an intravenous infusion.

Patients experience three responses to a positive tilt test: cardioinhibitory, vasodepressor, and mixed.[41,43] A cardioinhibitory response is a primary decrease in the heart rate to less than 40 beats per minute (bpm), occasionally with asystole lasting longer than 3 seconds, with a preceding or coincident decline in blood pressure. A vasodepressor response is a primary decline in blood pressure, with the heart rate not decreasing more than 10% of its peak. A mixed response, which is the most common response, includes a simultaneous variable fall in blood pressure and heart rate. **Table 5** summarizes the positive responses to tilt testing.

Tilt testing can be useful in patients with recurrent syncope suspected to be neurocardiogenic in origin. It is generally not useful in patients presenting with a convincing history of vasovagal syncope because it does not add to the diagnosis, and is best used as an adjunct after a careful history. A structured history is likely to be as or more useful than tilt testing in diagnosing vasovagal syncope, as outlined earlier. In patients with prior syncope, positive responses were reported in 49% and 66% of patients using passive and active tests, respectively. False-positive rates range from 9% with passive testing to 27% with active testing. Reproducibility ranges from 71% to 87%.[44–46]

Tilt testing can also be useful in diagnosing other causes of neurally mediated syncope, such as orthostatic hypotension, postural orthostatic tachycardia syndrome,[47] and carotid sinus syncope. Unusual diagnoses, such as hyperventilation syndrome[48] and psychogenic syncope,[49] can also be detected with tilt testing.

Electrophysiologic Testing

The role of electrophysiologic testing for syncope has decreased to such degree that it is seldom performed. It is largely restricted to patients with structural heart disease or abnormal electrocardiograms when noninvasive testing has not been rewarding.[50] The role of the electrophysiologic study is to induce an arrhythmia or show evidence of conduction system disease, which may have led to the syncopal event. The procedure is performed in an invasive laboratory with catheters positioned within the heart using fluoroscopic guidance. Intrinsic conduction intervals can be assessed, and programmed electrical stimulation can be performed in an attempt to induce tachycardias, both supraventricular and ventricular.

Table 5
Responses to a positive tilt table testing

Response Type	Heart Rate During Syncope	Blood Pressure Response
Type I (mixed)	≥40 beats per minute (bpm) or decreases to <40 bpm for <10 s ± asystole for <3 s	Blood pressure drop before heart rate drop
Type IIA (cardioinhibitory without asystole)	<40 bpm for >10 s or asystole for >3 s	Blood pressure drop before heart rate drop
Type IIB (cardioinhibitory with asystole)	<40 bpm for >10 s or asystole for >3 s	Blood pressure drops to <80 mm Hg systolic at or after rapid drop in heart rate
Type III (vasodepressor)	Heart rate does not change or drops <10% from its peak	Blood pressure drops and precipitates syncope

In patients with a structurally normal heart and electrocardiogram, the diagnostic yield of an electrophysiologic study is low.[51] However, in patients with structural heart disease, the diagnostic yield is approximately 50%.[51] Electrophysiologic testing is best directed at patients with structural heart disease, particularly previous myocardial infarction or left ventricular dysfunction.[50] Many of these patients have an indication for an implantable cardioverter defibrillator (ICD), obviating the need to consider electrophysiologic study.[52,53] The goal in these patients is to induce ventricular tachycardia. In patients with documented intermittent bradyarrhythmias and syncope, electrophysiologic testing has a low sensitivity.[54,55] In patients with conduction disease and a negative electrophysiologic study, long-term monitoring showed that the negative predictive value of an electrophysiologic study is poor, with 33% of patients experiencing at least one prolonged asystolic pause.[56] Induction of any arrhythmia suggests but does not prove that it caused clinical syncope.

Electrocardiographic Monitoring

The most common initial investigation in patients presenting with palpitations or syncope is short-term electrocardiographic monitoring via 3 or, in some cases, 12 surface electrodes. This monitoring is typically performed in the emergency room or inpatient setting with continuous telemetry monitoring. Unfortunately, the diagnostic yield of electrocardiographic monitoring is low. In one series, the reported diagnostic yield was 6.9%, with bradycardia or atrioventricular block observed in 40% of patients who had abnormalities detected, tachycardia in 43%, and acute myocardial infarction in 17%.[7] Electrocardiographic findings should be correlated with symptoms, because they may be unrelated to the presenting syncopal event. In one pooled analysis involving patients with symptoms of syncope or presyncope, a 4% correlation between symptoms and arrhythmias was seen with Holter monitoring for more than 12 hours.[51] Although presyncope is a more common event during ambulatory monitoring, it is less likely to be associated with an arrhythmia,[57,58] which is often a problem because presyncope is a common complaint and its role as a surrogate for syncope is doubtful.

Ambulatory electrocardiography or Holter monitoring for 24 to 48 hours is useful when an arrhythmic origin is suggested historically, or in unexplained syncope in patients at high risk for arrhythmia (ie, those with underlying structural heart disease or abnormal electrocardiogram). It establishes a "rhythm profile" in many patients but a firm diagnosis in only those with frequent symptoms. A Holter monitor is a portable battery-operated device that connects to the patient using bipolar electrodes and typically provides recordings of 2 but up to 12 electrocardiographic leads. Data are stored in the device, transformed into a digital format, and then analyzed using interpretive software. Markers for patient-activated events and time correlates are included for symptom–rhythm correlation (**Fig. 5**). Holter monitors have several limitations, the most important being a short monitoring period during which symptoms and arrhythmias may not occur. In one review, the overall diagnostic yield of Holter monitoring was 19%.[51] These studies reported symptoms that were not associated with arrhythmias in 15% of cases. Thus its major role is in patients with frequent symptoms as a "rule out" test at the primary care level.

Normal ambulatory electrocardiographic monitoring does not exclude an arrhythmic cause for syncope. If clinical suspicion is high, then further investigations such as prolonged monitoring or electrophysiological studies are required.

External Loop Recorder

An external loop recorder is an event monitor that continuously records and stores an external modified limb lead electrocardiogram with a 4- to 18-minute memory buffer

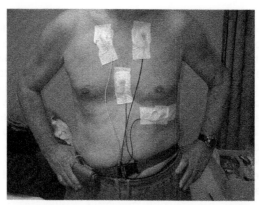

Fig. 5. Holter monitor. The most common form of monitoring involves 24 to 48 hours of monitoring, and records the entire period, which is reviewed by a technologists and interpreted by the physician. Holter monitoring plays a role in the primary care setting when symptoms are frequent.

(**Fig. 6**). After symptoms occur, the patient activates the event button, at which point the preceding 3 to 16 minutes and proceeding 1 to 2 minutes of cardiac rhythm are stored. The device memory is then "frozen" so the stored electrocardiograms can be downloaded and subsequently analyzed, either remotely over the telephone or when the device is returned. This monitor is ideal for patients with infrequent symptoms because it can be worn for weeks or even months at a time. The recording device is similar in size to a pager, with two leads attached to the chest by electrodes, which must be removed during bathing. Batteries function as the power source, and must be changed weekly. Occasionally, the rhythm strip obtained can be difficult to interpret, especially with respect to localizing P waves.

Long-term compliance can be challenging because of infrequent symptoms and electrode- or skin-related problems affecting the quality of electrocardiograms and

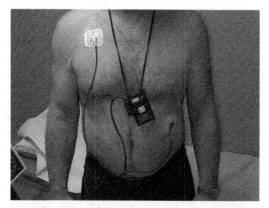

Fig. 6. External loop recorder. Minimal skin electrodes and lightweight portable technology enables a recording period of days to weeks. The device stores the preceding 5 to 20 minutes of single-lead electrocardiogram, which is recorded and transmitted over an analog telephone line to the monitoring center or physician's office. This device is best suited to patients whose symptoms are likely to recur within days to weeks and are able to manage the technology.

their subsequent interpretation. In symptomatic patients, additional reasons for not arriving at a diagnosis included device malfunction, patient noncompliance, and inability to activate the recorder.[59–61] The diagnostic yield for external loop recorders in three studies ranged from 24% to 47%, with highest yields in patients with palpitations.[59–61] In a retrospective database analysis, the diagnostic yields of Holter monitoring, memory loop recording, and autotriggered memory loop recording were 6%, 17%, and 36%, respectively, showing the additional benefit of automatic recording over patient-activated recordings.[62]

In a prospective randomized trial comparing external loop recorders to 48-hour Holter monitoring in patients with either presyncope or syncope, external loop recorders significantly increased the diagnostic yield from 22% to 55% because of the longer duration of monitoring.[63] However, the main limitation was the high rate of failure in the external loop recorder group, with device- or patient-related failure in 24% of patients.[63] In another study, multivariate predictors showed that patients who are unfamiliar with technology, live alone, or have a low motivation to reach a diagnosis have a lower diagnostic yield from external loop monitoring.[64]

An external loop recorder should be considered in motivated patients with frequent symptoms, likely to recur within 4 to 6 weeks, in whom an arrhythmic cause for syncope is suspected. Its major limitations include the infrequency of episodes and patient compliance with external electrodes.

Implantable Loop Recorders

An implantable loop recorder (ILR) is a programmable implanted device that allows for prolonged electrocardiographic monitoring in patients with infrequent recurrent syncope thought to be secondary to an arrhythmic cause. Similar to the external loop recorder, it is designed to obtain symptom–rhythm correlation, but, unlike the external loop recorder, it is implanted subcutaneously in the left chest and therefore devoid of surface electrodes and accompanying compliance issues. The ILR is also capable of monitoring for much longer periods than an external loop recorder. It is smaller than a conventional pacemaker generator and able to record a single ECG lead, without the need for a transvenous lead (**Fig. 7**). The battery life can be up to 36 months. The bipolar ECG signal is recorded and stored in a loop buffer. ILRs can automatically detect arrhythmias (bradyarrhythmias, tachyarrhythmias, and atrial

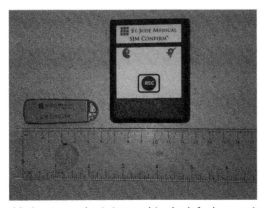

Fig. 7. The implantable loop recorder is inserted in the left chest region using local anesthetic, recording a single-lead ECG. The device stores 1- to 40-minute rhythm strips after automatic detection of tachycardia or bradycardia, or when patients experience symptoms.

fibrillation), and can be patient-activated after a patient experiences a presyncopal or syncopal event using a hand-held applicator. Data retrieval is manufacturer-specific and either occurs through a standard pacemaker programmer or via an analog telephone line and displayed on a Web site.

Several studies have established the efficacy of ILR in diagnosing syncope.[65–69] In a multicenter study of 206 patients with undiagnosed syncope, most had undergone noninvasive and invasive testing, including tilt testing and electrophysiologic studies.[65] Arrhythmia was diagnosed in 22% of patients and excluded in 42%, with no recurrent syncope in 31%. Bradycardia, leading to pacemaker implantation, was more common than tachycardia (17% vs 6%). Only 4% of patients did not properly activate the device, thereby failing to establish a symptom–rhythm correlation.

Other studies have examined the role of ILRs in select patient populations. In patients with ongoing seizures despite anticonvulsant therapy, Zaidi and colleagues[70,71] performed cardiac assessment, including head-up tilt testing and carotid sinus massage in all patients, and implantation of an ILR in 10 patients. Two of these patients had marked bradycardia preceding a seizure; one from sinus pauses and the other from heart block. This study suggested that atypical seizures may have a cardiovascular cause in as many as 42% of cases, and that cardiovascular assessment, including long-term electrocardiographic monitoring with an ILR, may play a role in select patients with atypical seizures.

In a series of studies from the International Study on Syncope of Uncertain Etiology (ISSUE) investigators, ILRs were implanted in three different groups of syncopal patients to assess cardiac rhythm after conventional testing.[56,72] Results from the first arm of the study found that the correlation between observations during tilt testing and cardiac rhythm during spontaneous syncope is poor and that bradycardia is more common in this population than previously recognized. Results from the second arm of the study confirmed that negative electrophysiologic testing does not exclude intermittent complete atrioventricular block, and that prolonged monitoring or consideration of permanent pacing is reasonable in this population. In the third arm of the study, ILR implantation showed a low incidence of ventricular arrhythmias and no sudden cardiac death in a higher-risk group with moderate structural heart disease.

ILR for prolonged monitoring has been compared with conventional testing in patients undergoing cardiac workup for unexplained syncope.[67,73] Early use of an ILR compared with conventional testing with an external loop recorder, tilt test, and electrophysiologic study led to a diagnosis in 55% versus 19% of patients. Bradycardia was much more likely to be detected with prolonged ILR monitoring than with conventional testing (40% vs 8%).

Another prospective, multicenter, observational study (ISSUE 2) assessed the efficacy of therapies based on ILR diagnosis of recurrent suspected neurocardiogenic syncope.[74] From this trial, the authors concluded that a strategy based on diagnostic information obtained from early ILR implant, with therapy delayed until documentation of syncope, allows for safe, specific, and effective therapy in patients with neurocardiogenic syncope. A prospective blinded version of the study recently completed enrollment.[75]

MANAGEMENT
Neurally Mediated Syncope

Treatment of neurally mediated syncope begins with reassurance focusing on a benign prognosis. Simple lifestyle modification includes adequate hydration, regular meals, and sufficient salt intake to help maintain intravascular volume. Fluid intake should be at least 2 to 3 L/d, with increased amounts necessary in warmer climates or if exercising. Salt tablets can be used to supplement intake if necessary. Avoidance of known triggers is of course important whenever possible. Medications that cause hypotension or volume depletion should be avoided. At the onset of symptoms, patients should sit or lie down with their legs elevated in an attempt to abort their episode. Venous support stockings can be helpful in patients who stand for prolonged periods. Orthostatic or tilt training, performed with a tilt table or standing against a wall under supervision, may also be useful.[76] Physical counterpressure maneuvers, which decrease lower extremity venous pooling, can also be helpful in aborting or delaying a syncopal episode in patients with a sufficiently long prodrome.[77]

A variety of medications have been used to treat neurally mediated syncope. The literature consists of small to medium-sized trials, often inadequately controlled and with conflicting results. β-blockers were thought to be useful in preventing syncope based on several observational studies.[78–80] The best evidence comes from the Prevention of Syncope Trial (POST),[81] which was a randomized controlled trial comparing metoprolol and placebo in 208 patients with recurrent syncope and a positive tilt test. β-blockers did not confer any benefit overall or in any prespecified subgroups. Vasoconstrictors, such as midodrine, have shown some benefit in small observational studies and clinical trials.[82–85] However, a randomized controlled trial with etilefrine, another alpha-agonist, showed no benefit.[86] Disopyramide, thought to be useful because of its anticholinergic and negative inotropic properties, was found to be ineffective in a placebo-controlled randomized trial.[87] Paroxetine, a selective serotonin uptake inhibitor, has also been studied. In a single controlled trial, paroxetine increased the likelihood of a negative tilt test at 1 month (38% vs 63%) and reduced the rate of recurrent syncope (53% vs 18%) during follow-up compared with placebo.[88] Pharmacotherapy for neurocardiogenic syncope is influenced by patient presentation and resting blood pressure. In the authors' experience, β-blockers are most useful in elderly people or patients with hypertension on peripheral-acting antihypertensives. Fludrocortisone is most often useful in young patients with low resting blood pressure, and alpha-agonists, such as midodrine, are used as second-line treatment because of their frequent dosing.

Cardiac pacing has also been studied in the treatment of neurocardiogenic syncope, which is usually associated with significant bradycardia or asystole. In patients with a significant cardioinhibitory component, pacing may be beneficial. However, varying degrees of peripheral vasodilatation (vasodepressor response) and hypotension usually occur, independent of heart rate slowing during neurally mediated syncope. Several unblinded studies showed the possible benefit of pacing compared with placebo or medical therapy,[89–91] although two double-blind randomized trials failed to show any benefit with pacing.[92,93] A meta-analysis of nine randomized trials suggested that a strong expectation response to pacing was the main mechanism of benefit of pacemaker implantation, with little physiologic benefit.[94] Cardiac pacing is generally reserved for patients for whom conservative measures fail, and is seldom performed.

In contrast to patients with neurocardiogenic syncope, those with a history consistent with carotid sinus hypersensitivity and a cardioinhibitory response to carotid sinus massage seem to benefit from pacing.[95]

Arrhythmias

Therapy is usually effective if arrhythmia is the underlying cause of syncope. If symptoms are caused by bradyarrhythmias, pacemaker implantation is usually highly successful.[96] The exception is when bradyarrhythmias occur as part of neurocardiogenic syncope, with a prominent vasodepressor response, as previously discussed. If symptoms are caused by tachyarrhythmias, treatment with antiarrhythmic therapy, catheter ablation, or ICD is usually highly effective.

In one study, patients treated with an ICD with unexplained syncope and inducible ventricular tachycardia/ventricular fibrillation (VT/VF) during electrophysiologic testing had a high rate of receiving appropriate shocks, with a similar incidence of appropriate ICD therapy, compared with patients with documented VT/VF.[97] In another study, electrophysiologic-guided therapy in patients with syncope and coronary artery disease found that those at high-risk had frequent appropriate ICD discharges.[98] In certain patient populations, ICD therapy may be indicated based on structural heart disease. Patients with left ventricular ejection (LVEF) of 30% or less and prior myocardial infarction[99]; LVEF of 35% or less and New York Heart Association class II or III heart failure[100]; or LVEF of 40% or less with nonsustained ventricular tachycardia and inducible ventricular tachycardia on electrophysiologic testing[101] should be considered for an ICD based on several primary and secondary prevention trials.

PROGNOSIS

The prognosis of patients with syncope largely depends on the underlying cause.[1,7,102] Patients can be categorized into different risk groups, with the highest mortality in those with underlying cardiac disease, approaching 50% at 5 years. Patients with neurocardiogenic syncope have similar outcomes to those who are free of syncope, confirming the benign prognosis in these patients. Therefore, aggressive investigations into the cause of syncope should be sought in patients with underlying structural heart disease.

SUMMARY

Syncope is a common presenting symptom, and is often a challenging diagnostic dilemma because of its various underlying causes. A careful initial clinical assessment with directed investigations is crucial in arriving at a presumptive diagnosis. Prolonged cardiac monitoring technologies have improved diagnostic accuracy in the more difficult cases.

REFERENCES

1. Soteriades ES, Evans JC, Larson MG, et al. Incidence and prognosis of syncope. N Engl J Med 2002;347(12):878–85.
2. Day SC, Cook EF, Funkenstein H, et al. Evaluation and outcome of emergency room patients with transient loss of consciousness. Am J Med 1982;73(1):15–23.
3. Doherty JU, Pembrook-Rogers D, Grogan EW, et al. Electrophysiologic evaluation and follow-up characteristics of patients with recurrent unexplained syncope and presyncope. Am J Cardiol 1985;55(6):703–8.
4. Morichetti A, Astorino G. Epidemiological and clinical findings in 697 syncope events [in Italian]. Minerva Med 1998;89(6):211–20.
5. Alshekhlee A, Shen WK, Mackall J, et al. Incidence and mortality rates of syncope in the United States. Am J Med 2009;122(2):181–8.
6. Sun BC, Emond JA, Camargo CA Jr. Direct medical costs of syncope-related hospitalizations in the United States. Am J Cardiol 2005;95(5):668–71.
7. Kapoor WN. Evaluation and outcome of patients with syncope. Medicine (Baltimore) 1990;69(3):160–75.
8. Grubb BP. Clinical practice. Neurocardiogenic syncope. N Engl J Med 2005; 352(10):1004–10.

9. Colman N, Nahm K, Ganzeboom KS, et al. Epidemiology of reflex syncope. Clin Auton Res 2004;14(Suppl 1):9–17.
10. Ganzeboom KS, Colman N, Reitsma JB, et al. Prevalence and triggers of syncope in medical students. Am J Cardiol 2003;91(8):1006–8, A1008.
11. Serletis A, Rose S, Sheldon AG, et al. Vasovagal syncope in medical students and their first-degree relatives. Eur Heart J 2006;27(16):1965–70.
12. Gregoratos G, Cheitlin MD, Conill A, et al. ACC/AHA Guidelines for implantation of Cardiac Pacemakers and Antiarrhythmia Devices: Executive Summary— a report of the American College of Cardiology/American Heart Association Task Force on Practice Guidelines (Committee on Pacemaker Implantation). Circulation 1998;97(13):1325–35.
13. Kenny RA, Ingram A, Bayliss J, et al. Head-up tilt: a useful test for investigating unexplained syncope. Lancet 1986;1(8494):1352–5.
14. Bonyhay I, Freeman R. Sympathetic nerve activity in response to hypotensive stress in the postural tachycardia syndrome. Circulation 2004;110(20):3193–8.
15. Fu Q, Vangundy TB, Galbreath MM, et al. Cardiac origins of the postural orthostatic tachycardia syndrome. J Am Coll Cardiol 2010;55(25):2858–68.
16. Stewart JM. Autonomic nervous system dysfunction in adolescents with postural orthostatic tachycardia syndrome and chronic fatigue syndrome is characterized by attenuated vagal baroreflex and potentiated sympathetic vasomotion. Pediatr Res 2000;48(2):218–26.
17. Raj SR, Robertson D. Blood volume perturbations in the postural tachycardia syndrome. Am J Med Sci 2007;334(1):57–60.
18. Mosqueda-Garcia R, Furlan R, Tank J, et al. The elusive pathophysiology of neurally mediated syncope. Circulation 2000;102(23):2898–906.
19. Kosinski D, Grubb BP, Temesy-Armos P. Pathophysiological aspects of neurocardiogenic syncope: current concepts and new perspectives. Pacing Clin Electrophysiol 1995;18(4 Pt 1):716–24.
20. Morillo CA, Eckberg DL, Ellenbogen KA, et al. Vagal and sympathetic mechanisms in patients with orthostatic vasovagal syncope. Circulation 1997;96(8): 2509–13.
21. Shy GM, Drager GA. A neurological syndrome associated with orthostatic hypotension: a clinical-pathologic study. Arch Neurol 1960;2:511–27.
22. Shibao C, Grijalva CG, Raj SR, et al. Orthostatic hypotension-related hospitalizations in the United States. Am J Med 2007;120(11):975–80.
23. Robertson D, Robertson RM. Causes of chronic orthostatic hypotension. Arch Intern Med 1994;154(14):1620–4.
24. Brignole M, Alboni P, Benditt D, et al. Guidelines on management (diagnosis and treatment) of syncope. Eur Heart J 2001;22(15):1256–306.
25. Linzer M, Yang EH, Estes NA III, et al. Diagnosing syncope. Part 1: value of history, physical examination, and electrocardiography. Clinical Efficacy Assessment Project of the American College of Physicians. Ann Intern Med 1997;126(12):989–96.
26. Krahn AD, Klein GJ, Yee R, et al. The use of monitoring strategies in patients with unexplained syncope—role of the external and implantable loop recorder. Clin Auton Res 2004;14(Suppl 1):55–61.
27. Brignole M, Menozzi C, Bartoletti A, et al. A new management of syncope: prospective systematic guideline-based evaluation of patients referred urgently to general hospitals. Eur Heart J 2006;27(1):76–82.
28. Lempert T, Bauer M, Schmidt D. Syncope: a videometric analysis of 56 episodes of transient cerebral hypoxia. Ann Neurol 1994;36(2):233–7.

29. Sheldon R, Rose S, Ritchie D, et al. Historical criteria that distinguish syncope from seizures. J Am Coll Cardiol 2002;40(1):142–8.
30. Adams R. Cases of disease of the heart, accompanied with pathological observations [abstract]. Dublin Hospital Reports 1827;4:353.
31. Stokes W. Observations on some cases of permanently slow pulse [abstract]. Dublin Quarterly Journal of Medical Science 1846;2:73.
32. Del Rosso A, Ungar A, Maggi R, et al. Clinical predictors of cardiac syncope at initial evaluation in patients referred urgently to a general hospital: the EGSYS score. Heart 2008;94(12):1620–6.
33. Sheldon R, Rose S, Connolly S, et al. Diagnostic criteria for vasovagal syncope based on a quantitative history. Eur Heart J 2006;27(3):344–50.
34. Waxman MB, Wald RW, Sharma AD, et al. Vagal techniques for termination of paroxysmal supraventricular tachycardia. Am J Cardiol 1980;46(4):655–64.
35. Sugrue DD, Gersh BJ, Holmes DR Jr, et al. Symptomatic "isolated" carotid sinus hypersensitivity: natural history and results of treatment with anticholinergic drugs or pacemaker. J Am Coll Cardiol 1986;7(1):158–62.
36. Davies AJ, Kenny RA. Frequency of neurologic complications following carotid sinus massage. Am J Cardiol 1998;81(10):1256–7.
37. Brignole M, Alboni P, Benditt DG, et al. Guidelines on management (diagnosis and treatment) of syncope—update 2004. Europace 2004;6(6):467–537.
38. Kapoor WN, Karpf M, Maher Y, et al. Syncope of unknown origin. The need for a more cost-effective approach to its diagnosis evaluation. JAMA 1982;247(19):2687–91.
39. Recchia D, Barzilai B. Echocardiography in the evaluation of patients with syncope. J Gen Intern Med 1995;10(12):649–55.
40. Benditt DG, Ferguson DW, Grubb BP, et al. Tilt table testing for assessing syncope. American College of Cardiology. J Am Coll Cardiol 1996;28(1):263–75.
41. Brignole M, Menozzi C, Del Rosso A, et al. New classification of haemodynamics of vasovagal syncope: beyond the VASIS classification. Analysis of the pre-syncopal phase of the tilt test without and with nitroglycerin challenge. Vasovagal Syncope International Study. Europace 2000;2(1):66–76.
42. Sheldon R, Killam S. Methodology of isoproterenol-tilt table testing in patients with syncope. J Am Coll Cardiol 1992;19(4):773–9.
43. Sutton R, Petersen M, Brignole M, et al. Proposed classification for tilt induced vasovagal syncope. Eur J Cardiac Pacing Electrophysiol 1992;2:180–3.
44. Kapoor WN, Smith MA, Miller NL. Upright tilt testing in evaluating syncope: a comprehensive literature review. Am J Med 1994;97(1):78–88.
45. Natale A, Akhtar M, Jazayeri M, et al. Provocation of hypotension during head-up tilt testing in subjects with no history of syncope or presyncope. Circulation 1995;92(1):54–8.
46. Petersen ME, Williams TR, Gordon C, et al. The normal response to prolonged passive head up tilt testing. Heart 2000;84(5):509–14.
47. Grubb BP, Kosinski DJ, Boehm K, et al. The postural orthostatic tachycardia syndrome: a neurocardiogenic variant identified during head-up tilt table testing. Pacing Clin Electrophysiol 1997;20(9 Pt 1):2205–12.
48. Naschitz JE, Gaitini L, Mazov I, et al. The capnography-tilt test for the diagnosis of hyperventilation syncope. QJM 1997;90(2):139–45.
49. Petersen ME, Williams TR, Sutton R. Psychogenic syncope diagnosed by prolonged head-up tilt testing. QJM 1995;88(3):209–13.
50. Krahn AD, Yee R, Klein GJ, et al. Inappropriate sinus tachycardia: evaluation and therapy. J Cardiovasc Electrophysiol 1995;6:1124–8.

51. Linzer M, Yang EH, Estes NA III, et al. Diagnosing syncope. Part 2: unexplained syncope. Clinical Efficacy Assessment Project of the American College of Physicians. Ann Intern Med 1997;127(1):76–86.

52. Olshansky B, Poole JE, Johnson G, et al. Syncope predicts the outcome of cardiomyopathy patients: analysis of the SCD-HeFT study. J Am Coll Cardiol 2008;51(13):1277–82.

53. Fuster V, Ryden LE, Cannom DS, et al. ACC/AHA/ESC 2006 guidelines for the management of patients with atrial fibrillation-executive summary: a report of the American College of Cardiology/American Heart Association Task Force on practice guidelines and the European Society of Cardiology Committee for Practice Guidelines (Writing Committee to Revise the 2001 Guidelines for the Management of Patients with Atrial Fibrillation). Eur Heart J 2006;27(16):1979–2030.

54. Fujimura O, Yee R, Klein GJ, et al. The diagnostic sensitivity of electrophysiologic testing in patients with syncope caused by transient bradycardia. N Engl J Med 1989;321(25):1703–7.

55. Krahn AD, Klein GJ, Norris C, et al. The etiology of syncope in patients with negative tilt table and electrophysiological testing. Circulation 1995;92(7):1819–24.

56. Brignole M, Menozzi C, Moya A, et al. Mechanism of syncope in patients with bundle branch block and negative electrophysiological test. Circulation 2001; 104(17):2045–50.

57. Kapoor WN. Evaluation and management of the patient with syncope. JAMA 1992;268(18):2553–60.

58. Krahn AD, Klein GJ, Yee R, et al. Predictive value of presyncope in patients monitored for assessment of syncope. Am Heart J 2001;141(5):817–21.

59. Brown AP, Dawkins KD, Davies JG. Detection of arrhythmias: use of a patient-activated ambulatory electrocardiogram device with a solid-state memory loop. Br Heart J 1987;58(3):251–3.

60. Cumbee SR, Pryor RE, Linzer M. Cardiac loop ECG recording: a new noninvasive diagnostic test in recurrent syncope. South Med J 1990;83(1):39–43.

61. Linzer M, Pritchett EL, Pontinen M, et al. Incremental diagnostic yield of loop electrocardiographic recorders in unexplained syncope. Am J Cardiol 1990; 66(2):214–9.

62. Reiffel JA, Schwarzberg R, Murry M. Comparison of autotriggered memory loop recorders versus standard loop recorders versus 24-hour Holter monitors for arrhythmia detection. Am J Cardiol 2005;95(9):1055–9.

63. Sivakumaran S, Krahn AD, Klein GJ, et al. A prospective randomized comparison of loop recorders versus Holter monitors in patients with syncope or presyncope. Am J Med 2003;115(1):1–5.

64. Gula LJ, Krahn AD, Massel D, et al. External loop recorders: determinants of diagnostic yield in patients with syncope. Am Heart J 2004;147(4):644–8.

65. Krahn AD, Klein GJ, Fitzpatrick A, et al. Predicting the outcome of patients with unexplained syncope undergoing prolonged monitoring. Pacing Clin Electrophysiol 2002;25(1):37–41.

66. Krahn AD, Klein GJ, Yee R, et al. Final results from a pilot study with an implantable loop recorder to determine the etiology of syncope in patients with negative noninvasive and invasive testing. Am J Cardiol 1998;82(1):117–9.

67. Krahn AD, Klein GJ, Yee R, et al. Randomized assessment of syncope trial: conventional diagnostic testing versus a prolonged monitoring strategy. Circulation 2001;104(1):46–51.

68. Krahn AD, Klein GJ, Yee R, et al. Use of an extended monitoring strategy in patients with problematic syncope. Reveal Investigators. Circulation 1999;99(3):406–10.

69. Edvardsson N, Frykman V, van Mechelen R, et al. Use of an implantable loop recorder to increase the diagnostic yield in unexplained syncope: results from the PICTURE registry. Europace 2011;13(2):262–9.

70. Zaidi A, Clough P, Cooper P, et al. Misdiagnosis of epilepsy: many seizure-like attacks have a cardiovascular cause. J Am Coll Cardiol 2000;36(1):181–4.

71. Zaidi A, Clough P, Mawer G, et al. Accurate diagnosis of convulsive syncope: role of an implantable subcutaneous ECG monitor. Seizure 1999;8(3):184–6.

72. Moya A, Brignole M, Menozzi C, et al. Mechanism of syncope in patients with isolated syncope and in patients with tilt-positive syncope. Circulation 2001; 104(11):1261–7.

73. Krahn AD, Klein GJ, Yee R, et al. Cost implications of testing strategy in patients with syncope: randomized assessment of syncope trial. J Am Coll Cardiol 2003; 42(3):495–501.

74. Brignole M, Sutton R, Menozzi C, et al. Early application of an implantable loop recorder allows effective specific therapy in patients with recurrent suspected neurally mediated syncope. Eur Heart J 2006;27(9):1085–92.

75. Brignole M. International study on syncope of uncertain aetiology 3 (ISSUE 3): pacemaker therapy for patients with asystolic neurally-mediated syncope: rationale and study design. Europace 2007;9(1):25–30.

76. Di Girolamo E, Di Iorio C, Leonzio L, et al. Usefulness of a tilt training program for the prevention of refractory neurocardiogenic syncope in adolescents: a controlled study. Circulation 1999;100(17):1798–801.

77. van Dijk N, Quartieri F, Blanc JJ, et al. Effectiveness of physical counterpressure maneuvers in preventing vasovagal syncope: the Physical Counterpressure Manoeuvres Trial (PC-Trial). J Am Coll Cardiol 2006;48(8):1652–7.

78. Cox MM, Perlman BA, Mayor MR, et al. Acute and long-term beta-adrenergic blockade for patients with neurocardiogenic syncope. J Am Coll Cardiol 1995; 26(5):1293–8.

79. Natale A, Sra J, Dhala A, et al. Efficacy of different treatment strategies for neurocardiogenic syncope. Pacing Clin Electrophysiol 1995;18(4 Pt 1):655–62.

80. Ventura R, Maas R, Zeidler D, et al. A randomized and controlled pilot trial of beta-blockers for the treatment of recurrent syncope in patients with a positive or negative response to head-up tilt test. Pacing Clin Electrophysiol 2002;25(5): 816–21.

81. Sheldon R, Connolly S, Rose S, et al. Prevention of Syncope Trial (POST): a randomized, placebo-controlled study of metoprolol in the prevention of vasovagal syncope. Circulation 2006;113(9):1164–70.

82. Klingenheben T, Credner S, Hohnloser SH. Prospective evaluation of a two-step therapeutic strategy in neurocardiogenic syncope: midodrine as second line treatment in patients refractory to beta-blockers. Pacing Clin Electrophysiol 1999;22(2):276–81.

83. Mitro P, Trejbal D, Rybar AR. Midodrine hydrochloride in the treatment of vasovagal syncope. Pacing Clin Electrophysiol 1999;22(11):1620–4.

84. Samniah N, Sakaguchi S, Lurie KG, et al. Efficacy and safety of midodrine hydrochloride in patients with refractory vasovagal syncope. Am J Cardiol 2001;88(1):A7, 80–3.

85. Ward CR, Gray JC, Gilroy JJ, et al. Midodrine: a role in the management of neurocardiogenic syncope. Heart 1998;79(1):45–9.

86. Raviele A, Brignole M, Sutton R, et al. Effect of etilefrine in preventing syncopal recurrence in patients with vasovagal syncope: a double-blind, randomized,

placebo-controlled trial. The Vasovagal Syncope International Study. Circulation 1999;99(11):1452–7.

87. Morillo CA, Leitch JW, Yee R, et al. A placebo-controlled trial of intravenous and oral disopyramide for prevention of neurally mediated syncope induced by head-up tilt. J Am Coll Cardiol 1993;22(7):1843–8.

88. Di Girolamo E, Di Iorio C, Sabatini P, et al. Effects of paroxetine hydrochloride, a selective serotonin reuptake inhibitor, on refractory vasovagal syncope: a randomized, double-blind, placebo-controlled study. J Am Coll Cardiol 1999;33(5):1227–30.

89. Ammirati F, Colivicchi F, Santini M. Permanent cardiac pacing versus medical treatment for the prevention of recurrent vasovagal syncope: a multicenter, randomized, controlled trial. Circulation 2001;104(1):52–7.

90. Connolly SJ, Sheldon R, Roberts RS, et al. The North American Vasovagal Pacemaker Study (VPS). A randomized trial of permanent cardiac pacing for the prevention of vasovagal syncope. J Am Coll Cardiol 1999;33(1):16–20.

91. Sutton R, Brignole M, Menozzi C, et al. Dual-chamber pacing in the treatment of neurally mediated tilt-positive cardioinhibitory syncope: pacemaker versus no therapy: a multicenter randomized study. The Vasovagal Syncope International Study (VASIS) Investigators. Circulation 2000;102(3):294–9.

92. Connolly SJ, Sheldon R, Thorpe KE, et al. Pacemaker therapy for prevention of syncope in patients with recurrent severe vasovagal syncope: Second Vasovagal Pacemaker Study (VPS II): a randomized trial. JAMA 2003;289(17):2224–9.

93. Raviele A, Giada F, Menozzi C, et al. A randomized, double-blind, placebo-controlled study of permanent cardiac pacing for the treatment of recurrent tilt-induced vasovagal syncope. The vasovagal syncope and pacing trial (SYNPACE). Eur Heart J 2004;25(19):1741–8.

94. Sud S, Massel D, Klein GJ, et al. The expectation effect and cardiac pacing for refractory vasovagal syncope. Am J Med 2007;120(1):54–62.

95. Kenny RA, Richardson DA, Steen N, et al. Carotid sinus syndrome: a modifiable risk factor for nonaccidental falls in older adults (SAFE PACE). J Am Coll Cardiol 2001;38(5):1491–6.

96. Rattes MF, Klein GJ, Sharma AD, et al. Efficacy of empirical cardiac pacing in syncope of unknown cause. CMAJ 1989;140(4):381–5.

97. Pires LA, May LM, Ravi S, et al. Comparison of event rates and survival in patients with unexplained syncope without documented ventricular tachyarrhythmias versus patients with documented sustained ventricular tachyarrhythmias both treated with implantable cardioverter-defibrillators. Am J Cardiol 2000;85(6):725–8.

98. Mittal S, Iwai S, Stein KM, et al. Long-term outcome of patients with unexplained syncope treated with an electrophysiologic-guided approach in the implantable cardioverter-defibrillator era. J Am Coll Cardiol 1999;34(4):1082–9.

99. Moss AJ, Zareba W, Hall WJ, et al. Prophylactic implantation of a defibrillator in patients with myocardial infarction and reduced ejection fraction. N Engl J Med 2002;346(12):877–83.

100. Bardy GH, Lee KL, Mark DB, et al. Amiodarone or an implantable cardioverter-defibrillator for congestive heart failure. N Engl J Med 2005;352(3):225–37.

101. Buxton AE, Lee KL, Fisher JD, et al. A randomized study of the prevention of sudden death in patients with coronary artery disease. Multicenter Unsustained Tachycardia Trial Investigators. N Engl J Med 1999;341(25):1882–90.

102. Klein GJ, Gersh BJ, Yee R. Electrophysiological testing. The final court of appeal for diagnosis of syncope? Circulation 1995;92(5):1332–5.

Infectious Diseases and Impaired Consciousness

Michael R. Wilson, MD[a], Karen L. Roos, MD[b],*

KEYWORDS

- Neuroinfectious diseases • Infectious disease
- Disorders of consciousness • Impaired consciousness

Any of a number of neuroinfectious diseases can cause a disorder of consciousness. The priority in the care of the patient is to identify an infectious disease that is treatable. The disorder of consciousness may be caused by a septic encephalopathy, bacterial meningoencephalitis, viral encephalitis, tick-borne bacterial disease, fungal meningitis, tuberculous meningitis, a focal infectious mass lesion, such as a brain abscess, or an autoimmune-mediated disorder as a complication of infection (**Box 1**).

SEPTIC ENCEPHALOPATHY

Infection is one of many systemic conditions associated with an alteration in the patient's level of consciousness. Sepsis has a nationwide annual incidence of 750,000 and is defined as the host reaction to infection characterized by a systemic inflammatory response.[1] Although the pathogenesis of sepsis remains incompletely understood, it involves an imbalance of proinflammatory and anti-inflammatory responses to an infection. Multiorgan failure frequently accompanies this cascade of events and largely explains the stubbornly high mortality of almost 30% associated with sepsis.

Although the multiorgan failure seen in septic patients frequently results in altered levels of consciousness, there is increasing awareness that many septic patients exhibit alterations in consciousness even before organ failure occurs. This syndrome, which involves impaired attention, orientation, concentration, and anxiety, has been termed septic encephalopathy. Unlike the asterixis, tremor, and multifocal myoclonus seen in patients with liver, kidney, or endocrine failure, patients with early septic encephalopathy typically lack these findings; however, like other aspects of sepsis, septic encephalopathy can also progress, resulting in delirium and coma. As it can

[a] Harvard-Partners Neurology Residency, Massachusetts General Hospital, Brigham and Women's Hospital, Boston, MA, USA
[b] Department of Neurology, Indiana University School of Medicine, Suite 1711 550 North University Boulevard, Indianapolis, IN 46202, USA
* Corresponding author.
E-mail address: kroos@iupui.edu

Neurol Clin 29 (2011) 927–942
doi:10.1016/j.ncl.2011.07.013   **neurologic.theclinics.com**
0733-8619/11/$ – see front matter © 2011 Elsevier Inc. All rights reserved.

Box 1
Differential diagnosis for infectious causes of impaired consciousness

Systemic Causes

- Septic encephalopathy (systemic site of infection should be suggested by patient's history, examination, radiographic and laboratory data)
- Organ dysfunction (eg, hepatic, renal)
- Toxic ingestion
- Electrolyte abnormalities, hypoglycemia or hyperglycemia

Focal Cerebral Dysfunction

- Brain abscess (bacterial, tuberculoma, fungal, parasitic)
- Tumor
- Granuloma
- Subdural empyema
- Demyelination
- Ischemic or hemorrhagic stroke

Diffuse Cerebral Dysfunction

- Viral encephalitis
- Bacterial meningitis
- Fungal meningoencephalitis
- Autoimmune encephalitis
- Postinfectious encephalomyelitis
- Seizure

Complications of Neuroinfectious disease

- Status epilepticus
- Hydrocephalus
- Hemorrhage (subdural, subarachnoid, intracerebral)
- Vasculopathy or vasculitis resulting in stroke
- Venous sinus thrombosis

---

be difficult to sort out the competing causes of altered levels of consciousness (eg, hypoxemia, hypotension, peripheral organ failure, focal central nervous system [CNS] infections and drugs of abuse) in the septic patient, estimated rates of septic encephalopathy vary, ranging from 8% to 70%.[2]

The degree of septic encephalopathy correlates with mortality, although it remains unclear whether the two are causally linked.[3] The pathophysiology of septic encephalopathy remains unknown, but animal and human studies have suggested contributions from amino acid derangements, inflammatory cytokines, microcirculatory failure, blood-brain barrier disruption, abnormal neurotransmitters and the direct impact of bacteria and/or their endotoxins on the CNS.[4,5]

That sepsis appears to have a real impact on neuronal health has been recently demonstrated by a large, prospective cohort study looking at the long-term cognitive and functional disability of elderly sepsis survivors.[6] Iwashyna and colleagues[6] found that rates of moderate and severe cognitive impairment increased 10% among severe sepsis survivors compared with no increase in cognitive impairment among elderly admitted to the hospital for nonsepsis indications. Given the high incidence of sepsis nationwide, this constitutes an important public health issue in the acute and chronic settings.

BACTERIAL MENINGOENCEPHALITIS

Bacterial meningitis begins as an acute purulent infection within the subarachnoid space. The multiplication and lysis of bacteria with the subsequent release of bacterial cell wall components in the subarachnoid space is the inciting event for an inflammatory response that leads to the neurologic complications of cerebral edema, arteritis with ischemic and hemorrhagic infarctions, obstructive and communicating hydrocephalitis, seizure activity, and venous sinus thrombosis. One or more of these complications of the inflammatory response results in an altered level of consciousness.

The most common causative organisms of community-acquired bacterial meningitis in individuals ages 15 to 50 years are *Streptococcus pneumoniae* and *Neisseria meningitidis*. Patients with the predisposing conditions of otitis media, mastoiditis, or sinusitis are at risk for meningitis caused by *Streptococcus* spp, gram-negative anaerobes, Enterobacteriaceae, *Staphylococcus aureus,* and *Haemophilus* spp. *Listeria monocytogenes* is a causative organism of bacterial meningitis in adults older than 55 and in patients with impaired cell-mediated immunity. This includes patients with hematological malignancies, organ transplantation, cancer and cancer chemotherapy, human immunodeficiency virus (HIV) infection, chronic corticosteroid therapy, and pregnant women.[7] In the neurosurgical patient, the most common causative organisms of bacterial meningitis are staphylococci, gram-negative bacilli, and anaerobes.

Clinical Presentation

The clinical presentation of bacterial meningitis is that of fever, headache, vomiting, and stiff neck. These symptoms may be followed either rapidly by a progressive alteration in the level of consciousness or can be present for a few days before there is a disorder of consciousness. Seizure activity occurs in approximately 40% of patients. Raised intracranial pressure is an expected complication of bacterial meningitis and is the most common cause of a disorder of consciousness in this disease.

Diagnosis

In the patient with an altered level of consciousness and fever, adjunctive and empiric antimicrobial therapy for bacterial meningitis is initiated immediately after a set of blood cultures is obtained (**Fig. 1**). The initiation of antimicrobial therapy should not await a head CT scan and a lumbar puncture. Antimicrobial therapy for several hours before lumbar puncture does not significantly alter the cerebrospinal fluid (CSF) white blood cell count or glucose concentration so that a diagnosis of bacterial meningitis is not suspected, and it is not likely to sterilize the CSF so that the organism cannot be identified by Gram's stain or grown in culture. Empiric therapy of bacterial meningitis in children and adults up to age 50 should include a combination of dexamethasone and either a third-generation (ceftriaxone) or fourth-generation (cefepime) cephalosporin plus vancomycin. See **Table 1** for the recommended doses of antimicrobial agents. In patients with the predisposing condition of otitis media, mastoiditis, or sinusitis, metronidazole is added to empiric therapy. Ampicillin should be added for coverage of *Listeria monocytogenes* in individuals older than 55 years and in individuals with impaired cell-mediated immunity. Gentamicin is added to ampicillin in critically ill

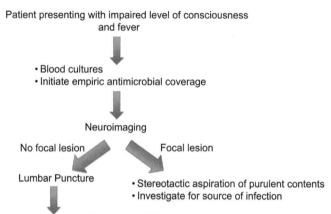

Patient presenting with impaired level of consciousness and fever

• Blood cultures
• Initiate empiric antimicrobial coverage

Neuroimaging

No focal lesion   Focal lesion

Lumbar Puncture
                       • Stereotactic aspiration of purulent contents
                       • Investigate for source of infection

• Modify empiric therapy based on results of spinal fluid analysis
• Consider autoimmune causes if infectious work-up negative
• Consider complications such as non-convulsive status epilepticus or
  increased intracranial pressure

Fig. 1. Diagnostic and treatment algorithm.

patients with *Listeria monocytogenes* meningitis. Empiric therapy in the neurosurgical patient should include a combination of vancomycin plus meropenem or vancomycin plus ceftazidime. Metronidazole should be added to this regimen in patients with ventriculostomies to cover anaerobes. In addition, acyclovir is added to empiric therapy to cover for the possibility of herpes simplex virus encephalitis and doxycycline is added during tick season for tick-borne bacterial infections.

The classic cerebrospinal fluid abnormalities in bacterial meningitis are as follows: (1) increased opening pressure (>180 mm H_2O in 90%); (2) a pleocytosis of polymorphonuclear leukocytes; (3) a decreased glucose concentration (<45 mg/dL); and (4) an increased protein concentration. The CSF should be examined by Gram's stain and bacterial culture. The 16S rRNA conserved sequence broad-based bacterial polymerase chain reaction (PCR) can detect small numbers of viable and nonviable organisms in CSF. There also are a number of meningeal pathogen-specific bacterial PCRs that are increasingly available.

Treatment

Once the meningeal pathogen is isolated and the sensitivity of the organism to the antibiotic is confirmed by in vitro testing, antimicrobial therapy is modified accordingly (see **Table 1**).

Of note, recent work has demonstrated that an increased dosing schedule of vancomycin is more likely to achieve therapeutic concentrations within the CSF. Vancomycin's passage through the blood-brain barrier is facilitated by meningeal inflammation, and adjunctive dexamethasone administration can limit this. In a prospective study, Ricard and colleagues[8] measured vancomycin concentrations in the serum and CSF of adults in medical intensive care units who had confirmed pneumococcal meningitis and who were treated with dexamethasone and intravenous antibiotics, including vancomycin (60 mg/kg per day after a loading dose of 15 mg/kg). At this dosage, all patients achieved vancomycin levels in the CSF much greater than the minimal inhibitory concentration of vancomycin for *S pneumoniae*, and all tolerated it well. Present recommendations are that patients receive 45 to 60 mg/kg per day in an 8-hour dosing schedule.

Table 1	
Recommended doses for antibiotic therapy in bacterial meningitis	
Antibiotic Agent	**Total Daily Dosage (Dosing Interval in Hours)**
Ampicillin	Neonate: 150 mg/kg/d (q8h) Infants and children: 300 mg/kg/d (q6h) Adult: 12 g/d (q4–6h)
Cefepime	Infants and children: 150 mg/kg/d (q8h) Adult: 6 g/d (q8h)
Cefotaxime	Neonate: 100–150 mg/kg/d (q8–12h) Infants and children: 225–300 mg/kg/d (q6–8h) Adult: 8–12 g/d (q4–6h)
Ceftazidime	Children: 125–150 mg/kg/d (q8h) Adult: 6 g/d (q8h)
Ceftriaxone	Infants and children: 80–100 mg/kg/d (q12h) Adult: 4 g/d (q12h)
Gentamicin	Neonate: 5 mg/kg/d (q12h) Infants and children: 7.5 mg/kg/d (q8h) Adult: 5 mg/kg/d (q8h)
Meropenem	Infants and children: 120 mg/kg/d (q8h) Adult: 6 g/d (q8h)
Metronidazole	Infants and children: 30 mg/kg/d (q6h) Adult dose: 1500–2000 mg/d (q6h)
Nafcillin	Neonates: 75 mg/kg/d (q8–12h) Infants and children: 200 mg/kg/d (q6h) Adult: 9–12 g/d (q4h)
Penicillin G	Neonates: 0.15–0.2 mU/kg/d (q8–12h) Infants and children: 0.3 mU/kg/d (q4–6h) Adult: 24 million units/d (q4–6h)
Rifampin	Infants and children: 10–20 mg/kg/d (q12–24h) Adults: 600–1200 mg/d (q12h)
Vancomycin	Neonates: 20–30 mg/kg/d (q8–12h) Infants and children: 60 mg/kg/d (q6h) Adults: 45–60 mg/kg/d (q6–12h)
Chemoprophylaxis *Neisseria meningitidis*	Rifampin 600 mg twice daily for 2 days or Ceftriaxone 250 mg intramuscularly

Before or with the first dose of antibiotic therapy, dexamethasone is administered in a dose of 10 mg and given every 6 hours for 4 days. A prospective, randomized, multicenter, double-blind trial of adjunctive dexamethasone therapy for bacterial meningitis in 301 adults in 5 European countries over 9 years demonstrated that dexamethasone improves the outcome in adults with acute bacterial meningitis, and reduces mortality.[9] A follow-up study by this group was recently published in which they compared national mortality and disability rates in the Netherlands before and after the dexamethasone dosing regimen became successfully implemented nationwide.[10] Unfavorable outcomes at hospital discharge decreased from 50% to 39%, and death rates were reduced from 30% to 20%.

Meningitis caused by *S pneumoniae* and *H influenzae* is treated with intravenous antibiotics for 10 to 14 days. Meningitis caused by *N meningitidis* is treated for 5 to 7 days. Patients with suspected or confirmed meningococcal meningitis have to be isolated for the first 24 hours after initiation of antibiotic therapy, and treated with rifampin 600 mg every 12 hours for 2 days after they finish a course of intravenous antimicrobial therapy to eradicate nasopharyngeal colonization. Meningitis caused by *Listeria monocytogenes* is treated for 3 to 4 weeks. All patients with pneumococcal meningitis should have their CSF reexamined 48 hours after antibiotic therapy has been initiated to determine if the CSF culture is negative, given the emergence of penicillin-resistant and cephalosporin-resistant pneumococcal organisms. Empiric therapy for postoperative meningitis should include a combination of vancomycin and meropenem based on the possibility that methicillin-resistant *Staphylococcus aureus* is the causative organism. Meropenem is added for gram-negative coverage. When the results of culture and sensitivities are known, antimicrobial therapy can be modified accordingly.

VIRAL ENCEPHALITIS

Herpes simplex virus type 1 (HSV-1) is the most common cause of acute sporadic viral encephalitis. Reactivation of latent trigeminal ganglionic infection with replication of herpes simplex virus leads to encephalitis with inflammatory and necrotizing lesions in the inferior and medial temporal lobes, the orbital frontal cortex, and the limbic structures.[11,12] In addition, another herpesvirus, varicella zoster virus, is increasingly identified as the etiologic agent of encephalitis.

A number of arthropod-borne viruses (arboviruses) can cause encephalitis, including West Nile virus, St. Louis encephalitis virus, La Crosse virus, Japanese encephalitis virus, eastern equine encephalitis virus, western equine encephalitis virus, Venezuelan equine encephalitis virus, dengue virus, Powassan virus, and Colorado tick fever virus. Rabies virus may also cause encephalitis. In patients who are immunosuppressed from organ transplantation, immunosuppressive therapy, cancer and cancer chemotherapy, encephalitis may be caused by HSV-1, varicella zoster virus, human herpesvirus type 6 (HHV-6), cytomegalovirus (CMV), or Epstein-Barr virus (EBV).

Clinical Presentation

Encephalitis caused by HSV-1 begins with fever, hemicranial or generalized headache, difficulty with memory, behavioral abnormalities, word-finding difficulty, and focal seizure activity. Encephalitis caused by varicella zoster virus typically presents with fever, headache, and an altered level of consciousness or focal neurologic deficits, due to ischemic and hemorrhagic infarctions and demyelinating lesions. Varicella zoster virus encephalitis may be a complication of shingles, follow the cutaneous eruption of zoster by several months, or occur in the absence of a history of shingles. HHV-6 may cause an encephalitis in immunocompromised patients with focal features that resemble HSV-1.

The arthropod-borne viruses may cause a mild febrile illness with headache, an aseptic meningitis, or an encephalitis. Arthropod-borne viral encephalitis, in general, is often preceded by an influenzalike prodrome of malaise, myalgias, and fever. This is followed by headache, nausea, vomiting, confusion, seizures, and a progressive deterioration in the level of consciousness. West Nile virus encephalitis may be associated with an acute flaccid paralysis, a poliomyelitis-like syndrome. The Flaviviruses, which include West Nile virus, St. Louis encephalitis virus, and Japanese encephalitis virus, infect the basal ganglia and substantia nigra and may be associated with symptoms of parkinsonism. Most dengue virus infections result in relatively mild illness, but dengue virus may cause a reduced level of consciousness and seizures.[13]

Classic rabies caused by the bite of a rapid dog may present as an encephalitis. Rabies caused by the bite of a bat presents with focal neurologic deficits (hemiparesis), choreiform movements, myoclonus, seizure, and hallucinations.[14]

Diagnosis

The diagnosis of encephalitis as the etiology of a disorder of consciousness is made by magnetic resonance imaging (MRI) and spinal fluid analysis. The characteristic MRI abnormality of HSV-1 encephalitis is a high signal intensity lesion on T2-weighted and fluid-attenuated inversion recovery (FLAIR) images in the medial and inferior temporal lobe extending up into the insula. Examination of the CSF demonstrates an increased opening pressure, a lymphocytic pleocytosis of 5 to 500 cells/mm^3, a mild to moderate increase in the protein concentration, and a normal or mildly decreased glucose concentration. The CSF PCR for HSV DNA is most likely to be positive on days 3 to 10 after symptom onset; therefore if the HSV PCR is negative on CSF obtained within the first 24 to 72 hours after symptom onset, spinal fluid analysis should be repeated and the PCR performed again. In addition, spinal fluid should be sent for antibodies against herpes simplex virus. Antibodies against herpes simplex virus appear in the spinal fluid approximately 8 to 12 days after symptom onset and they can increase markedly during the first 2 to 4 weeks of infection. A serum-to-CSF antibody ratio of less than 20:1 is considered diagnostic of herpes simplex virus infection.

The best test to send on CSF for the diagnosis of West Nile virus encephalitis and for varicella zoster virus encephalitis are immunoglobulin M (IgM) antibodies. In addition, there is a PCR for West Nile virus nucleic acid that can be sent on CSF and there is a PCR for varicella zoster virus DNA that can be sent on CSF. However these PCRs are not as sensitive as the IgM. In varicella zoster virus encephalitis, the MRI may demonstrate large and small ischemic and hemorrhagic infarctions of the cortical and subcortical gray matter and white matter as well as lesions typical of demyelination. In West Nile virus encephalitis and encephalitis caused by the other flaviviruses, St. Louis encephalitis virus and Japanese encephalitis virus, on T2-weighted and FLAIR MRI images, hyperintense lesions may be seen in the substantia nigra, basal ganglia, and thalamus.

EBV may cause encephalitis during acute EBV infection and in immunocompromised patients. During primary infection and in immunocompromised patients, the detection of RBV DNA in the CSF is evidence that EBV is the causative virus of the encephalitis; however, EBV DNA is found in peripheral blood latently infected mononuclear cells and can be present in any inflammatory or infectious CNS disorder. Thus, a positive PCR for EBV DNA in an immunocompetent patient with encephalitis should be interpreted cautiously, and in the context of EBV serology.

To make a diagnosis of arboviral encephalitis, send acute and convalescent sera to detect a fourfold or greater increase in viral antibody titer in sera over the course of 4 weeks.

Treatment

HSV-1 encephalitis is treated with intravenous acyclovir 10 mg/kg every 8 hours for 3 weeks. Varicella zoster virus encephalitis is treated with intravenous acyclovir 10 mg/kg every 8 hours for a minimum of 14 days. The therapy of arboviral encephalitis is primarily supportive care with management of the neurologic complications of seizures and increased intracranial pressure, but there are ongoing studies to investigate human intravenous immunoglobulin (IVIg) for West Nile virus encephalitis. In immunosuppressed patients, HHV-6 variant A encephalitis is treated with foscarnet 60 mg/kg every 8 hours and HHV-6 variant B can be treated with either foscarnet or ganciclovir 5 mg/kg every 12 hours. CMV encephalitis is treated with a combination of ganciclovir 5 mg/kg intravenously every 12 hours plus foscarnet 60 mg/kg intravenously every 8 hours for a minimum of 2 to 3 weeks followed by maintenance therapy. Acyclovir-resistant herpes simplex virus isolates have been identified in immunosuppressed and immunocompromised patients; therefore, in the patient with herpes simplex virus encephalitis who is not improving on acyclovir therapy, consideration can be given to switching the patient to foscarnet.

HUMAN IMMUNODEFICIENCY VIRUS

The course of HIV has changed dramatically since the introduction of highly active antiretroviral therapy (HAART). HAART has affected not only the systemic, but also the neurologic complications of HIV and its associated opportunistic infections.[15] Although many of the opportunistic infections that affect the CNS are discussed elsewhere in this article (eg, CMV encephalitis, crytopccoccal meningitis, and tuberculous meningitis), it is important to emphasize that HIV itself can alter the level of consciousness both when untreated and in the setting of HAART.[16] Acute HIV infection typically causes fever, lethargy, flulike illness, headache, pharyngitis, generalized rash, lymphadenopathy, and gastrointestinal disturbances; however, patients can also present with an aseptic meningitis or a fulminant meningoencephalitis.[17] Thus, primary HIV infection needs to be on the differential diagnosis of patients presenting with a clinical picture consistent with viral encephalitis or meningitis.

Untreated, however, HIV frequently causes a progressive, subcortical dementia that can develop insidiously over weeks but also appear more clinically fulminant over a period of days. Patients typically complain initially of short-term memory loss, inability to concentrate, and slowness of thinking. In its final stage, HIV dementia manifests with wide-eyed mutism, quadriparesis, and incontinence.[18] Characteristic imaging changes on MR include diffuse, nonenhancing T2/FLAIR hyperintensities throughout the subcortical white matter. The CSF profile is characterized by a mild to moderately elevated protein concentration and a mild to moderate lymphocytic pleocytosis. HIV dementia is most commonly seen in patients with CD4 counts less than 200 cells per mm^3. Patients typically make significant gains in cognition with institution of HAART therapy.

Although the incidence of HIV dementia has dropped dramatically in the HAART era, new reasons for a rapid decline in consciousness independent of opportunistic infections are being described. With the introduction of HAART, patients with advanced HIV are vulnerable to an immune reconstitution inflammatory syndrome (IRIS). IRIS is typically directed against an inadequately controlled systemic opportunistic infection like tuberculosis and can result in a dramatic worsening of symptoms and even death. More recent recognition has been given to IRIS syndromes affecting the CNS (ie, neuro IRIS), against CNS opportunistic infections like toxoplasmosis, tuberculosis, and progressive multifocal leukoencephalopathy, but also in the setting of advanced HIV without any known opportunistic infections. The latter can present with a rapid decrease in the level of consciousness together with imaging and CSF findings that are consistent with untreated HIV dementia. Patients can become quite disabled, and it can take months to achieve full neurologic recovery.[19,20]

Although patients frequently achieve full systemic virologic suppression with initiation of HAART, the varying degrees to which the different antiretroviral medications penetrate the CNS and the ability of HIV to mutate independently in the immune-privileged CNS has resulted in cases of full serologic viral suppression but active replication of HIV in the CNS. This phenomenon of HIV escape in the CNS can manifest as an acute to subacute decline in mental status together with neuroimaging and CSF profiles consistent with changes seen in HIV dementia.[21,22]

INFLUENZA A VIRUS

Influenza A is a member of the Orthomyxoviridae family and is an enveloped negative-strand RNA virus that is spread primarily by inhalation of infectious droplets. Although it has been reported, influenza A is not typically neuroinvasive.[23] Despite this, neurologic complications have been well recognized as a consequence of influenza infection, especially when a number of patients developed a potentially influenza-associated encephalopathy known as encephalitis lethargica in the 1918 pandemic.

The new triple-reassortant influenza A (H1N1) virus that swept the globe in 2009 also caused rare neurologic side effects that typically altered the patient's level of consciousness. This most recent H1N1 strain most commonly affected children, and the neurologic complications were seen most commonly in children as well. These ranged from seizures, acute necrotizing encephalopathy (ANE), meningoencephalitis, acute disseminated encephalomyelitis (ADEM), and transverse myelitis.[24,25] Although many of the patients with neurologic complications had normal neuroimaging and CSF profiles, the imaging changes seen in the patients with ANE included subcortical hemorrhages and bilateral, symmetric restricted diffusion in the basal ganglia.[26] Fortunately, it does not appear that the severity or frequency of these syndromes is in excess of prior influenza A virus outbreaks. Although patients who developed ANE had a high mortality rate, most of the other patients with neurologic complications made a full recovery.

TICK-BORNE BACTERIAL INFECTIONS

Rickettsia rickettsii is transmitted by the bite of a tick and causes Rocky Mountain spotted fever. In addition, 2 human ehrlichioses may also cause a syndrome of fever and an altered level of consciousness. Human monocytic ehrlichioses is caused by *Ehrlichia chaffeensis*, and human granulocytic anaplasmosis is caused by *Anaplasma phagocytophilum*.

Clinical Presentation

Rocky Mountain spotted fever begins with fever, malaise, headache, myalgias, and a rash. The rash beings on the wrist and ankles and then spreads to the trunk, face, palms, and soles. The rash is initially a maculopapular rash that then becomes petechial and finally a purpuric rash. A disorder of consciousness may develop during the course of the illness.[27] This is most often a delirium or confusion but patients may progress to coma.

The human ehrlichioses may present with high fever, intense headache, and a disorder of consciousness ranging from mild lethargy to coma.

Diagnosis

The tick-borne bacterial infections are difficult to diagnose because of the lack of availability of good serologic tests. Acute and convalescent sera should be sent to detect a fourfold increase in antibody titers. Detectable antibodies may not be present in the acute sample and therefore serial samples should be sent on a weekly basis to detect antibodies. In both Rocky Mountain spotted fever and in human monocytic ehrlichioses, spinal fluid analysis demonstrates a lymphocytic pleocytosis and a normal glucose concentration. In human granulocytic anaplasmosis, spinal fluid analysis may demonstrate a mild CSF pleocytosis.[28]

Treatment

Rocky Mountain spotted fever is treated with doxycycline 100 mg intravenously every 12 hours for at least 7 days and until the patient has been afebrile for at least 48 hours. Human monocytic ehrlichioses and human granulocytic anaplasmosis are also treated with doxycycline 100 mg twice daily for a minimum of 5 to 7 days and for at least 48 hours after defervescence.

FUNGAL MENINGITIS

Fungal meningitis can cause a disorder of consciousness in both immunocompetent and immunosuppressed individuals. An individual's risk of fungal meningitis is determined by his or her risk of having acquired a fungus through residence in an endemic area, travel history, or occupational and recreational activities. Histoplasma capsulatum is a fungus that is endemic to the Ohio and Mississippi River Valleys and is acquired by inhalation. Cryptococcus neoformans is acquired through direct exposure to pigeon droppings. Coccidioides immitis is a fungus that is endemic to the desert areas of the southwest United States and infection is acquired by inhalation of airborne arthroconidia.

Clinical Presentation

The most common symptoms of fungal meningitis are headache that is typically present for weeks, rather than days, fever and malaise, nausea and vomiting, and meningismus. As the disease progresses, a disorder of consciousness may develop, as well as cranial nerve palsies.

Diagnosis

The diagnosis of fungal meningitis is made by examination of the CSF, which demonstrates the following abnormalities: (1) normal or slightly elevated opening pressure; (2) lymphocytic pleocytosis; (3) elevated protein concentration; and (4) a decreased glucose concentration. Fungi can be demonstrated on India ink stain of CSF and grown in culture; however, it can take serial lumbar punctures or a high cisternal puncture to obtain fluid from which the fungus can be identified. The cryptococcal antigen is a highly sensitive and specific test for cryptococcal meningitis. The CSF histoplasma polysaccharide antigen is positive in patients with meningitis caused by Histoplasma capsulatum; however, there are cross reactions with Coccidioides immitis, Cryptococcus neoformans, and Candida.[29] The recommended CSF test for the diagnosis of meningitis caused by Coccidioides immitis is the compliment fixation antibody test.[30]

The management of cryptococcal meningitis is divided into primary therapy (induction and consolidation) and maintenance (suppressive) therapy.[31] Primary therapy is with amphotericin B (0.7–1 mg/kg per day) plus flucytosine (100 mg/kg per day in 4 divided doses) for at least 4 weeks for patients with meningoencephalitis without neurologic complications and with negative CSF yeast culture results after 2 weeks of treatment. Induction therapy should be extended for a total of 6 weeks in patients with neurologic complications. Induction therapy is followed by consolidation therapy with fluconazole 400 mg per day for 8 weeks. For patients with HIV infection, chronic suppressive therapy with fluconazole is recommended.[31] The treatment of meningitis caused by H capsulatum typically requires a course of amphotericin to a target dose of 30 mg/kg. Meningitis caused by C immitis is treated with either high-dose fluconazole,

1000 mg daily as monotherapy, or intravenous amphotericin B (0.5–0.7 mg/kg per day) for longer than 4 weeks. Intrathecal amphotericin B (0.25–.075 mg per day 3 times weekly) may be required to eradicate the infection. Lifelong therapy with fluconazole is recommended to prevent relapse.

In the management of the patient with fungal meningitis, careful attention must be given to the development of increased intracranial pressure as well as to the development of hydrocephalus. Either or both of these may cause a disorder of consciousness. Intracranial pressure should be measured at the time of initial lumbar puncture. Reduce the opening pressure by 50% and repeat the lumbar puncture daily until the CSF pressure has stabilized for more than 2 days. Intracranial pressure should be measured by lumbar puncture any time during the course of the illness when the patient has a change in mental status or a change in the neurologic examination. If the practice of daily lumbar punctures does not lead to a stabilization in the CSF pressure, or if for any reason it is impractical to do, a ventriculostomy should be inserted and CSF removed through the ventriculostomy.

TUBERCULOUS MENINGITIS

Similar to fungal infections, a person becomes infected with *Mycobacterium tuberculosis* when they inhale aerosolized droplet nuclei containing tubercle bacilli. Tuberculous meningitis does not typically develop during the course of primary infection, but immunocompetent individuals with untreated *M tuberculosis* infection have a lifetime risk of developing central nervous system disease, which greatly increases should they develop an immunosuppressed state.

Clinical Presentation

Tuberculous meningitis presents either as a subacute or chronic meningitis characterized by fever, night sweats, and headache that are present for weeks before the patient presents for diagnosis or a fulminant meningoencephalitis with an altered level of consciousness, raised intracranial pressure, seizure activity, and stroke. The British Medical Research Counsel divides the clinical course of tuberculous meningitis into 3 stages. In the first stage, the level of consciousness is normal and there are no focal neurologic signs. In the second stage, the patient is confused but not comatose and may have focal neurologic deficits, such as hemiparesis and a single cranial nerve palsy. In the third stage, the patient is febrile and stuperous or comatose, and may have focal neurologic deficits and multiple cranial nerve palsies.[32]

Diagnosis

The most common neuroimaging abnormality of tuberculous meningitis is meningeal enhancement after the administration of a contrast agent and hydrocephalus. The characteristic CSF abnormalities in tuberculous meningitis are as follows: (1) an elevated opening pressure, (2) a lymphocytic pleocytosis, (3) a mildly decreased glucose concentration, and (4) an elevated protein concentration. It is the combination of the CSF lymphocytic pleocytosis and a mildly decreased glucose concentration associated with the clinical presentation of fever and headache that suggest tuberculous meningitis. In addition, fulminant tuberculous meningitis should be a consideration in the patient with a clinical presentation more typical of bacterial meningitis with fever, headache, stiff neck, and an altered level of consciousness. In both bacterial meningitis and tuberculous meningitis, there will be enhancement of the meninges on neuroimaging after the administration of a contrast agent. These two diseases can be differentiated typically by the CSF formula. Early in tuberculous meningitis, however, the CSF may have a predominance of polymorphonuclear leukocytes rather than lymphocytes and look more typical of a bacterial meningitis. As a general rule, the CSF glucose concentration is markedly decreased in bacterial meningitis and only mildly to moderately decreased in tuberculous meningitis. For the diagnosis of tuberculous meningitis, spinal fluid should be examined by acid-fast smear and culture. There are a number of PCRs available to detect *M tuberculosis* DNA in CSF.

Treatment

The treatment of tuberculous meningitis is with a combination of isoniazid (300 mg per day), rifampin (10 mg/kg per day, up to 600 mg per day), and pyrazinamide (25–35 mg/kg per day) for 2 months, followed by isoniazid and rifampin for an additional 9 to 12 months. In patients with a high probability of multidrug-resistant *M tuberculosis* meningitis, therapy is initiated with a combination of isoniazid, rifampin, pyrazinamide, and either streptomycin (1 g daily by intramuscular injection) or ethambutol (15–25 mg/kg per day) for 2 months. This is followed by isoniazid and rifampin to complete a 9-month to 18-month course of therapy. During therapy, the CSF should be monitored and therapy continued until cultures are negative for 6 months.[33]

In a review of the literature on adjunctive corticosteroid therapy for tuberculous meningitis from 1966 to 1996 using MedLine, adjunctive corticosteroid therapy had a significant benefit in improving survival and reducing sequelae for patients with stage 2 disease (characterized by lethargy or confusion but not coma) and less benefit in early disease or late disease (coma), and more benefit with longer regimens.[34]

INTRACRANIAL MASS LESIONS

Either a brain abscess or a rapidly expanding subdural empyema can cause an altered level of consciousness. Empiric antimicrobial therapy is initiated with a combination of a third-generation or fourth-generation cephalosporin plus vancomycin and metronidazole. Diagnosis is made by stereotactic aspiration of the purulent contents. Once the organism and its antimicrobial sensitivities have been identified, antimicrobial therapy is modified accordingly. In addition, a search for the infectious source must be undertaken. Underlying etiologies for brain abscess include poor dentition, mastoiditis, sinusitis, or otitis media resulting in direct invasion, hematogenous spread from bacterial endocarditis or another remote site, or presence of a foreign body.

POSTINFECTIOUS ENCEPHALOMYELITIS

Postinfectious encephalomyelitis is an acute monophasic, inflammatory, and demyelinating disorder of the CNS that follows infection. Patients may present with a disorder of consciousness or with focal neurologic deficits. On T2-weighted and FLAIR MRI, there are asymmetric areas of increased signal abnormality in the subcortical white matter, brainstem, cerebellum, and periventricular white matter. There may be lesions in gray matter as well. On T1 imaging after gadolinium, the lesions enhance. During the acute illness, all the lesions are in the same stage and during the recovery phase of the illness there will be partial resolution of existing lesions without the formation of new lesions. Spinal fluid analysis demonstrates a lymphocytic or mononuclear cell pleocytosis, an elevated protein concentration, and a normal glucose concentration. Myelin basic protein and oligoclonal bands may be detected. Treatment is with high-dose intravenous methylprednisolone 1000 mg per day for 3 to 5 days. Patients who do not respond to IV methylprednisolone can be treated with either plasma exchange therapy or IVIg therapy.

IMMUNE-MEDIATED ENCEPHALITIS

When a patient presents with a clinical syndrome consistent with encephalitis, immune-mediated causes are an increasingly important part of the differential diagnosis. In the California Encephalitis Project, the rate of noninfectious causes was 10%.[34] A significant portion of these cases were caused by an array of autoimmune and paraneoplastic conditions. There have been numerous excellent reviews of these conditions.[35,36] However, 2 etiologies that fall into the recently recognized category of diseases caused by antibodies directed against neuronal extracellular membrane antigens deserve special mention here: anti–voltage-gated potassium channel (VGKC) and anti–N-methyl-D-aspartate receptor (NMDAR) encephalitides. Autoimmune encephalitis caused by antibodies against neuronal antigens are important to recognize, as several of these diseases may respond to appropriate treatment, including immunotherapy.

Anti-NMDAR encephalitis was first described in 2007 in women with ovarian teratomas. Initially, patients present with psychosis, memory and language deficits, and seizures, progressing to a state of unresponsiveness that can resemble catatonia. Other prominent features include abnormal movements (eg, orofacial dyskinesias, complex choreoathetosis, dystonic postures) as well as autonomic instability and hypoventilation. Children and young adults are most commonly affected. Although many patients have normal neuroimaging, a significant percentage develop T2 FLAIR hyperintensities, less commonly with patchy areas of enhancement. Almost all patients have a mild CSF lymphocytic pleocytosis. Although a tumor is frequently found, there are numerous presumably autoimmune cases in which a tumor is not identified. With treatment (both immunosuppression and tumor resection), more than 75% of patients make a good recovery.[37] A recent, retrospective, single-institution study looked at all patients between the ages of 18 and 35 years admitted to a medical intensive care unit (ICU) over the past 5 years. Seven patients diagnosed with encephalitis of unknown etiology were identified, and archived CSF and blood samples were tested for the presence of anti-NMDAR antibodies. Six of the 7 patients tested positive for anti-NMDAR antibodies, representing 1% of that hospital's young adult ICU admissions.[38]

Patients with VGKC-Ab–associated encephalopathy typically present subacutely with memory loss, confusion, and seizures. A low serum sodium concentration is common. MRI can reveal T2 hyperintensities in the medial temporal lobes. With immunosuppressive treatment, patients frequently achieve significant cognitive improvement. As in anti-NMDAR encephalitis, clinical improvement is accompanied by a drop in antibody titers. The frequency of VGKC-Ab–associated encephalopathy has been estimated relative to other well-described paraneoplastic causes of limbic encephalitis, including anti-Hu, anti-Ma, and anti-Ta antibodies. Over a 6-year period, 284 patients with suspected limbic encephalitis presented to a single hospital, and 67 were found to have a paraneoplastic antibody: 40% had the VGKC-Ab whereas 31% had anti-Hu, 15% had anti-Ma, and 13% had anti-Ta antibodies.[39]

NONCONVULSIVE STATUS EPILEPTICUS

Nonconvulsive status epilepticus (NCSE) is an increasingly recognized cause of a prolonged decreased level of consciousness in the setting of CNS infection, especially viral and immune-mediated encephalitis. It especially needs to be considered if a patient's level of consciousness appears to be out of proportion to his or her disease burden as assessed by CSF profile, neuroimaging, and other studies. Fifteen percent of patients with encephalitis develop status epilepticus (SE)[40,41]; however, it is not known what percentage of these patients have NCSE. Refractory NCSE can be quite prolonged. A recent case of NCSE lasting 6 months in a young woman with anti-NMDA receptor encephalitis ultimately resulted in a full functional recovery after removal of her ovarian teratoma.[42]

A study of more than 1000 patients evaluated by the California Encephalitis Project looked at clinical characteristics of 3 groups of patients with encephalitis: those with treatment-refractory SE requiring general anesthetic coma (4% of patients), those with treatment-sensitive SE (40% of patients), and those who did not have seizures (56% of patients). They found that patients with treatment-refractory SE were younger (median age was 10 years) and more likely to have fever and prodromal respiratory or gastro-intestinal symptoms. They were also less likely to have CSF pleocytosis (47%) or abnormal neuroimaging (16%). Although a likely viral cause was determined in 28% of these patients, the increased rate of a normal CSF profile and normal neuroimaging suggests that autoimmune encephalitides also play a role. With regard to prognosis, 28% of these patients died within 2 years and 56% were neurologically impaired or undergoing rehabilitation after 2 years of follow-up.

REFERENCES

1. Angus DC, Linde-Zwirble WT, Lidicker J, et al. Epidemiology of severe sepsis in the United States: analysis of incidence, outcome, and associated cost of care. Crit Care Med 2001;29:1303–10.
2. Green R, Scott LK, Minagar A, et al. Sepsis associated encephalopathy (SAE): a review. Front Biosci 2004;9:1637–41.
3. Sprung CL, Peduzzi PN, Shatney CH, et al. Impact of encephalopathy on mortality in the sepsis syndrome. The Veterans Administration Systemic Sepsis Cooperative Study Group. Crit Care Med 1990;18:8010–806.
4. Streck EL, Comin CM, Barichello T, et al. The septic brain. Neurochem Res 2008; 33:2171–7.
5. Pytel P, Alexander JJ. Pathogensis of septic encephalopathy. Curr Opin Neurol 2009;22:283–7.
6. Iwashyna TJ, Wesley Ely E, Smith DM. Long-term cognitive impairment and func-tional disability among survivors of severe sepsis. JAMA 2010;304:1787–94.
7. Armstrong D, Wong B. Central nervous system infections in immunocompro-mised hosts. Annu Rev Med 1982;33:293–308.
8. Ricard JD, Wolff M, Lacherade JC, et al. Levels of vancomycin in cerebrospinal fluid of adult patients receiving adjunctive corticosteroids to treat pneumococcal meningitis: a prospective multicenter observational study. Clin Infect Dis 2007;44: 250–5.
9. de Gans J, van de Beek D, European Dexamethasone in Adulthood Bacterial Meningitis Study Investigators. Dexamethasone in adults with bacterial menin-gitis. N Engl J Med 2002;347:1549–56.
10. Brouwer MC, Heckenberg SG, de Gans J, et al. Nationwide implementation of adjunctive dexamethasone therapy for pneumococcal meningitis. Neurology 2010;75:1533–9.
11. Stroop WG, Schaefer DC. Production of encephalitis restricted to the temporal lobes by experimental reactivation of herpes simplex virus. J Infect Dis 1986; 153:721.
12. Barnett EM, Jacobsen G, Evans G, et al. Herpes simplex encephalitis in the temporal cortex and limbic system after trigeminal nerve inoculation. J Infect Dis 1994;169:782.

13. Solomon T, Dung NM, Vaughn DW, et al. Tick-borne diseases in the United States. N Engl J Med 1993;329:936–47.
14. Hemachudha T, Rupprecht CE. Rabies. In: Roos KL, editor. Principles of neurologic infectious diseases. New York: McGraw-Hill; 2005. p. 151–74.
15. Sacktor N. The epidemiology of human immunodeficiency virus-associated neurological disease in the era of highly active antiretroviral therapy. J Neurovirol 2002;8:115–21.
16. Ho EL, Jay CA. Altered mental status in HIV-infected patients. Emerg Med Clin North Am 2010;28:311–23.
17. Newton PJ, Newsholme W, Brink NS. Acute meningoencephalitis and meningitis due to primary HIV infection. BMJ 2002;325:1225–7.
18. Navia BA, Jordan BD, Price RW. The AIDS dementia complex: I. Clinical features. Ann Neurol 1986;19:517–24.
19. McCombe JA, Auer RN, Maingat FG, et al. Neurologic immune reconstitution inflammatory syndrome in HIV/AIDS: outcome and epidemiology. Neurology 2009;72:835–41.
20. Venkataramana A, Pardo CA, McArthur JC, et al. Immune reconstitution syndrome in the CNS of HIV infected patients. Neurology 2006;67:383–8.
21. Canestri A, Lescure F, Jaureguiberry S, et al. Nationwide implementation of adjunctive dexamethasone therapy for pneumococcal meningitis. Neurology 2010;75:1533–9.
22. Edén A, Fuchs D, Hagberg L, et al. HIV-1 viral escape in cerebrospinal fluid of subjects on suppressive antiretroviral treatment. J Infect Dis 2010;202:1819–25.
23. de Jong MD, Cam BV, Qui PT, et al. Fatal avian influenza A (H5N1) in a child presenting with diarrhea followed by coma. N Engl J Med 2005;352:686–91.
24. Rellosa N, Bloch K, Shane AL, et al. Neurologic manifestations of pediatric novel H1N1 influenza infection. Pediatr Infect Dis J 2011;30:165–7.
25. Denholm JT, Neal A, Yan B, et al. Acute encephalomyelitis syndromes associated with H1N1. Neurology 2010;75:2246–8.
26. Fugate JE, Lam EM, Rabinstein AA, et al. Acute hemorrhagic leukoencephalitis and hypoxic brain injury associated with H1N1 influenza. Arch Neurol 2010;67: 756–8.
27. Spach DH, Liles WC, Campbell GL, et al. Tick-borne diseases in the United States. N Engl J Med 1993;329:936–47.
28. Sexton DJ, Dasch GA. Rickettsial and ehrlichial infections. In: Roos KL, editor. Principles of neurologic infectious diseases. New York: McGraw-Hill; 2005. p. 327–42.
29. Christin L, Sugar AM. Fungal infections. In: Roos KL, editor. entral nervous system infectious diseases and therapy. New York: Marcel-Dekker; 1997. p. 167–92.
30. Treseler CB, Sugar AM. Fungal meningitis. Infect Dis Clin North Am 1990;4: 789–808.
31. Perfrect JR, Dismukes WE, Dromer F, et al. Clinical practice guidelines for the management of cryptococcal disease: 2010 update by the Infectious Diseases Society of America. Clin Infect Dis 2010;50:291–322.
32. Medical Research Council. Streptomycin in Tuberculosis Trials Committee. Lancet; 1948.
33. Garcia-Monco JC. CNS tuberculosis and myocbacteriosis. In: Roos KL, editor. Principles of neurologic infectious diseases. New York: McGraw-Hill; 2005. p. 195–213.
34. Glaser CA, Honarmand S, Anderson LJ, et al. Beyond viruses: clinical profiles and etiologies associated with encephalitis. Clin Infect Dis 2006;43:1565–77.

35. Rosenbloom MH, Smith S, Akdal G, et al. Immunologically mediated dementias. Curr Neurol Neurosci Rep 2009;9:359–67.
36. Darnell RB, Posner JB. Paraneoplastic syndromes affecting the nervous system. Semin Oncol 2006;33:270–98.
37. Dalmau J, Gleichman AJ, Hughes EG, et al. Anti-NMDA-receptor encephalitis: case series and analysis of the effects of antibodies. Lancet Neurol 2008;7: 1091–8.
38. Prüss H, Dalmau J, Harms L, et al. Retrospective analysis of NMDA receptor antibodies in encephalitis of unknown origin. Neurology 2010;75:1735–9.
39. Jaruis S, Hoffman LA, Stich O, et al. Relative frequency of VGKC and 'classical' paraneoplastic antibodies in patients with limbic encephalitis. J Neurol 2008;255: 1100–1.
40. Misra UK, Kalita J, Nair PP. Status epilepticus in central nervous system infections: an experience from a developing country. Am J Med 2008;121:618–23.
41. Glaser CA, Gilliam S, Honarmand S, et al. Refractory status epilepticus in suspected encephalitis. Neurocrit Care 2008;9:74–82.
42. Johnson N, Henry C, Fessler AJ, et al. Anti-NMDA receptor encephalitis causing prolonged non-convulsive status epilepticus. Neurology 2010;75:1480–2.

Central Nervous System Complications After Transplantation

Rajat Dhar, MD, FRCPC(C)[a],*, Theresa Human, PharmD, BCPS[b]

KEYWORDS

- Organ transplantation • Bone marrow transplant • Seizures
- Opportunistic infections • Brain diseases • Metabolic
- Drug toxicity

The ability to transplant visceral organs and hematopoietic stem cells into donors with organ failure and other life-threatening diseases has revolutionized modern medicine. Advances in transplant techniques and immunosuppression have facilitated graft and patient survival, resulting in improved quality of life for many transplant recipients.[1] Transplantation uniquely combines: (1) unstable recipients with organ failure and other comorbidities; (2) complex surgical procedures with high risk for hemodynamic instability and perioperative physiologic derangements; (3) postoperative organ dysfunction, sepsis, and polypharmacy; and (4) a prolonged state of immunosuppression. This complex milieu places transplant recipients at high risk for several neurologic complications. The spectrum of neurologic morbidity includes frequent postoperative alterations in mental status as well as seizures and cerebrovascular events. This risk persists with recipients at risk for opportunistic central nervous system (CNS) infections and delayed CNS malignancies (especially lymphoma). A significant proportion of these complications can be attributed to the effects of drug toxicity or the immunosuppressed state they induce. Events are often multifactorial, with several interacting factors contributing to encephalopathy and seizures. The frequency, type, and cause of such complications are reviewed, considering solid organ transplants (heart, lung, liver, kidneys, and intestinal) as well as hematopoietic stem cell transplantation (HSCT). The number of each organs transplanted annually in the United States, common indications for transplantation, and organ-specific technical issues that contribute to neurologic complications, as well as patient survival at 1 and 5 years, are summarized in **Table 1**.

The authors have nothing to disclose.

[a] Division of Neurocritical Care, Department of Neurology, Washington University in St Louis School of Medicine, Campus Box 8111, 660 South Euclid Avenue, St Louis, MO 63110, USA
[b] Neurology/Neurosurgery Intensive Care Unit, Department of Pharmacy, Barnes-Jewish Hospital, 216 South Kingshighway Boulevard, St Louis, MO 63110, USA
* Corresponding author.
E-mail address: dharr@neuro.wustl.edu

Table 1
Specific details of various solid organ and hematopoietic transplants

Organ	Heart	Lung	Liver	Kidneys[b]	Intestinal[a]	HSCT
Number transplanted in United States (2008)	2085	1473	5817[b]	16,067[b]	69	Not reported
Common indications for transplantation	Idiopathic CM Ischemic CM Congenital HD HOCM	COPD including 1-antitrypsin deficiency Cystic fibrosis Interstitial lung disease Primary PH Sarcoidosis	Hepatitis B/C Alcoholic cirrhosis PBC/PSC Autoimmune hepatitis Cryptogenic cirrhosis Malignancy, amyloid Acute liver failure (eg, acetaminophen)	Dialysis caused by: diabetes glomerulonephritis renovascular polycystic kidney disease	Short-bowel syndrome (TPN-dependent) caused by: mesenteric thrombosis Crohn disease neoplasm radiation	Leukemia MDS Lymphoma Aplastic anemia Myeloma Sickle cell Malignancy SCID
Organ-specific technical issues	Cardiac bypass Aortic cannulation Manipulation of heart (introduces air) Postoperative arrhythmias	Phrenic nerve injury May require bypass Reperfusion pulmonary edema Hypoxemia + PH	Fluid and electrolyte shifts, blood loss Anastomotic leak or stenosis Air embolism	Femoral nerve injury Lumbosacral plexopathy	Bacterial translocation Malnutrition Hepatic cholestasis	Conditioning including myeloablative chemotherapy ± TBI GVHD[c]
Markers of posttransplant organ function	Off circulatory support Cardiac index/BP	Oxygenation Extubation	Making bile (bilirubin) Synthetic function (eg, INR)	Making urine Creatinine	Decreasing G tube returns/increasing ileostomy output	Engrafting (rising cell counts)
Patient survival (%)[d]	88 at 1 y 75 at 5 y	83 at 1 y 54 at 5 y	88 at 1 y 74 at 5 y	95 at 1 y 82 at 5 y	89 at 1 y 58 at 5 y	Varies with disease 10%–85% at 5 y
Specific neurocomplications	Embolic stroke, HIE	HIE	CPM ICH related to coagulopathy	Hypertension-related ischemic stroke or ICH	Wernicke encephalopathy	Early infections ICH Tumor recurrence

Abbreviations: BP, blood pressure; CM, cardiomyopathy; COPD, chronic obstructive pulmonary disease; CPM, central pontine myelinolysis; GVHD, graft-versus-host disease; HD, heart disease; HIE, hypoxic-ischemic encephalopathy; HOCM, hypertrophic obstructive cardiomyopathy; ICH, intracranial hemorrhage; INR, international normalized ratio; MDS, myelodysplastic syndrome; PBC, primary biliary cirrhosis; PH, pulmonary hypertension; PSC, primary sclerosing cholangitis; SCID, severe combined immunodeficiency; TBI, total-body irradiation; TPN, total parenteral nutrition.
[a] May be performed in combination with liver transplant.
[b] Includes living and deceased donors.
[c] Allogeneic HSCT only.
[d] Survival for 2006 to 2007 (1 y) and 2002 to 2007 (5 y).
Data from Wolfe RA, Roys EC, Merion RM. Trends in organ donation and transplantation in the United States, 1999–2008. Am J Transplant 2010;10:961–72. (Survival for deceased donors).

INCIDENCE

The frequency at which patients experience neurologic complications after organ or bone marrow transplants has been reviewed in several studies.[2–21] However, most are retrospective and have not used rigorous definitions of specific complications, meaning that at best they represent broad approximations of incidence and likely underestimate less severe sequelae. Studies included in **Table 2** were restricted to contemporary clinical series (excluding autopsy series, which are inherently biased toward a higher incidence of severe complications) that examined either acute/early postoperative or both early and delayed complications (specifically encephalopathy, seizures, and ischemic/hemorrhagic strokes). We focused on studies of adult recipients but some studies combined adult and pediatric patients.

Timing of neurologic events provides significant guidance on which causes to consider; for example, most cases of metabolic encephalopathy and seizures occur in the first few weeks after transplantation, whereas most opportunistic infections occur 1 month or more after transplant. Drug toxicity tends to occur early (contributing to the high rate of seizures and altered mental status observed after transplant) but can occur at any point while the patient is on immunosuppressant therapy. The total rate of complications is variable because investigators include a variety of other neurologic symptoms, including headache, tremor, and peripheral nervous system dysfunction in this figure. Serious complications occur in roughly 10% to 30% of transplant recipients. The spectrum of neurologic morbidity may also be shifting, with a declining incidence of severe acute complications with refined operative techniques and postoperative care (including lower-intensity immunosuppressive regimens); as transplant patients survive longer, they become more at risk for delayed complications such as opportunistic infections and malignancies.

Encephalopathy remains the most common complication in these series, with rates as high as 43% (generally highest after liver, intestinal, and lung transplant); it predominantly occurs in the immediate postoperative period, out until hospital discharge and often extending length of stay.[6,11,13,21] Encephalopathy may be attributed to many disease processes both systemic and CNS, and each patient may harbor multiple contributing processes. It may be useful to divide the presentation of altered mental states after transplant into those not waking up after surgery and those developing delirium and other alterations in mentation after initial awakening.

FAILURE TO AWAKEN

When a patient does not recover normal alertness after transplant surgery, a review of operative and perioperative factors often reveals relevant abnormalities. The operative records should be reviewed for evidence of hypotension (related to excess blood loss, cardiac arrhythmias or cardiac arrest, time on cardiac bypass, and postreperfusion syndrome in liver transplantation[22]). Air embolism can also occur during organ or vascular manipulation and may present with perioperative mental status changes, seizures and cardiovascular collapse[23]; head computed tomography (CT) may reveal air within intracranial vessels. Pulmonary complications may lead to significant arterial desaturation precipitating or worsening cerebral hypoxia. Global hypoxia or cerebral hypoperfusion may lead to a condition of hypoxic-ischemic encephalopathy (HIE), with widespread ischemic damage to susceptible brain regions.[24] Many patients with persistent encephalopathy after surgery have significant graft dysfunction, including primary nonfunction resulting in persistent hypoxemia (lung), hypotension (cardiac), hepatic encephalopathy (liver), or uremia (kidney); some require retransplantation (then associated with a higher rate of neurologic morbidity).[25–27] Hypotension

Table 2
Incidence of neurologic complications after organ and hematopoietic transplantation

Organ	Study	Type	Number	Follow-up: Acute/Chronic	Encephalopathy (%)	Seizures (%)	Cerebrovascular (%)	Total Neurologic Complications (%)
Heart	Mayer et al,[2] 2002	R	191	Acute	2.1	6.8	7.3	36 (including PN)
Heart	Perez-Miralles et al,[3] 2005	R	322[a]	Both	n/a	1.9	3.5% stroke, 0.6% ICH	13.7
Heart	Zierer et al,[4] 2007	R	200	Acute	5	7	3.5 stroke, 2 ICH	23
Heart	van de Beek et al,[5] 2008	R	313	Acute	9	2.6	2.2 stroke, 0.6 ICH	19
Heart	Munoz et al,[6] 2010	R	384	Both	1.3	1.5	5 stroke, 1.6 ICH 0.8 HIE	20
Lung	Goldstein et al,[7] 1998	R	100	Both	3%	10	5%	26
Lung	Zivkovic et al,[8] 2009	R	132	Both	25	8	5 stroke, 1.5 ICH	68
Lung	Mateen et al,[9] 2010	R	120	Both	24	5.8	10.8	79
Liver	Vecino et al,[10] 1999	P	43	Both	16	7	9	53 including HA
Liver	Bronster et al,[11] 2000	R	463	Both	12	8	0.6 stroke, 1.5 ICH	20
Liver	Lewis and Howdle,[12] 2003	R	711	Acute	10	6	1.7 stroke, 2 ICH	26
Liver	Saner et al,[13] 2007	R	168	Both (1 y)	19	5.4	2.4	27
Liver	Dhar et al,[14] 2008	R	101	Acute	28	4	No cases	31
Intestinal	Zivkovic et al,[15] 2010	R	54	Both	43	17	4	85 including HA

Renal	Yardimci et al,[16] 2008	R	132	Both	0.8 (caused by hyponatremia)	2	1.5 (1 case of CVST)	13.6 including HA
HSCT	Graus et al,[17] 1996	R	425[b]	Both	3 metabolic	3.7	3.8 ICH (mostly SDH), 0.5 strokes	11
HSCT	Antonini et al,[18] 1998	P	115[b]	Acute (90 d)	7	7	0.9 ICH	56 including PN[c]
HSCT	Sostak et al,[19] 2003	P	71	Both (1 y)	3 metabolic	1.4	4 stroke, 2.8 SDH	18
HSCT	Denier et al,[20] 2006	R	361[d]	Both	2.8[e]	5[f]	1.7 ICH	16
HSCT	Siegal et al,[21] 2007	P	302	Both (1 y)	14.6 (PRES in 7)	9	0.3	9 at 30 d 23 at 1 y

Abbreviations: CVST, cerebral venous sinus thrombosis; HA, headache; HSCT, hematopoietic stem cell transplant; ICH, intracerebral hemorrhage; n/a, not applicable; P, prospective; PN, peripheral neuropathy; R, retrospective; SDH, subdural hematoma; stroke, ischemic stroke.

[a] Excluded those who died in first month.
[b] All had leukemia, in Antonini (1998) all were allogeneic.
[c] 27 (24%) had major complications (excluding tremor and headache).
[d] Allogeneic in 245.
[e] More frequent in allogeneic than autologous HSCT.
[f] Mainly infections.

and shock associated with multiorgan failure or sepsis may be responsible for the high incidence of anoxic/ischemic changes seen in autopsy series of patients dying after organ transplantation.[28–31]

Anesthetic and sedative drugs given intraoperatively and in the intensive care unit (ICU) can accumulate and contribute to delayed awakening, especially in combination with hepatic and renal dysfunction, altering drug metabolism and elimination. Benzodiazepines, opioids, and barbiturates can lead to prolonged sedation in this setting. Occasionally neuromuscular blocking agents can have persistent effects, resulting in paralysis even a day or more postoperatively.[32] This state can easily be excluded by train-of-four testing using a peripheral nerve stimulator on the median, ulnar, or facial nerves, and reversed with neostigmine (given along with glycopyrrolate).

An algorithm for the assessment of failure to awaken after organ transplantation is provided in **Fig. 1**. Those patients with impaired premorbid function (including preexisting encephalopathy and more severe underlying disease) are at higher risk for neurologic complications after transplant.[14,33] Close attention should be paid to the often evolving medical status of the transplant recipient. Impaired graft function (as

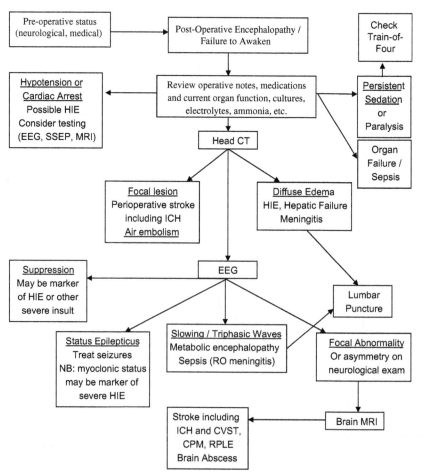

Fig. 1. Algorithm for the evaluation of a patient with posttransplant encephalopathy, including failure to awaken from surgery.

assessed by the organ-specific factors outlined in **Table 1**), presence of other organ dysfunction (eg, posttransplant renal failure), and sepsis/multiorgan failure syndrome all contribute to postoperative encephalopathy.[34] It is unclear whether a distinct syndrome of encephalopathy specifically related to allograft rejection exists, separate from the adverse effects induced by metabolic disturbances resulting from graft dysfunction (eg, uremia). The term rejection encephalopathy has been proposed to encapsulate mental status changes in renal transplant recipients with acute rejection, postulated to result from cytokine release but also associated with acute hypertension.[35] A thorough evaluation for reversible causes should be undertaken in any patient with failure to awaken after organ transplantation. It may be worthwhile reviewing complex patient cases with the transplant surgeon, anesthesiologist, and the ICU pharmacist to identify potential operative insults and ongoing factors accounting for encephalopathy.

Primary neurologic disorders presenting as failure to recover consciousness include HIE, multiple embolic strokes (especially after cardiac transplant), cerebral air embolism, and rarely meningitis. Central pontine myelinolysis (CPM) related to perioperative fluid and sodium shifts can produce a locked-in or comatose state and is seen in a small percentage of liver transplant recipients (discussed later).[28] In those patients with signs of hepatic dysfunction (caused by liver allograft failure or hepatic dysfunction after HSCT or other transplants), consider checking arterial ammonia levels. Although not predictive of severity or outcome, high levels may point to hepatic encephalopathy as a contributing factor in postoperative mental status changes. Idiopathic hyperammonemia after HSCT is described later. Uremia from graft dysfunction (seen in 20%–40% of renal transplant recipients)[36] or acute kidney injury after cardiac, liver, and other transplant surgeries (related to hypotension, medications, or sepsis) may be treated with dialysis, resulting in amelioration of altered mental status. If encephalopathy persists once reversible metabolic disturbances have been identified and reversed (or excluded), then CNS injury should be considered. Further evaluation including magnetic resonance imaging (MRI), lumbar puncture, or electroencephalography (EEG) may be helpful in these cases.

ENCEPHALOPATHY

Alterations in awareness and arousal are frequent after transplantation, most occurring in the first 30 days postoperatively.[11] The spectrum of encephalopathy encompasses reduced levels of consciousness as severe as coma to delirium with diminished attention, or agitation and hallucinations.[37] The differential diagnosis of altered mentation after transplantation is shown in **Table 3**; many cases are multifactorial. The prognosis for patients with encephalopathy is largely governed by the underlying cause. Those with drug toxicity or metabolic causes (each accounting for roughly one-third of cases of encephalopathy) usually do well if the offending abnormality can be reversed, whereas those in whom reduced mental status heralds underlying CNS infection, HIE, or CPM (together accounting for one-third of cases) often do poorly.

Encephalopathy may be particularly common after liver transplantation, as a result of a combination of preoperative neurologic dysfunction, frequent perioperative metabolic derangements, and administration of neurotoxic medications, coupled with postoperative hepatic and renal dysfunction, altering drug metabolism.[23,38] Hepatic encephalopathy that was symptomatic at the time of transplantation was the strongest predictor of postoperative encephalopathy in 1 series.[14] Another study found higher rates of encephalopathy in patients with alcoholic liver disease, associated

Table 3
Cause of posttransplant encephalopathy

Cause of Encephalopathy	Timing	Evaluation
Drug toxicity (especially cyclosporine, tacrolimus)	Days to weeks	Serum drug levels may be increased or normal MRI may show RPLE
Organ and graft failure, sepsis, electrolyte disturbance (calcium, sodium, glucose, magnesium) (ie, metabolic encephalopathy [including HE])	Variable	Organ function panels (renal, hepatic, ABG) Electrolytes, cultures Arterial ammonia
Cerebrovascular: infarcts, intracranial hemorrhage, CVST, HIE	Perioperative or later	CT or MR Imaging ± MRV
CNS infections (meningitis, encephalitis, brain abscesses) and malignancies (including PTLD)	Usually delayed	CSF analysis (consider cryptococcal antigen, fungal and AFB cultures, PCR for viruses) MRI
Nonconvulsive seizures/status epilepticus	Variable	EEG
CPM (ODS)	Perioperative/acute	MRI (findings may be delayed)
Wernicke encephalopathy	Few weeks postoperatively	Ataxia/ophthalmoplegia (absent caloric responses) Malnutrition, MRI changes

Abbreviations: ABG, arterial blood gas; AFB, acid-fast bacilli (eg, Ziehl-Neelson) stain; CVST, cerebral venous sinus thrombosis; HE, hepatic encephalopathy; MRV, magnetic resonance venography; ODS, osmotic demyelination syndrome; PTLD, posttransplantation lymphoproliferative disorder; RPLE, reversible posterior leukoencephalopathy.

with higher ammonia levels.[39] Ammonia impairs synaptic function and produces astrocyte swelling related to glutamine accumulation, which may promote disruption of the blood-brain barrier.[40] This preexisting brain dysfunction makes such patients more susceptible to the unstable perioperative milieu, including the toxic effects of medications on the vulnerable brain.

AKINETIC MUTISM

A state of impaired verbal and motor responsiveness has been noted in transplant recipients.[23] Patients appear awake but do not speak and have minimal motor activity. This syndrome has been reported as a complication of cyclosporine and tacrolimus toxicity, improving after drug discontinuation,[41] but may also be seen with CPM or HIE.[42] A similar picture has been reported with amphotericin treatment of HSCT patients who received irradiation as part of conditioning.[43,44] Radiation may open the blood-brain barrier and thereby facilitate drug toxicity. There is also a case of akinetic mutism in a heart transplant recipient after receiving muromonab-CD3 (OKT3), which resolved once the drug was discontinued and CD3+ lymphocyte counts normalized.[45] A loss of speech (ie, mutism) without akinesia has also been reported in 1% of liver transplant recipients within the first 10 days after surgery, often in association with seizures, responsive to stopping cyclosporine or tacrolimus.[46,47] Any patient with mutism and altered awareness should be evaluated for neuroleptic malignant syndrome, which can be rapidly fatal if not recognized. This condition is related to neuroleptic exposure and associated with fever, rigidity, increased creatine kinase level, and dysautonomia.[48]

SEIZURES

Seizures are not only frightening to a patient, their family, and health care personnel, but they can lead to patient injury, hemodynamic instability, risk of aspiration, and dislodgement of catheters and monitoring devices. Contemporary series have revealed that seizures still occur in 5% to 10% of transplant patients, most often in the first few weeks (see **Table 1**). Many of the same processes listed in **Table 3** may also present with seizures, often associated with prodromal or postictal encephalopathy. Distinction of benign, transient causes (eg, metabolic or drug-related) from primary CNS disorders or severe systemic disease with organ/graft failure is imperative for determining prognosis. Systemic processes typically result in generalized convulsions, whereas focal-onset seizures (albeit often missed or unwitnessed) signal an underlying infectious or cerebrovascular CNS lesion. Seizures related to drug toxicity (the most common cause) are often preceded by subtle behavioral and mental status changes. Nonetheless, cyclosporine or tacrolimus levels are often normal in the face of drug-induced seizures.[49–52]

The stabilization and evaluation of a patient with new posttransplant seizures is outlined in **Fig. 2**. Although status epilepticus is rare, if a patient remains unresponsive after cessation of convulsive activity, an urgent electroencephalogram should be obtained.[53] EEG may also be useful to differentiate epileptic from nonepileptic movements. Tremors and myoclonus are both common complications of medications and metabolic derangements. EEG may be obtained to exclude seizures in an unresponsive patient with twitching movements. Multifocal myoclonus is a specific marker of metabolic encephalopathy (ie, nonepileptic),[54] whereas myoclonic status epilepticus is a reliable indicator of poor prognosis after HIE.[55] Awakening phenomenon with tremors or myoclonus can also be seen after emergence from anesthesia (especially with propofol) and can be mistaken for seizures.[56]

Most seizures after transplant respond to first-line treatment with benzodiazepines; unless a rapidly reversible cause is immediately apparent (eg, hypoglycemia or hyponatremia), then treatment with an antiepileptic drug (AED) should be initiated to prevent further seizures. Phenytoin had been commonly used because it is easily available in most hospital locations and can be loaded intravenously. However, phenytoin has significant limitations, both in terms of drug interactions (most seriously, induction of cyclosporine metabolism, necessitating higher doses and active titration to maintain therapeutic levels) and high degree of protein binding, which may be altered in the critically ill; free phenytoin levels should be obtained for drug monitoring in such situations.[57,58] For these reasons, levetiracetam (Keppra) has become an attractive alternative because it can be administered intravenously, does not undergo hepatic metabolism or induce immunosuppressant medications, and is free of serious toxicity. Most patients do not have seizure recurrence on low doses of levetiracetam (500 mg twice daily), and AED therapy can usually be safely discontinued after the acute period of risk has subsided (eg, a few weeks to a few months). AEDs should be continued longer/indefinitely in the presence of a structural CNS lesion or epileptiform electroencephalogram. The most important step in managing seizures after transplantation is reversal of any underlying cause (eg, stopping or reducing the dose of offending medications, correcting metabolic derangements, treating infections). The prognosis is good for patients with seizures related to a reversible cause (with late recurrence being rare) but poor for those in whom seizures herald a severe

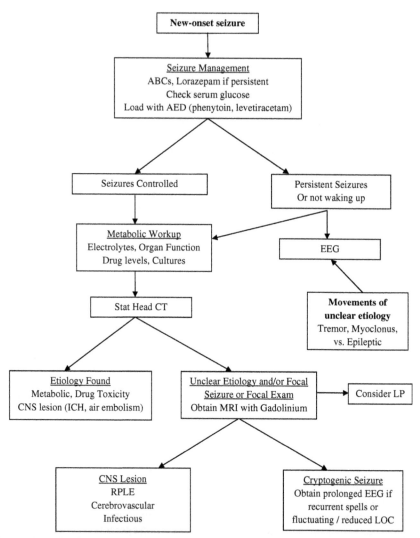

Fig. 2. Algorithm for the management and evaluation of a patient with seizures after transplantation. AED, antiepileptic drug; CVST, cerebral venous sinus thrombosis; EEG, electroencephalogram; ICH, intracranial hemorrhage; LOC, level of consciousness; LP, lumbar puncture; RPLE, reversible posterior leukoencephalopathy.

underlying CNS or systemic illness, in whom they may occur as part of an agonal decline.[52]

DRUG TOXICITY

The introduction of cyclosporine and subsequently other effective immunosuppressive agents revolutionized transplantation, minimizing rejection and improving graft survival.[59] Induction agents are sometimes used immediately after transplant (including thymoglobulin, OKT3, or basiliximab) followed by maintenance therapy with a calcineurin inhibitor (CNI) (cyclosporine or tacrolimus) often coupled with mycophenolate mofetil (MMF) and corticosteroids. CNIs and MMF are usually continued after discharge, whereas steroids are tapered to the lowest effective dose. These medications, although effective, have a narrow therapeutic window, and neurotoxicity was quickly recognized as a significant complication.[60,61] A list of common neurotoxic symptoms and the agents typically responsible for them is presented in **Table 4**.

A significant proportion of encephalopathy after transplantation can be attributed to drug toxicity, with figures ranging from 28% to 39%[8,11,14,15]; this peaks in the early postoperative period with high initial drug exposure.[11,15] Similarly, 29% to 61% of seizures in transplant recipients have been associated with drug toxicity.[11,52,58] The chief culprits amongst these agents are the CNIs. These agents work by binding to specific proteins called the immunophilins (cyclophilin for cyclosporine and FK506-binding protein for tacrolimus) to form a complex that inhibits calcineurin.[62] This process results in inhibition of the calcium-dependent signaling pathway necessary to activate T cells. Several mechanisms have been proposed to explain the neurotoxicity associated with CNIs.[63] Calcineurin is a critical regulator of neuronal excitability

Table 4
Symptom-based differential diagnosis of drug toxicities and their management

Symptom/Syndrome	Medication	Management
Tremor (usually postural)	CNI, steroids, sirolimus	Observe/may resolve over time
Headaches	CNI, MMF, sirolimus OKT3 (aseptic meningitis)	Try abortive agents (sumatriptan) Consider change to other CNI Exclude CNS lesion
Psychiatric (hallucinations, insomnia, anxiety)	CNI, steroids, MMF	Reduce dose if possible
Encephalopathy/Delirium	CNI, OKT3, steroids Also: benzodiazepines, opioids, and other medications	Hold CNI[a] May be multifactorial
Seizures	CNI, busulfan, OKT3 (rare) Also: imipenem, β-lactams, metronidazole, theophylline	Hold CNI[a] (see seizure algorithm)
Akinetic mutism	CNI, OKT3 Amphotericin B (with TBI)	Hold CNI[a] Consider CPM or HIE
Leukoencephalopathy (RPLE) including cortical blindness	CNI	Hold CNI[a]
Paresthesias/peripheral neuropathy	CNI, chemotherapy for HSCT or GVHD including thalidomide	Follow/minimize drug exposure Consider CIP
Myopathy	Steroids, GVHD (polymyositis)	Wean steroids if possible
Epidural lipomatosis (spinal cord or cauda equina compression)	Steroids	May require surgical decompression

Abbreviations: CIP, critical illness polyneuropathy; GVHD, graft-versus-host disease; TBI, total-body irradiation.
[a] Consider restarting at lower dose or changing to other CNI after symptoms resolve.

and function, including regulation of the blood-brain barrier and vasoconstriction/sympathetic activation.[64,65] Preexisting hepatic encephalopathy and perioperative hypotension may disrupt the blood-brain barrier, allowing more drug to reach cerebral tissue and affect neuronal function. Low cholesterol also allows higher unbound circulating drug to diffuse into the brain,[61] accentuating neurotoxic effects, which may include endothelial disruption and formation of vasogenic edema.[66]

Presentation of CNI Toxicity

A variety of neurologic symptoms may be seen with CNI toxicity. Minor complaints, including headache, paresthesias, and tremor, are seen in up to half of treated patients. Neuropsychiatric symptoms, including insomnia, anxiety, and agitation, may occur alone or presage the development of more overt delirium with hallucinations and delusions. Severe manifestations of toxicity include seizures, encephalopathy akinetic mutism, and the clinical-radiographic syndrome of reversible posterior leukoencephalopathy (RPLE), also termed posterior reversible encephalopathy syndrome (PRES).

RPLE is a serious neurologic syndrome with many causes, including CNI therapy. It is also a manifestation of hypertensive encephalopathy and eclampsia.[67] It has acute or subacute onset manifesting with subcortical vasogenic edema believed to result from disruption of the blood-brain barrier and capillary leakage. It typically preferentially affects the occipital and posterior temporal/parietal white matter symmetrically but variants are increasingly being recognized; for example, frontal lobe and brainstem/cerebellar involvement are not uncommon.[68] One large retrospective series found PRES in 0.5% of 4222 solid organ transplant patients, whereas another in HSCT found an incidence of 1.6%.[69,70] However, without prospective studies evaluating each patient with neurologic symptoms using MRI, the exact incidence is likely underrepresented by such estimates. For example, a prospective series in HSCT found PRES in 7% by 1 year, most diagnosed within the first 30 days.[21]

RPLE commonly presents with mental status changes, visual disturbances (including cortical blindness), and focal deficits (eg, hemiparesis, aphasia).[21] Seizures occur in most cases, either as the presenting symptom or in the setting of evolving encephalopathy.[68,71] An older series found RPLE in 4 of 17 patients with drug-induced seizures after liver transplant, whereas a contemporary series found MRI changes of RPLE in all 4 patients with tacrolimus-induced seizures.[52,72] Half the seizures after heart transplant in 1 series were attributed to RPLE.[73] Most RPLE occurs within 30 to 90 days of transplant, but late cases have been reported especially in renal transplant recipients, associated with hypertension.[69] Patients with liver disease may be at particularly high risk early after transplantation, given disruption of the blood-brain barrier from portosystemic encephalopathy, and are typically not hypertensive.

RPLE is diagnosed by synthesizing clinical features of toxicity with radiographic findings on CT (which may be negative or show subtle white matter hypodensity) or preferably MRI (**Box 1**). These findings may reveal the typical posterior white matter hyperintensity, best seen on fluid-attenuated inversion recovery (FLAIR) imaging (**Fig. 3**).[71] These regions are typically negative on diffusion-weighted imaging (DWI) (or show increased not decreased diffusion, differentiating them from acute infarction). They can also involve the cortical ribbon, frontal lobe, and deeper white matter. Brainstem involvement in RPLE may mimic CPM, whereas hemispheric white matter disease can be confused with extrapontine demyelination seen in cases of CPM or with demyelination from progressive multifocal leukoencephalopathy (PML). An approach to differentiating white matter disease is shown in **Table 5**. Hemorrhage may occur within regions of edema in severe cases, resulting in permanent deficits.

Box 1
Diagnostic criteria for CNI neurotoxicity

The development of seizures or encephalopathy in a patient receiving cyclosporine or tacrolimus with:

1. High serum trough levels of the drug at the time of symptom onset

2. Rapid increase in drug levels before symptoms

Human herpesvirus 6 (HHV-6) encephalitis (after HSCT) has also been reported to mimic RPLE with symmetric white matter involvement, but systemic symptoms are often present and cerebrospinal fluid (CSF) reveals a viral polymerase chain reaction (PCR).[74]

Risk Factors for Toxicity

Several factors seem to predispose patients to the neurotoxic effects of CNIs, including high drug levels,[51] rapid changes in levels (as seen with intravenous loading), concomitant administration of medications that inhibit drug metabolism (methylprednisolone, liposomal amphotericin B, and ganciclovir),[75,76] liver disease and low cholesterol,[61] hypertension, and hypomagnesemia.[69]

Although CNI toxicity is often dose related, clinical symptoms are not always associated with increased drug levels. Multiple studies have found no clear correlation between symptoms (including seizures) and increased drug levels.[49–51] Symptoms may develop with rapid increases in drug levels above a patient-specific threshold (not necessarily corresponding to the upper limit of the laboratory reference range). Furthermore, levels of drug metabolites (especially with cyclosporine) may contribute to toxicity.[49,77] Incidence of severe complications may now be lower compared with earlier studies with more cautious titration, avoidance of loading doses, and lower target levels used in modern studies.[78] High rates of neurotoxicity are still reported

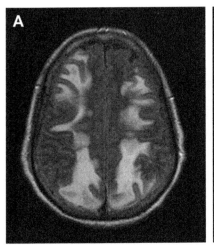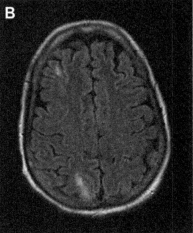

Fig. 3. MRI FLAIR sequence showing increased signal in the hemispheric white matter (A) with improvement 11 days after discontinuation of tacrolimus (B). (*From* Junna MR, Rabinstein AA. Tacrolimus induced leukoencephalopathy presenting with status epilepticus and prolonged coma. J Neurol Neurosurg Psychiatry 2007;78:1411; with permission.)

Table 5
Comparison of white matter diseases affecting transplant recipients

	RPLE	Osmotic Demyelination Syndrome	PML
Timing after transplant	Mostly acute (<4 wk) but can be delayed months to years	Acute (<2 wk), predominantly after liver transplant	Late (>6 mo)
Onset	Acute (d)	Acute (d)	Subacute (wk)
Location/Pattern	Posterior ± frontal white matter May also involve brainstem/cerebellum (usually symmetric)	Pons (CPM) ± external capsule/basal ganglia	Asymmetric, multifocal Subcortical white matter ± cerebellar peduncles
MRI (T2/DWI/Contrast)	High T2 signal, DWI negative Nonenhancing (imaging > clinical symptoms)	High T2 signal, DWI variable, Nonenhancing (imaging may lag behind clinical)	High T2 signal, DWI negative, nonenhancing
Disease	Disruption of BBB Vasogenic edema	Myelin edema and demyelination	Oligodendrocyte infection resulting in demyelination
Cause	CNI toxicity, hypertension	Shifts in sodium and osmolality	Reactivation of JC virus
Presenting features	Encephalopathy, seizures, headache, cortical blindness	Quadriparesis, pseudobulbar state, locked-in syndrome, confusion, EPS	Confusion, behavioral changes, focal deficits including visual
Diagnosis	High drug levels Reversibility on stopping CNI	Characteristic timing and location, abrupt increase in sodium	PCR for JC virus in CSF (70%) Brain biopsy
Prognosis	Reversible	Improvement possible in survivors	Progressive/often fatal
Treatment	Stop or reduce CNI	Supportive Reinstitution of hyponatremia?	Reduce immunosuppressants Cytarabine

Abbreviations: BBB, blood-brain barrier; EPS, extrapyramidal syndrome.
Data from Aksamit AJ. Demyelinating disorders. In: Wijdicks EF, editor. Neurologic complications in organ transplant recipients. Woburn (MA): Butterworth-Heinemann; 1999. p. 230.

in transplant settings in which high drug levels are targeted to prevent or manage rejection.[15]

Cyclosporine Versus Tacrolimus

Tacrolimus has largely supplanted cyclosporine for the prevention of rejection after organ transplantation. It has been shown to reduce the incidence of hypertension, hirsutism, and acute severe rejection in several transplants settings compared with cyclosporine.[79–81] However, it may be associated with higher rates of diabetes and gastrointestinal intolerance, as well as neurotoxicity, specifically headache and tremor. Comparative (but uncontrolled) series have not found a higher rate of serious neurotoxicity (ie, seizures, encephalopathy, RPLE) with 1 CNI over another,[13,14] with rates of 25% found with both agents in 1 study after liver transplant.[12] Lack of major neurotoxicity with novel agents such as sirolimus and everolimus make them appealing alternatives to CNI therapy either in cases with toxicity or as first-line agents[82,83]; such CNI-sparing regimens are being evaluated.[84] However, isolated cases of sirolimus-associated PRES have been reported in association with hypertension.[85,86]

Management of Suspected Drug Neurotoxicity

If drug neurotoxicity is suspected, then management revolves around dose reduction or discontinuation of the offending agent (the latter being preferred in cases of severe toxicity).[65] However, this strategy places allografts at risk for rejection while drug therapy is interrupted. There is no single standard approach to restarting immunosuppresants.[87] Most commonly 1 CNI is substituted for another, whereas in other cases the same agent is restarted at a lower dose once symptoms have resolved; recurrence of toxicity is low with either paradigm.[51] Sirolimus may also be initiated either as replacement therapy or in combination with continued low-dose CNI.[88,89] Generally neurologic symptoms are reversible after CNI discontinuation except in patients in whom late detection has permitted permanent brain injury to occur (eg, hemorrhage with RPLE).[90] For this reason, early recognition is critical. Whereas neurologic deficits with RPLE resolve within a few days of stopping the CNI, radiographic abnormalities may take a few weeks to fully disappear.[91]

OKT3 is an induction agent directed against the CD3 antigen on T cells, effectively blocking T-cell function.[92] It is used commonly for induction after organ transplantation or to halt acute rejection. Headache is frequent and may occur within hours of the first dose and last for days. Preemptive therapy with acetaminophen and antihistamines may be administered. Its major toxicity is aseptic meningitis related to cytokine release. CSF reveals pleocytosis and imaging may confirm meningeal enhancement.[93] Rarely progression to seizures, cerebral edema, and encephalopathy can occur.[94,95] A case of akinetic mutism has also been reported.[45] Treatment is supportive, including discontinuation of further doses if severe toxicity occurs.

CPM

CPM was first described in malnourished alcoholics experiencing rapid increases in serum sodium and osmolality.[96] It is now categorized under the rubric osmotic demyelination syndromes (ODSs),[97] because shifts in sodium and brain water are postulated to result in noninflammatory oligodendrocyte injury and intramyelin edema. This situation results in myelin loss, particularly within the central pons, but involvement of other brain regions (including the basal ganglia, external capsule, and thalamus, ie, extrapontine demyelination) in ODS is increasingly being recognized.[98]

CPM classically presents with quadriparesis, pseudobulbar palsy (dysarthria, dysphagia, alterations in affect), and mental status changes. If horizontal eye movements are abolished, it may result in a locked-in syndrome, with the patient appearing unresponsive to questioning or stimulation, unable to move or look to either side, but potentially fully awake.[99] Vertical eye movements and blinking should be preserved, allowing the patient a means of communicating. Extrapyramidal involvement may produce symptoms of catatonia, tremor, myoclonus, or an akinetic-rigid state.

In the transplant population, ODS has been reported almost exclusively after liver transplantation (although a single case in a child after intestinal transplant has been reported).[23,31,100] Its incidence is estimated at 1.2% to 2% in large series of liver transplant recipients.[11,12] Its pathogenesis is believed to be related to the significant perioperative fluid and sodium shifts (ie, rapid correction of the hyponatremia commonly seen in cirrhotic patients) that occur,[101,102] in association with preexisting hepatic encephalopathy, which is known to deplete myoinositol, an important mediator of cerebral osmotic homeostasis.[103] However, not all patients with CPM show large rises in sodium and not all patients present with the classic pontine syndrome with motor deficits. Instead, many may present with nonfocal postoperative alterations in consciousness.[104] Confusion and depressed level of consciousness may progress, reaching peak severity several days after transplant, whereas in severe cases it may present with failure to awaken postoperatively. CT imaging is relatively insensitive for detecting CPM, whereas the characteristic trident or bat-shaped increase in T2 signal within the central pons may be seen only on MRI several days after symptom onset (**Fig. 4**).[11,105]

Prognosis was assumed to be dismal for those with CPM because it was first noted in autopsy series or in those with locked-in syndrome. However, with MRI permitting detection of less severe cases, patient series have reported significant potential for independent recovery, albeit sometimes with residual motor or cognitive deficits.[106] There are no proven treatments for CPM, although the reintroduction of hyponatremia in the acute phase has been proposed to prevent further myelin injury.[107] Small series have also suggested the use of plasmapheresis or intravenous immunoglobulin.[108,109] Preferably, close attention should be paid to avoiding excessive swings in sodium or serum osmolality (including uremia) in the perioperative period to prevent morbidity from CPM.

STROKE

Development of focal neurologic deficits in a transplant patient most often signals a vascular or infectious CNS process. However, focal deficits may also be seen after seizures (ie, postictal Todd paresis), with drug neurotoxicity (ie, asymmetric RPLE) and with peripheral nerve dysfunction (eg, related to herpes zoster reactivation or perioperative compression neuropathy). Conversely, not infrequently focal and multifocal CNS lesions in transplant patients present with only nonfocal mental status changes or seizures.

Several factors account for the high risk that posttransplant patients have for cerebrovascular events, both ischemic and hemorrhagic (**Box 2**). Thrombocytopenia is common with HSCT and may result in acute spontaneous subdural bleeding (**Fig. 5**). A hypercoagulable state after chemotherapy or transplantation can trigger venous sinus thrombosis, which may present with multiple hemorrhagic lesions (**Fig. 6**). After cardiac transplant, emboli and hypotension contribute to multiple ischemic infarcts (**Fig. 7**).

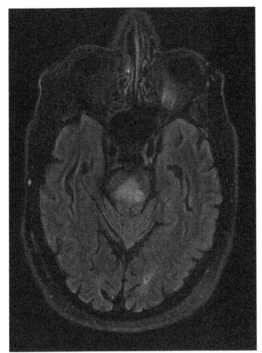

Fig. 4. MRI FLAIR sequence with a triangular hyperintensity within the central pons in a patient who experienced rapid correction of hyponatremia after liver transplantation.

Box 2
Risk factors for cerebrovascular events in posttransplant patients

Ischemic Stroke

- Perioperative hypotension
- Cardiac arrest
- Hypoxemia
- Embolic from cardiac/vascular manipulation (including air embolism)
- Postoperative arrhythmias (eg, atrial fibrillation)
- Septic infarcts (aspergillosis, endocarditis)
- Vasculitis (varicella-zoster virus [VZV], graft-versus-host disease [GVHD, discussed in next section])
- Vascular comorbidity (diabetes, hypertension)

Intracerebral hemorrhage

- Coagulopathy
  - Increased international normalized ratio in liver dysfunction
  - Thrombocytopenia after HSCT
- Fungal infections (especially aspergillosis), including mycotic aneurysms
- Venous sinus thrombosis (may be related to hypercoagulable state)
- Hypertensive intracerebral hemorrhage

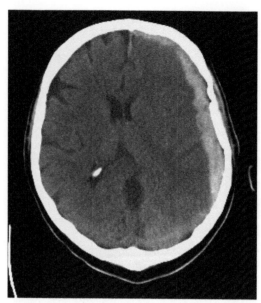

Fig. 5. Head CT with high-density subdural hematoma overlying the left hemisphere causing mass effect and midline shift. Patient was severely thrombocytopenic after bone marrow transplantation.

HSCT AND GVHD

HSCT involves transfer of stem cells from 1 person to another (allogeneic) or (after procurement and storage) back to the donor (autologous).[110] This process allows reconstitution of marrow and immune function after ablation of native bone marrow (and it is hoped the underlying disease process or malignancy) with toxic myeloablative conditioning regimens (typically involving a combination of cyclophosphamide and total-body irradiation [TBI]). However, without hematopoiesis or immune function until engraftment of new stem cells occurs, patients are susceptible to infections and bleeding. Busulfan is used in some TBI-sparing regimens but can acutely precipitate seizures in approximately 10% of recipients.[111] Regimen toxicity can also result in veno-occlusive disease of the liver, causing hepatomegaly, jaundice, and hepatic encephalopathy in severe cases.[112,113]

Allogeneic stem cells provide the benefit of showing potent graft-versus-tumor effect to eradicate refractory neoplasms. However, the most significant and frequent complication of allogeneic HSCT is GVHD.[114] This immune-mediated multiorgan disorder is related to attack by donor leukocytes on recipient tissues. It most commonly affects the skin (rash), oral mucosa, lungs, intestinal tract (diarrhea, abdominal pain), and liver (increased bilirubin level).[115] Acute GVHD is seen in 20% to 40% of allogeneic HSCT recipients and is the rationale for prophylaxis of allogeneic recipients with potent immunosuppression (typically methotrexate early after HSCT and maintenance therapy with cyclosporine or tacrolimus).[116] GVHD can be treated with high doses of corticosteroids much like solid organ rejection. Bowel involvement may induce thiamine deficiency, precipitating the subacute mental status changes of Wernicke encephalopathy.[117,118]

The peripheral nervous system may be involved in chronic GVHD, with inflammatory myopathies being most common.[119] CNS involvement in chronic GVHD is

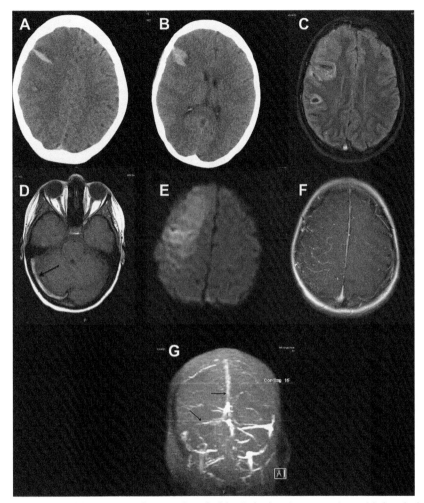

Fig. 6. 19-year-old patient with acute lymphoblastic leukemia presenting with headaches then seizures and left hemiparesis 2 weeks after bone marrow transplantation (platelet count was normal). Head CT shows several hemorrhages in the right frontal lobe and small hemorrhage in the left frontal lobe (A, B). FLAIR sequence on MRI confirms hemorrhagic lesions (C). T1 sequence without contrast reveals high signal in the right transverse sinus consistent with thrombus (arrow, D). There is also right frontal DWI hyperintensity consistent with venous infarction (E). Contrast-enhancing T1 sequence shows engorgement of cerebral veins in the right hemisphere (F). Magnetic resonance venography confirms loss of venous flow in right transverse sinus and patchy loss in the superior sagittal sinus (arrows, G).

controversial.[120] This diagnosis should be entertained only after exclusion of the multiple other potential causes for CNS symptoms in these complex patients. Some cases have been described with a vasculitis-like picture or an immune-mediated encephalitis.[121] Patients may develop cognitive or focal neurologic deficits months to years after HSCT, often after a reduction in immunosuppression. To substantiate the diagnosis of CNS GVHD there must be both evidence of chronic GVHD in other organs and a clear response to immunosuppressive therapy (eg, pulse steroids).

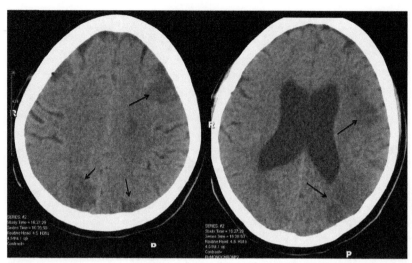

Fig. 7. Multiple embolic or watershed infarcts on head CT in a patient 4 days after cardiac transplant (*arrows* depict hypodense regions of subacute infarction). Patient was confused and had mild aphasia. Echocardiography was normal.

CSF may show increased protein levels, oligoclonal bands, and a variable pleocytosis. MRI may show white matter lesions not dissimilar to multiple sclerosis.[122] Opportunistic infections must be assiduously excluded by thorough CSF testing, MRI, and sometimes even biopsy. Autologous HSCT does not confer a risk of GVHD and these patients are at low risk of ongoing complications once engraftment occurs and cell counts normalize. Complications also occur more often with nonrelated HSCT donors and more often in those with underlying chronic myelogenous leukemia.[17,20,123]

IDIOPATHIC HYPERAMMONEMIA

A rare but often fatal syndrome has been described in 0.5% of HSCT recipients during the period of severe neutropenia.[124] Onset is acute, with lethargy, confusion, and tachypnea, usually progressing to seizures and coma. Ammonia levels are characteristically increased (often more than 200 μmol/L), associated with respiratory alkalosis, but normal or only mildly increased liver enzyme levels. Brain imaging may reveal marked cerebral edema, similar to Reye syndrome.[125] Urea cycle defects including ornithine transcarbamylase deficiency should be excluded by measurement of urinary amino acids and orotic acid. High ammonia levels may also be seen in liver failure, multiple myeloma, and valproate drug therapy.[126] Attempts at treatment have included dialysis or sodium benzoate to remove and trap ammonia but mortality remains high.[127]

CNS POSTTRANSPLANTATION LYMPHOPROLIFERATIVE DISORDER

Lymphoma is the most common brain tumor seen in transplant recipients. The CNS may be the primary site of involvement or associated with systemic posttransplantation lymphoproliferative disorder (PTLD).[128] Most cases of PTLD are associated with Epstein-Barr virus (EBV) infection and occur a few years after solid organ transplantation (although some may occur within the first year).[129] Tumor involvement is more often parenchymal than leptomeningeal (a pattern similar to that seen in patients with AIDS and different from nonimmunocompromised cohorts). Most patients have multiple (often periventricular) enhancing lesions, which may resemble toxoplasmosis (**Fig. 8**); increased uptake on single-photon emission CT (SPECT) may be useful to differentiate. Presentation is usually subacute, with headache, mental status changes, and sometimes focal deficits or seizures. CSF cytology is often negative. Corticosteroids should be held pending biopsy because prebiopsy administration compromises histopathologic diagnosis and may cause tumor cell lysis, with radiographic disappearance of tumor. Steroids should be started after diagnosis to reduce edema pending local radiation or chemotherapy. Reduction in immunosuppression may also be instituted concurrently.

CNS INFECTIONS

More potent and effective immunosuppressive regimens have reduced the risk of graft rejection but increased the susceptibility of transplant recipients to a variety of opportunistic CNS infections. Furthermore, because of the blunted host immune response and less pathogenic nature of these organisms, presentation of these potentially life-threatening infections may be nonspecific and far from acute or obvious. Headache and low-grade fever may be the only signs of CNS involvement, whereas mental status changes comprise the most common neurologic symptoms even in those with focal or multifocal abscesses.[130] Neck stiffness is conspicuously absent in most cases. An outline of the common infections, their modes of presentation, and means of diagnosis and treatment is provided in **Table 6**.

CNS involvement is often metastatic from another site, as part of systemic dissemination; symptoms of the primary infection or systemic involvement may be present (eg, pneumonia with *Aspergillus* and *Nocardia*, diarrhea with *Listeria*). Sites such as skin and bone may also be involved (eg, with *Cryptococcus* and *Nocardia*) and blood cultures or serum PCR may be useful for diagnosis (eg, candidemia). Spread can also occur directly from sinuses, as is seen with rhinocerebral forms of zygomycoses. Sinus imaging may reveal characteristic central calcifications and any suspicious sinusitis should be cultured for fungi.[131]

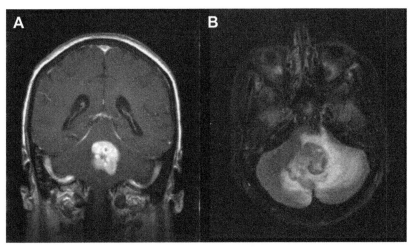

Fig. 8. Primary CNS lymphoma manifesting as large enhancing mass (*A*) centered on the left cerebellar peduncle. There is significant surrounding edema on FLAIR sequence (*B*).

Table 6
Opportunistic infections affecting transplant recipients

Disease	Organism/Details	Primary Site/Source	Meningitis	Encephalitis	Mass Lesion(s) Abscess	Diagnosis	Treatment
Listeria	L monocytogenes GP bacillus	Gastrointestine (contaminated milk or cheese)	X	Brainstem		CSF and blood Cx	Ampicillin ± gentamicin
Nocardiosis	Nocardia asteroides GP branching filamentous rod	Lung (inhalation)	±		X	Sputum, skin, or brain: acid-fast stain and Cx	TMP-SMX
Aspergillosis	Aspergillus fumigatus A flavus Angioinvasive fungus	Lung (inhalation)		Septic infarcts/hemorrhages	X	Galactomannan test (serum) Lung or brain histology, Cx	Voriconazole or amphotericin + flucytosine
Candidiasis	Candida albicans and others Pseudohyphae	Disseminated (skin, lungs) Candidemia	±		X (Mycotic aneurysms)	Blood Cx Brain/lung/skin histology. Cx	Amphotericin
Cryptococcosis	Cryptococcus neoformans Encapsulated yeast	Lung (skin/soft tissue)	X		X	Blood and CSF for antigen, India ink (CSF)	Amphotericin ± flucytosine
CMV, EBV, VZV, HHV-6, HSV	Herpes viruses	Reactivation or primary infection ± pneumonitis, hepatitis, skin	X	Limbic encephalitis (HHV-6, HSV)	PTLD with EBV	CSF and blood: viral PCR (CSF pleocytosis may be absent)	Acyclovir ganciclovir or foscarnet (CMV/HHV-6)
PML	JC virus (polyomavirus)	Reactivation			X PML	PCR for JC virus Biopsy	Cytarabine?
Toxoplasmosis	Toxoplasma gondii Parasite	Reactivation (or transmission from allografts)	X		X	Serology and PCR (CSF, blood) Brain biopsy	Pyrimethamine Sulfadiazine Folinic acid
Tuberculosis	Mycobacterium tuberculosis	Lung (primary or reactivation)	X Basilar		X Tuberculoma	CSF (or sputum): AFB stain, PCR and Cx (delayed) low CSF glucose	INH + rifampin + pyrazinamide + ethambutol ± steroids

Abbreviations: AFB, acid-fast bacilli; Cx, culture; GI, gastrointestinal; GP, gram positive; HSV, herpes simplex virus; INH, isoniazid; TMP-SMX, trimethoprim-sulfamethaxole.

CNS infections can also represent reactivation of latent infections, as is the case for many herpes viruses and the JC virus (causing PML, **Fig. 9**). The spectrum of infections encountered in transplant recipients has also been changing with the contemporary practice of prophylaxis for certain common pathogens; sulfa prophylaxis has reduced the rates of *Listeria*, *Toxoplasma*, and *Nocardia*, whereas cytomegalovirus (CMV) screening and preemptive treatment have reduced consequences of CMV reactivation.

The period of highest risk for infections is typically between 1 and 6 months after solid organ transplantation. Nosocomial infections such as pneumonia and wound infections predominate in the early posttransplant period and opportunistic infections are uncommon, because maximal immunosuppression has not yet been attained (except with HSCT). Early infections may rarely be caused by transmission from a contaminated donor allograft; neurologic morbidity from transmission of West Nile, rabies, and lymphocytic choriomeningitis viruses has been reported in transplant recipients.[132–134] Transmission of toxoplasmosis is common in cardiac transplants if the donor is seropositive and recipient seronegative.[135] If the patient is doing well after 6 months (without rejection or GVHD), the intensity of immunosuppression may be reduced, minimizing ongoing risk for infections. High risk of infection remains beyond 6 months for those with rejection, poor graft function, or GVHD, who require ongoing immunosuppression including repeated courses of high-dose steroids. These patients remain susceptible to CNS infections months to years after transplant.

Any transplant patient with new headache or mental status change more than 1 month after solid organ transplant requires thorough evaluation for underlying infection. Any CNS lesion in a transplant patient must be assumed to be potentially infectious. As with clinical presentation, CSF may be unrevealing or nonspecific. CSF

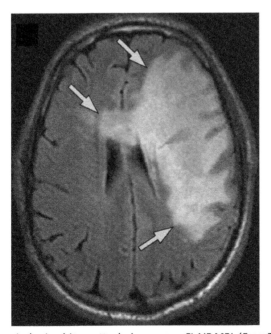

Fig. 9. PML. Left hemispheric white matter lesion seen on FLAIR MRI. (*From* Tan CS, Koralnik IJ. Progressive multifocal leukoencephalopathy and other disorders caused by JC virus: clinical features and pathogenesis. Lancet Neurol 2010;9:430; with permission.)

protein levels may be increased but CSF cell counts may be only minimally increased or even normal. Imaging may be less dramatic even with abscesses, with minimal enhancement and less edema (especially after HSCT, with complete failure of immune response).

SUMMARY

Neurologic complications contribute to significant morbidity after solid organ transplant and HSCT. Encephalopathy is the most common neurologic presentation in the early posttransplant period and may be related to serious organ or graft dysfunction, drug neurotoxicity, or CNS lesions (including vascular, infectious, or demyelinating). Mental status changes may be accompanied by seizures, which are especially common in the setting of immunosuppressant drug toxicity causing RPLE. Prognosis for transplant patients with mental status changes is largely governed by the underlying cause and its reversibility. Many cases of opportunistic CNS infections and major organ dysfunction are fatal, although drug toxicity can usually be reversed if promptly recognized and managed by dose reduction or discontinuation. All patients presenting with encephalopathy, seizures, focal neurologic deficits, or even a new headache should undergo comprehensive evaluation, including laboratory testing, brain imaging, and possibly CSF analysis.

REFERENCES

1. Tome S, Wells JT, Said A, et al. Quality of life after liver transplantation. A systematic review. J Hepatol 2008;48:567–77.
2. Mayer TO, Biller J, O'Donnell J, et al. Contrasting the neurologic complications of cardiac transplantation in adults and children. J Child Neurol 2002;17:195–9.
3. Perez-Miralles F, Sanchez-Manso JC, Almenar-Bonet L, et al. Incidence of and risk factors for neurologic complications after heart transplantation. Transplant Proc 2005;37:4067–70.
4. Zierer A, Melby SJ, Voeller RK, et al. Significance of neurologic complications in the modern era of cardiac transplantation. Ann Thorac Surg 2007;83:1684–90.
5. van de Beek D, Kremers W, Daly RC, et al. Effect of neurologic complications on outcome after heart transplant. Arch Neurol 2008;65:226–31.
6. Munoz P, Valerio M, Palomo J, et al. Infectious and non-infectious neurologic complications in heart transplant recipients. Medicine (Baltimore) 2010;89:166–75.
7. Goldstein LS, Haug MT III, Perl J, et al. Central nervous system complications after lung transplantation. J Heart Lung Transplant 1998;17:185–91.
8. Zivkovic SA, Jumaa M, Barisic N, et al. Neurologic complications following lung transplantation. J Neurol Sci 2009;280:90–3.
9. Mateen FJ, Dierkhising RA, Rabinstein AA, et al. Neurological complications following adult lung transplantation. Am J Transplant 2010;10:908–14.
10. Vecino MC, Cantisani G, Zanotelli ML, et al. Neurological complications in liver transplantation. Transplant Proc 1999;31:3048–9.
11. Bronster DJ, Emre S, Boccagni P, et al. Central nervous system complications in liver transplant recipients–incidence, timing, and long-term follow-up. Clin Transplant 2000;14:1–7.
12. Lewis MB, Howdle PD. Neurological complications of liver transplantation in adults. Neurology 2003;61:1174–8.
13. Saner FH, Sotiropoulos GC, Gu Y, et al. Severe neurological events following liver transplantation. Arch Med Res 2007;38:75–9.

14. Dhar R, Young GB, Marotta P. Perioperative neurological complications after liver transplantation are best predicted by pre-transplant hepatic encephalopathy. Neurocrit Care 2008;8:253–8.
15. Zivkovic SA, Eidelman BH, Bond G, et al. The clinical spectrum of neurologic disorders after intestinal and multivisceral transplantation. Clin Transplant 2010;24:164–8.
16. Yardimci N, Colak T, Sevmis S, et al. Neurologic complications after renal transplant. Exp Clin Transplant 2008;6:224–8.
17. Graus F, Saiz A, Sierra J, et al. Neurologic complications of autologous and allogeneic bone marrow transplantation in patients with leukemia: a comparative study. Neurology 1996;46:1004–9.
18. Antonini G, Ceschin V, Morino S, et al. Early neurologic complications following allogeneic bone marrow transplant for leukemia: a prospective study. Neurology 1998;50:1441–5.
19. Sostak P, Padovan CS, Yousry TA, et al. Prospective evaluation of neurological complications after allogeneic bone marrow transplantation. Neurology 2003;60: 842–8.
20. Denier C, Bourhis JH, Lacroix C, et al. Spectrum and prognosis of neurologic complications after hematopoietic transplantation. Neurology 2006;67:1990–7.
21. Siegal D, Keller A, Xu W, et al. Central nervous system complications after allogeneic hematopoietic stem cell transplantation: incidence, manifestations, and clinical significance. Biol Blood Marrow Transplant 2007;13:1369–79.
22. Aggarwal S, Kang Y, Freeman JA, et al. Postreperfusion syndrome: hypotension after reperfusion of the transplanted liver. J Crit Care 1993;8:154–60.
23. Starzl TE, Schneck SA, Mazzoni G, et al. Acute neurological complications after liver transplantation with particular reference to intraoperative cerebral air embolus. Ann Surg 1978;187:236–40.
24. Singh N, Yu VL, Gayowski T. Central nervous system lesions in adult liver transplant recipients: clinical review with implications for management. Medicine (Baltimore) 1994;73:110–8.
25. Pokorny H, Gruenberger T, Soliman T, et al. Organ survival after primary dysfunction of liver grafts in clinical orthotopic liver transplantation. Transpl Int 2000;13(Suppl 1):S154–7.
26. Varotti G, Grazi GL, Vetrone G, et al. Causes of early acute graft failure after liver transplantation: analysis of a 17-year single-centre experience. Clin Transplant 2005;19:492–500.
27. Marasco SF, Vale M, Pellegrino V, et al. Extracorporeal membrane oxygenation in primary graft failure after heart transplantation. Ann Thorac Surg 2010;90: 1541–6.
28. Blanco R, De Girolami U, Jenkins RL, et al. Neuropathology of liver transplantation. Clin Neuropathol 1995;14:109–17.
29. Prayson RA, Estes ML. The neuropathology of cardiac allograft transplantation. An autopsy series of 18 patients. Arch Pathol Lab Med 1995;119:59–63.
30. McCarron KF, Prayson RA. The neuropathology of orthotopic liver transplantation: an autopsy series of 16 patients. Arch Pathol Lab Med 1998;122: 726–31.
31. Idoate MA, Martinez AJ, Bueno J, et al. The neuropathology of intestinal failure and small bowel transplantation. Acta Neuropathol 1999;97:502–8.
32. Watling SM, Dasta JF. Prolonged paralysis in intensive care unit patients after the use of neuromuscular blocking agents: a review of the literature. Crit Care Med 1994;22:884–93.

33. Kanwal F, Chen D, Ting L, et al. A model to predict the development of mental status changes of unclear cause after liver transplantation. Liver Transpl 2003;9: 1312–9.
34. Young GB, Bolton CF, Austin TW, et al. The encephalopathy associated with septic illness. Clin Invest Med 1990;13:297–304.
35. Gross ML, Pearson RM, Kennedy J, et al. Rejection encephalopathy. Lancet 1982;2:1217.
36. Schnuelle P, Gottmann U, Hoeger S, et al. Effects of donor pretreatment with dopamine on graft function after kidney transplantation: a randomized controlled trial. JAMA 2009;302:1067–75.
37. Beresford TP. Neuropsychiatric complications of liver and other solid organ transplantation. Liver Transpl 2001;7:S36–45.
38. Adams DH, Ponsford S, Gunson B, et al. Neurological complications following liver transplantation. Lancet 1987;1(8539):949–51.
39. Buis IC, Wiesner RH, Krom RA, et al. Acute confusional state following liver transplantation for alcoholic liver disease. Neurology 2002;59:601–5.
40. Haussinger D, Kircheis G, Fischer R, et al. Hepatic encephalopathy in chronic liver disease: a clinical manifestation of astrocyte swelling and low-grade cerebral edema? J Hepatol 2000;32:1035–8.
41. Sierra-Hidalgo F, Martinez-Salio A, Moreno-Garcia S, et al. Akinetic mutism induced by tacrolimus. Clin Neuropharmacol 2009;32:293–4.
42. Laureno R, Karp BP. Cyclosporine mutism. Neurology 1997;48:296–7.
43. Devinsky O, Lemann W, Evans AC, et al. Akinetic mutism in a bone marrow transplant recipient following total-body irradiation and amphotericin B chemo-prophylaxis. A positron emission tomographic and neuropathologic study. Arch Neurol 1987;44:414–7.
44. Walker RW, Rosenblum MK. Amphotericin B-associated leukoencephalopathy. Neurology 1992;42:2005–10.
45. Pittock SJ, Rabinstein AA, Edwards BS, et al. OKT3 neurotoxicity presenting as akinetic mutism. Transplantation 2003;75:1058–60.
46. Bronster DJ, Boccagni P, O'Rourke M, et al. Loss of speech after orthotopic liver transplantation. Transpl Int 1995;8:234–7.
47. Bianco F, Fattapposta F, Locuratolo N, et al. Reversible diffusion MRI abnormalities and transient mutism after liver transplantation. Neurology 2004;62:981–3.
48. Garrido SM, Chauncey TR. Neuroleptic malignant syndrome following autologous peripheral blood stem cell transplantation. Bone Marrow Transplant 1998;21:427–8.
49. Lane RJ, Roche SW, Leung AA, et al. Cyclosporin neurotoxicity in cardiac transplant recipients. J Neurol Neurosurg Psychiatry 1988;51:1434–7.
50. Wijdicks EF, Wiesner RH, Dahlke LJ, et al. FK506-induced neurotoxicity in liver transplantation. Ann Neurol 1994;35:498–501.
51. Wijdicks EF, Wiesner RH, Krom RA. Neurotoxicity in liver transplant recipients with cyclosporine immunosuppression. Neurology 1995;45:1962–4.
52. Wijdicks EF, Plevak DJ, Wiesner RH, et al. Causes and outcome of seizures in liver transplant recipients. Neurology 1996;47:1523–5.
53. Junna MR, Rabinstein AA. Tacrolimus induced leukoencephalopathy presenting with status epilepticus and prolonged coma. J Neurol Neurosurg Psychiatry 2007;78:1410–1.
54. Mahoney CA, Arieff AI. Uremic encephalopathies: clinical, biochemical, and experimental features. Am J Kidney Dis 1982;2:324–36.

55. Young GB, Gilbert JJ, Zochodne DW. The significance of myoclonic status epilepticus in postanoxic coma. Neurology 1990;40:1843–8.
56. Walder B, Tramer MR, Seeck M. Seizure-like phenomena and propofol: a systematic review. Neurology 2002;58:1327–32.
57. Keown PA, Laupacis A, Carruthers G, et al. Interaction between phenytoin and cyclosporine following organ transplantation. Transplantation 1984;38:304–6.
58. Glass GA, Stankiewicz J, Mithoefer A, et al. Levetiracetam for seizures after liver transplantation. Neurology 2005;64:1084–5.
59. Calne RY, White DJ, Thiru S, et al. Cyclosporin A in patients receiving renal allografts from cadaver donors. Lancet 1978;2:1323–7.
60. Berden JH, Hoitsma AJ, Merx JL, et al. Severe central-nervous-system toxicity associated with cyclosporin. Lancet 1985;1:219–20.
61. de Groen PC, Aksamit AJ, Rakela J, et al. Central nervous system toxicity after liver transplantation. The role of cyclosporine and cholesterol. N Engl J Med 1987;317:861–6.
62. Ho S, Clipstone N, Timmermann L, et al. The mechanism of action of cyclosporin A and FK506. Clin Immunol Immunopathol 1996;80:S40–5.
63. Gijtenbeek JM, van den Bent MJ, Vecht CJ. Cyclosporine neurotoxicity: a review. J Neurol 1999;246:339–46.
64. Dawson TM. Immunosuppressants, immunophilins, and the nervous system. Ann Neurol 1996;40:559–60.
65. Bechstein WO. Neurotoxicity of calcineurin inhibitors: impact and clinical management. Transpl Int 2000;13:313–26.
66. Bunchman TE, Brookshire CA. Smooth muscle cell proliferation by conditioned media from cyclosporine-treated endothelial cells: a role of endothelin. Transplant Proc 1991;23:967–8.
67. Hinchey J, Chaves C, Appignani B, et al. A reversible posterior leukoencephalopathy syndrome. N Engl J Med 1996;334:494–500.
68. Lee VH, Wijdicks EF, Manno EM, et al. Clinical spectrum of reversible posterior leukoencephalopathy syndrome. Arch Neurol 2008;65:205–10.
69. Bartynski WS, Tan HP, Boardman JF, et al. Posterior reversible encephalopathy syndrome after solid organ transplantation. AJNR Am J Neuroradiol 2008;29:924–30.
70. Wong R, Beguelin GZ, de Lima M, et al. Tacrolimus-associated posterior reversible encephalopathy syndrome after allogeneic haematopoietic stem cell transplantation. Br J Haematol 2003;122:128–34.
71. Furukawa M, Terae S, Chu BC, et al. MRI in seven cases of tacrolimus (FK-506) encephalopathy: utility of FLAIR and diffusion-weighted imaging. Neuroradiology 2001;43:615–21.
72. Emiroglu R, Ayvaz I, Moray G, et al. Tacrolimus-related neurologic and renal complications in liver transplantation: a single-center experience. Transplant Proc 2006;38:619–21.
73. Navarro V, Varnous S, Galanaud D, et al. Incidence and risk factors for seizures after heart transplantation. J Neurol 2010;257:563–8.
74. Gewurz BE, Marty FM, Baden LR, et al. Human herpesvirus 6 encephalitis. Curr Infect Dis Rep 2008;10:292–9.
75. Henricsson S, Lindholm A, Aravoglou M. Cyclosporin metabolism in human liver microsomes and its inhibition by other drugs. Pharmacol Toxicol 1990;66:49–52.
76. Paterson DL, Singh N. Interactions between tacrolimus and antimicrobial agents. Clin Infect Dis 1997;25:1430–40.

77. Trull AK, Tan KK, Roberts NB, et al. Cyclosporin metabolites and neurotoxicity. Lancet 1989;2:448.
78. Wijdicks EF, Dahlke LJ, Wiesner RH. Oral cyclosporine decreases severity of neurotoxicity in liver transplant recipients. Neurology 1999;52:1708–10.
79. Webster A, Woodroffe RC, Taylor RS, et al. Tacrolimus versus cyclosporin as primary immunosuppression for kidney transplant recipients. Cochrane Database Syst Rev 2005;4:CD003961.
80. Hachem RR, Yusen RD, Chakinala MM, et al. A randomized controlled trial of tacrolimus versus cyclosporine after lung transplantation. J Heart Lung Transplant 2007;26:1012–8.
81. Penninga L, Moller CH, Gustafsson F, et al. Tacrolimus versus cyclosporine as primary immunosuppression after heart transplantation: systematic review with meta-analyses and trial sequential analyses of randomised trials. Eur J Clin Pharmacol 2010;66:1177–87.
82. Maramattom BV, Wijdicks EF. Sirolimus may not cause neurotoxicity in kidney and liver transplant recipients. Neurology 2004;63:1958–9.
83. van de Beek D, Kremers WK, Kushwaha SS, et al. No major neurologic complications with sirolimus use in heart transplant recipients. Mayo Clin Proc 2009;84:330–2.
84. Harper SJ, Gelson W, Harper IG, et al. Switching to sirolimus-based immune suppression after liver transplantation is safe and effective: a single-center experience. Transplantation 2011;91(1):128–32.
85. Bodkin CL, Eidelman BH. Sirolimus-induced posterior reversible encephalopathy. Neurology 2007;68:2039–40.
86. Moskowitz A, Nolan C, Lis E, et al. Posterior reversible encephalopathy syndrome due to sirolimus. Bone Marrow Transplant 2007;39:653–4.
87. Guarino M, Benito-Leon J, Decruyenaere J, et al. EFNS guidelines on management of neurological problems in liver transplantation. Eur J Neurol 2006;13:2–9.
88. Sevmis S, Karakayali H, Emiroglu R, et al. Tacrolimus-related seizure in the early postoperative period after liver transplantation. Transplant Proc 2007;39:1211–3.
89. Vivarelli M, Dazzi A, Cucchetti A, et al. Sirolimus in liver transplant recipients: a large single-center experience. Transplant Proc 2010;42:2579–84.
90. Casanova B, Prieto M, Deya E, et al. Persistent cortical blindness after cyclosporine leukoencephalopathy. Liver Transpl Surg 1997;3:638–40.
91. Singh N, Bonham A, Fukui M. Immunosuppressive-associated leukoencephalopathy in organ transplant recipients. Transplantation 2000;69:467–72.
92. Wilde MI, Goa KL. Muromonab CD3: a reappraisal of its pharmacology and use as prophylaxis of solid organ transplant rejection. Drugs 1996;51:865–94.
93. Adair JR, Athwal DS, Bodmer MW, et al. Humanization of the murine anti-human CD3 monoclonal antibody OKT3. Hum Antibodies Hybridomas 1994;5:41–7.
94. Shihab F, Barry JM, Bennett WM, et al. Cytokine-related encephalopathy induced by OKT3: incidence and predisposing factors. Transplant Proc 1993;25:564–5.
95. Parizel PM, Snoeck HW, van den HL, et al. Cerebral complications of murine monoclonal CD3 antibody (OKT3): CT and MR findings. AJNR Am J Neuroradiol 1997;18:1935–8.
96. Adams RD, Victor M, Mancall EL. Central pontine myelinolysis: a hitherto undescribed disease occurring in alcoholic and malnourished patients. AMA Arch Neurol Psychiatry 1959;81:154–72.

97. King JD, Rosner MH. Osmotic demyelination syndrome. Am J Med Sci 2010; 339:561–7.
98. Wright DG, Laureno R, Victor M. Pontine and extrapontine myelinolysis. Brain 1979;102:361–85.
99. Messert B, Orrison WW, Hawkins MJ, et al. Central pontine myelinolysis. Considerations on etiology, diagnosis, and treatment. Neurology 1979;29:147–60.
100. Estol CJ, Faris AA, Martinez AJ, et al. Central pontine myelinolysis after liver transplantation. Neurology 1989;39:493–8.
101. Wszolek ZK, McComb RD, Pfeiffer RF, et al. Pontine and extrapontine myelinolysis following liver transplantation. Relationship to serum sodium. Transplantation 1989;48:1006–12.
102. Abbasoglu O, Goldstein RM, Vodapally MS, et al. Liver transplantation in hyponatremic patients with emphasis on central pontine myelinolysis. Clin Transplant 1998;12:263–9.
103. Haussinger D, Laubenberger J, vom DS, et al. Proton magnetic resonance spectroscopy studies on human brain myo-inositol in hypo-osmolarity and hepatic encephalopathy. Gastroenterology 1994;107:1475–80.
104. Wijdicks EF, Blue PR, Steers JL, et al. Central pontine myelinolysis with stupor alone after orthotopic liver transplantation. Liver Transpl Surg 1996;2:14–6.
105. Miller GM, Baker HL Jr, Okazaki H, et al. Central pontine myelinolysis and its imitators: MR findings. Radiology 1988;168:795–802.
106. Menger H, Jorg J. Outcome of central pontine and extrapontine myelinolysis (n = 44). J Neurol 1999;246:700–5.
107. Soupart A, Ngassa M, Decaux G. Therapeutic relowering of the serum sodium in a patient after excessive correction of hyponatremia. Clin Nephrol 1999;51:383–6.
108. Zhang ZW, Kang Y, Deng LJ, et al. Therapy of central pontine myelinolysis following living donor liver transplantation: report of three cases. World J Gastroenterol 2009;15:3960–3.
109. Ludwig KP, Thiesset HF, Gayowski TJ, et al. Plasmapheresis and intravenous immune globulin improve neurologic outcome of central pontine myelinolysis occurring post orthotopic liver transplant (February). Ann Pharmacother 2011. [Epub ahead of print].
110. Copelan EA. Hematopoietic stem-cell transplantation. N Engl J Med 2006;354: 1813–26.
111. De La Camara R, Tomas JF, Figuera A, et al. High dose busulfan and seizures. Bone Marrow Transplant 1991;7:363–4.
112. Baglin TP, Harper P, Marcus RE. Veno-occlusive disease of the liver complicating ABMT successfully treated with recombinant tissue plasminogen activator (rt-PA). Bone Marrow Transplant 1990;5:439–41.
113. MacQuillan GC, Mutimer D. Fulminant liver failure due to severe veno-occlusive disease after haematopoietic cell transplantation: a depressing experience. QJM 2004;97:581–9.
114. Perreault C, Gyger M, Boileau J, et al. Acute graft-versus-host disease after allogeneic bone marrow transplantation. Can Med Assoc J 1983;129:969–74.
115. Deeg HJ, Storb R. Graft-versus-host disease: pathophysiological and clinical aspects. Annu Rev Med 1984;35:11–24.
116. Chao NJ, Chen BJ. Prophylaxis and treatment of acute graft-versus-host disease. Semin Hematol 2006;43:32–41.
117. Bleggi-Torres LF, de Medeiros BC, Werner B, et al. Neuropathological findings after bone marrow transplantation: an autopsy study of 180 cases. Bone Marrow Transplant 2000;25:301–7.

118. Choi YJ, Park SJ, Kim JS, et al. Wernicke's encephalopathy following allogeneic hematopoietic stem cell transplantation. Korean J Hematol 2010;45:279–81.

119. Stevens AM, Sullivan KM, Nelson JL. Polymyositis as a manifestation of chronic graft-versus-host disease. Rheumatology (Oxford) 2003;42:34–9.

120. Grauer O, Wolff D, Bertz H, et al. Neurological manifestations of chronic graft-versus-host disease after allogeneic haematopoietic stem cell transplantation: report from the Consensus Conference on Clinical Practice in chronic graft-versus-host disease. Brain 2010;133:2852–65.

121. Sostak P, Padovan CS, Eigenbrod S, et al. Cerebral angiitis in four patients with chronic GVHD. Bone Marrow Transplant 2010;45:1181–8.

122. Matsuo Y, Kamezaki K, Takeishi S, et al. Encephalomyelitis mimicking multiple sclerosis associated with chronic graft-versus-host disease after allogeneic bone marrow transplantation. Intern Med 2009;48:1453–6.

123. de Brabander C, Cornelissen J, Smitt PA, et al. Increased incidence of neurological complications in patients receiving an allogenic bone marrow transplantation from alternative donors. J Neurol Neurosurg Psychiatry 2000;68:36–40.

124. Davies SM, Szabo E, Wagner JE, et al. Idiopathic hyperammonemia: a frequently lethal complication of bone marrow transplantation. Bone Marrow Transplant 1996;17:1119–25.

125. Metzeler KH, Boeck S, Christ B, et al. Idiopathic hyperammonemia (IHA) after dose-dense induction chemotherapy for acute myeloid leukemia: case report and review of the literature. Leuk Res 2009;33:e69–72.

126. Clay AS, Hainline BE. Hyperammonemia in the ICU. Chest 2007;132:1368–78.

127. del Rosario M, Werlin SL, Lauer SJ. Hyperammonemic encephalopathy after chemotherapy. Survival after treatment with sodium benzoate and sodium phenylacetate. J Clin Gastroenterol 1997;25:682–4.

128. Buell JF, Gross TG, Hanaway MJ, et al. Posttransplant lymphoproliferative disorder: significance of central nervous system involvement. Transplant Proc 2005;37:954–5.

129. Cavaliere R, Petroni G, Lopes MB, et al. Primary central nervous system post-transplantation lymphoproliferative disorder: an International Primary Central Nervous System Lymphoma Collaborative Group Report. Cancer 2010;116:863–70.

130. van de Beek D, Patel R, Daly RC, et al. Central nervous system infections in heart transplant recipients. Arch Neurol 2007;64:1715–20.

131. Yoon JH, Na DG, Byun HS, et al. Calcification in chronic maxillary sinusitis: comparison of CT findings with histopathologic results. AJNR Am J Neuroradiol 1999;20:571–4.

132. Fischer SA, Graham MB, Kuehnert MJ, et al. Transmission of lymphocytic choriomeningitis virus by organ transplantation. N Engl J Med 2006;354:2235–49.

133. Iwamoto M, Jernigan DB, Guasch A, et al. Transmission of West Nile virus from an organ donor to four transplant recipients. N Engl J Med 2003;348:2196–203.

134. Srinivasan A, Burton EC, Kuehnert MJ, et al. Transmission of rabies virus from an organ donor to four transplant recipients. N Engl J Med 2005;352:1103–11.

135. Luft BJ, Naot Y, Araujo FG, et al. Primary and reactivated toxoplasma infection in patients with cardiac transplants. Clinical spectrum and problems in diagnosis in a defined population. Ann Intern Med 1983;99:27–31.

Coma in the Pregnant Patient

Peter W. Kaplan, MB, FRCP

KEYWORDS
- Pregnancy • Coma • Cardiac • Stroke
- Hepatic and endocrine failures • Seizures • Eclampsia

Pregnancy presents unique challenges of caring for at least 2 patients simultaneously, offering different vulnerabilities and therapeutic priorities. Pregnant women may go into coma for the same reasons that face the general population, but also encounter conditions unique to or more common in this state. For example, pregnancy is subject to gestational hypertension, eclampsia, and HELLP (Hemolysis, Elevated Liver enzymes, Low Platelet count) syndrome. There are several particular pregnancy-related organ failures including acute renal, hepatic, or pulmonary failure. Vascular risks include cerebral venous sinus thrombosis and pituitary apoplexy.

This article reviews these subjects by etiology and syndrome, covering vascular, ictal, and endocrine causes, infections, and syndromes with multiple risks for coma such as eclampsia that can induce hypertension, hematological disturbances with intracranial bleeding, and seizures, all of which may cause coma.

COMA IN PREGNANCY: OVERVIEW

The management of coma in general can be found in other articles or texts, given that the considerations in coma treatment are generally similar to those facing patients who are not pregnant. Coma represents such a dire state that even concerns such as radiation exposure are usually outweighed by the need for maternal diagnosis and management. In nonurgent settings, clearly there would be great reluctance in ordering radiation imaging. With coma in pregnancy, in effect, no investigations are categorically excluded (eg, cerebral angiogram, spiral computed tomography [CT], or even brain biopsy), because with the prospect of potentially treatable causes, a mother's life is accorded priority.

VASCULAR COMPLICATIONS IN PREGNANCY
Cerebrovascular Disease in Pregnancy

Stroke causes coma relatively infrequently. For ischemic strokes as a whole, the older literature reflects incidence rates in pregnancy and the puerperium, of 5 to 210 per

Department of Neurology, Johns Hopkins Bayview Medical Center, 301 Building, 4940 Eastern Avenue, Baltimore, MD 21224, USA
E-mail address: pkaplan@jhmi.edu

Neurol Clin 29 (2011) 973–994
doi:10.1016/j.ncl.2011.07.010
0733-8619/11/$ – see front matter © 2011 Elsevier Inc. All rights reserved.

100,000 deliveries.[1–9] When compared with the nonpregnant population, this would represent a 13-fold increase.[10] Estimates of nonhemorrhagic stroke by Sharshar and colleagues[11] derived from public maternities state an incidence of 4.4 per 100,000 deliveries (95% confidence interval, 2.4–7.1). Although studies before 1965 failed to distinguish between bland stroke and intracranial hemorrhage (ICH), more recent data indicate that pregnancy does not significantly increase the risk of *nonhemorrhagic* stroke.[12–16] Predisposing causes in pregnancy are believed to include rapid hormonal changes in the postpartum period and decreases in blood volume,[11,17] but most infarcts arise from arterial occlusions (60%–80% of ischemic strokes).[10] These occlusions usually occur sometime between the second trimester and the first week postpartum. Maximal risk for intracranial venous thrombosis occurs in the first month postpartum.[10,14] Eclampsia and chronic hypertension also cause ICHs, and infarction or ICH increase the risk of maternal mortality by 8.5%.[18] Rarer causes of stroke include thrombocytopenic purpura, pituitary apoplexy, cerebral abscess (which can cause bleeding directly or from the associated vasculitis), and inflammatory processes. Other pregnancy-specific causes include amniotic embolism,[19] peripartum cardiomyopathy,[20] and postpartum cerebral angiopathy. During the last trimester and first weeks of pregnancy there may be hypercoagulable states, with increases in clotting factors VII, VIII, IX, and X, fibrinogen, and plasminogen, and decreases in antithrombin III, protein C, and protein S,[21–23] while estrogens may increase blood viscosity.[22] An increase in cardiac output of 30% to 50% during pregnancy along with increases in blood volume may favor thrombus formation. These findings are reviewed by Bódis and colleagues,[24] Donaldson,[25] and Digre and Varner.[26]

Head CT or magnetic resonance imaging (MRI) provide the location and cause of stroke, and are instrumental in guiding management. Other tests may include cardiac echo, carotid duplex, and coagulopathy studies.

Antiphospholipid Antibody Syndrome

The antiphospholipid antibody (APA) syndrome is a condition encompassing recurrent venous thromboses affecting organs and the limbs, along with cerebral arteries, and may result in fetal death. APA causes stroke, but rarely results in coma. There are certain similarities to preeclampsia-eclampsia, with endothelial damage, platelet activation, and thomboxane-mediated vasoconstriction. The process involves the coagulation cascade and affects inhibition of protein C-protein S and antithrombin III activity, as well as platelet activation.[27] Focal problems include cerebral infarction from thrombotic and venous occlusion. More general disturbances include raised intracranial pressure, encephalopathy, blindness, and anterior ischemic optic neuropathy. Symptoms encompass headache and confusion. Antibodies contribute to the pathogenesis, and include the lupus anticoagulant antibody, anticardiolipin antibody, and anti-B_2 glycoprotein. Treatment often involves immunosuppression and anticoagulation.

CARDIAC CAUSES OF STROKE IN PREGNANCY
Peripartum Cardiomyopathy

Peripartum cardiomyopathy is defined as an unexplained cardiac failure occurring during the last month of pregnancy to the first sixth postpartum month. Coma may occur from global cerebral hypoperfusion or by strokes. Cardiac stroke and coma has a high mortality and often recurs,[28] is seen in 1 in 3000 to 4000 pregnancies in the United States, and rises to 1 in 350 pregnancies in Haiti. Both viral and autoimmune causes of cardiomyopathy have been invoked. There is a predilection to thrombus formation in the left ventricle, accounting for much of the risk for embolic stroke (up to 10% of patients).[7,9] A raised intrathoracic pressure with Valsalva maneuvers in labor and delivery can route an embolism through a patent foramen ovale.[29] A patient clinically manifests signs of focal ischemia, but with brainstem involvement or cerebral swelling and raised intracranial pressure, there may be herniation and coma. Investigations include cardiac echo. Management often involves anticoagulation.

Heart Valve Abnormalities

Another frequent cause of cardioembolic strokes is from heart valve abnormalities that can present in pregnancy and the puerperium, and rarely result in coma.[30,31] Prosthetic heart valves or chronic atrial fibrillation may induce stroke in pregnancy or in the peripartum period. With tetralogy of Fallot, left ventricular dysfunction, severe pulmonary hypertension, and pulmonic regurgitation with right ventricular dysfunction can result in syncope, coma, or even sudden death,[32] with an overall mortality of up to 50%.[33] In normal childbirth and with Valsalva maneuvers, right atrial pressure rises and the foramen ovale may open, enabling pelvic and peripheral vein emboli to pass to the lung. Echocardiography helps with diagnosis, while management usually involves anticoagulation.

Cerebral Venous Thrombosis

Cerebral edema and hence coma can arise after occlusion of cerebral veins which, in turn, decreases brain tissue perfusion with cerebral infarction. There may be secondary hemorrhagic transformation. Onset is generally acute, often with paralysis and seizures. Coma may be heralded by intense headache, encephalopathy, or psychosis. In one series there was headache in 82%, papilledema in 56%, focal deficits in 42%, seizures in 39%, and coma in 31%.[34] Purported causes include fibrinogen activation with increased platelet adhesiveness, and a decrease in fibrinolytic activity and platelet count. Cerebral venous thrombosis (CVT) (**Box 1**) may arise from impingement on the sagittal sinus, prothrombotic states, dehydration, or trauma. Rarely CVT occurs with sickle cell disease, APA syndrome, factor V Leiden, prothrombin mutations, and antithrombin III deficiency.[34] Hypercoagulable factors may cause result in

---

Box 1
Possible causes of cerebral venous thrombosis

Dehydration

Sepsis

Trauma

Eclampsia

Antithrombin III

Protein C or S

Factor V Leiden deficiencies

Leiden mutation

Sickle cell disease

Antiphospholipid antibodies

Prothrombinase gene mutation

Hemocystinuria

CVT and not arterial clots, affecting the sagittal, petrosal, straight or transverse sinuses, and cortical veins, often causing central nervous system (CNS) hemorrhage. Fundoscopic examination may reveal papilledema and hence resemble pseudotumor cerebri. Diagnosis is indicated by the venous drainage infarction pattern seen on cerebral imaging. Head MRI or CT can demonstrate clot in the sinuses, producing a bright triangle or "delta sign" on MRI. MRI and CT venograms are now available, but the gold standard is still angiography.[34]

Treatment often includes heparin. In a randomized prospective trial, 8 of 20 patients recovered; 3 died in the placebo group.[35] Absolute risk reduction was 70% with heparin.[36] Vacuum catheters introducing recombinant tissue plasminogen activator may rapidly unblock occlusions. One series showed an 80% return to independent living at 3 years, but often with visual field defects, seizures, weakness, or headaches.[37] A poor outcome is still seen in 13%.[37,38]

A deep venous thrombosis causes diencephalic impairment, confusion, or coma, often with abnormal pupil reflexes and eye movements. Outcome often is poor.[39]

For diagnosis, diffusion-weighted MRI shows cerebral venous congestion and hemorrhage near the midline. MR angiography/venography can distinguish deep CVT from bithalamic lesions.[40]

Treatment involves intravenous unfractionated heparin and then oral anticoagulation for at least 6 months.[39] In 624 CVT patients there were 8% deaths, increasing with ICH, infection, and age.[38]

Postpartum Cerebral Angiopathy

Postpartum cerebral angiopathy (PCA) produces reversible narrowing of large and medium-sized cerebral arteries. Although characterized as benign, ICH and nonhemorrhagic strokes may occur,[41] and vasospasm may arise from intimal hyperplasia, sympathomimetic medications, and other endothelial factors.[42,43] PCA usually occurs after a normal pregnancy (in contrast to preeclampsia-eclampsia) and also involves posterior watershed leukoencephalopathy, hypertension, and visual complaints.[44] Treatment may include lowering blood pressure, steroids, and magnesium.[43,45,46] It may be difficult to differentiate between PCA and postpartum unheralded eclampsia or posterior reversible encephalopathy syndrome (PRES).

Amniotic Fluid Embolism

Amniotic fluid embolism (AFE) may account for up to 30% of maternal deaths.[47] AFE occurs when amniotic fluid enters uterine veins and is forced into the maternal circulation, causing hemodynamic collapse, disseminated intravascular coagulopathy (DIC), focal cerebral hypoperfusion, thrombosis or hemorrhage, and focal or multifocal neurologic signs, including coma.

Pulmonary and cardiac problems occur with air embolism. Larger bubbles may go to the brain through pulmonary or cardiac shunts, causing strokes.[48]

Cerebral Vascular Malformations and Aneurysms

Cerebral angiomata rarely rupture during pregnancy to the extent of inducing coma, and may in fact regress.[49] Although there is no greater risk in pregnancy for initial bleed, rebleed risk does increase.[50] Bleed risk rises with age, and is greater for arterial aneurysms (AAs) than for arteriovenous malformations (AVMs), which increasingly rupture in the second and third trimesters, but curiously not more so in labor and delivery.

Head CT angiography or MRI angiography are the cornerstones of diagnosis, while treatment involves surgical clipping or endovascular coiling of the aneurysm. Nonruptured AVMs are treated after delivery and are managed similarly to nonruptured AA.

Subarachnoid Hemorrhage

Subarachnoid hemorrhage (SAH) is often caused by rupture of an AVM or aneurysm, leading to blood entry into the subarachnoid space. Patients present with severe headache, vomiting, neck stiffness, focal neurologic signs, and coma. Loss of consciousness may be transient and brief at the ictus, or prolonged with high-grade hemorrhages, often with a poor prognosis.

Aneurysmal SAH causes about 4% of all maternal deaths and is ranked third among nonobstetric causes.[51] There may be a fivefold increase in ruptured intracranial aneurysms in pregnancy[52] and a quadrupling of hemorrhage rate from AVMs.[53] SAH is a leading cause of maternal death.[54] Cerebral aneurysms increasingly rupture during the course of pregnancy and early in the postpartum period, reaching 55% in the third trimester.[17] Aneurysms can be managed with clipping or coiling during pregnancy until the baby reaches term.[55] Cesarean section may be needed with brainstem compromise or coma. SAH during pregnancy may be mistaken for eclampsia.[55]

Choriocarcinoma

Metastatic choriocarcinoma rarely causes SAH, ICH, or subdural hemorrhage.[56] Trophoblastic tissue may invade blood vessels and induce aneurysmal dilatation, which may cause rupture. This disorder is seen in 1 in 50,000 pregnancies, and may result in brain metastases.[57] Elevated levels of β–human chorionic gonadotropin may help in diagnosis.

Rarer causes of ICH include septic emboli, DIC, and other bleeding diatheses.

Subdural Hematomas

Subdural hematomas may appear in patients who are anticoagulated for cardiac reasons such as with artificial heart valves, and may be precipitated by head trauma.

Moyamoya Disease

Moyamoya in Japanese means "puff of smoke." Moyamoya disease (MD) occurs with large cerebral vessel occlusions, usually early in life, but in adults, following carotid stenosis. The tangled collateral vessels produce the angiographic appearance suggestive of a puff of smoke. Women are 50-fold more likely to have MD, predisposed to it by smoking and oral contraceptives. Patients may present with headache, focal weakness, ICH from the thin-walled aneurysmal vessels, infarctions, and seizures. Angiography typically reveals MD. Encephalomyosynangiosis surgery may improve cerebral function but without decreasing morbidity or mortality.[58]

MD may worsen in the third trimester, possibly because of the underlying risk presented by hypertension. Of 30 pregnant patients with MD, 4 had transient cerebral ischemia, but all recovered; one had intraventricular hemorrhage (IVH) at 30 weeks' gestation, with a poor outcome. Some patients may be able to have vaginal deliveries without problems,[59] but most physicians favor cesarean section to avoid hyperventilation-induced cerebral ischemia and hypertension during labor. The goal is to avoid hyperventilation, hypoventilation, hypercapnea, and hypothermia.[60]

EVALUATION OF STROKE IN PREGNANCY

Stroke assessment during pregnancy is largely the same as that for nonpregnant woman. For causes of stroke, see **Box 2**. Shielding the uterus, maternal head CT results in a uterine exposure of less than 1 mrad, below the threshold causing fetal harm.[61] Animal studies do not show fetal damage with MRI scanning. There are some rare reports of an increased rate of ocular abnormalities after MRI in mid

Box 2
Current causes of stroke in pregnancy

1. Arterial occlusive disease
   a. Thrombotic cause:
      i. Atherosclerotic
      ii. Fibromuscular dysplasia
      iii. Arterial dissection
      iv. Hemocystinuria
      v. Moyamoya disease
   b. Embolic source
      i. Cardiac
         1. Peripartum cardiomyopathy
         2. Mitral valve prolapse
         3. Rheumatic heart disease
         4. Endocarditis (bacterial and nonbacterial)
         5. Paradoxic embolus
         6. Atrial fibrillation
2. Peripartum cerebral angiopathy
3. Cerebral venous and sinus thrombosis
   a. Hypercoagulable state
   b. Infectious
4. Drug abuse: cocaine and others
5. Hypotensive disorders
   a. Watershed infarction
   b. Sheehan pituitary necrosis
6. Hematological disorders
   a. Lupus anticoagulant
   b. Thrombocytopenic purpura
   c. Sickle cell disease
   d. Protein C, protein S, antithrombin III deficiency
7. Arteritis
   a. Systemic lupus erythematosus
   b. Infectious arteritis (syphilis, tuberculosis, meningococcal)
   c. Cerebral angiitis
   d. Takayasu arteritis
8. Intracerebral hemorrhage
   a. Eclampsia and hypertensive disorders
   b. Venous thrombosis
   c. Metastatic choriocarcinoma
   d. Arteriovenosus malformation

e. Vasculitis

f. Cocaine abuse

9. Subarachnoid hemorrhage

a. Aneurysm (saccular, mycotic)

b. Arteriovenous malformation

c. Eclampsia

d. Vasculitis

e. Metastatic choriocarcinoma

f. Venous thrombosis

g. Cocaine abuse

10. Other

a. Carotid cavernosus fistula

b. Dural vascular malformation

Data from Digre KB, Varner MW. Diagnosis and treatment of cerebrovascular disorders in pregnancy. In: Adams HP Jr, editor. Handbook of cerebrovascular diseases. New York: Marcel Dekker; 1993. p. 255–86; and Donaldson JQ. Neurologic emergencies in pregnancy. Obstet Gynecol Clin North Am 1991;18(2):199–212.

gestation.[62] There is, however, a clinical consensus that MR angiography and venography are safe in late pregnancy in contrast to the first 2 trimesters. Conventional angiography is used to diagnose vasculitis and cerebral venous thrombosis, and may uncover aneurysms in SAH.[61] Angiography may result in less than 1 mrad to the fetus. Intravenous contrast with iodine confers a slight risk of fetal hypothyroidism when used in the third trimester.[63]

Echocardiography may reveal a right to left shunt or patent foramen ovale.[63]

With ICH, recent approaches have been more active and based on neurosurgical criteria, with intervention during pregnancy. Immediate surgery is advocated with Hunt and Hess grades I to III, avoiding hypotensive therapy. Hypothermia has been used safely. Some favor treating asymptomatic aneurysms only if they are larger than 7 mm. As noted, many contemporary neurosurgeons favor resection of ruptured AVMs, whereas others favor waiting because the risk of bleeding from an AVM is lower than that for aneurysms. Vaginal delivery is still advocated over cesarean section, particularly if surgery is performed before the third trimester. If bleeding occurs in the second trimester, surgical intervention may follow cesarean section. Raised intracranial pressures have additionally been treated with steroids, but diuretics are often avoided. Vasospasm is usually managed with hypervolemia treatment and hypertension. Nicardipine and nimodipine (calcium channel blockers) may decrease vasospasm, but can cause fetal acidosis and hypoperfusion; teratogenesis has been demonstrated in animals.[33]

PREECLAMPSIA-ECLAMPSIA
Definition

Preeclampsia is defined by pregnancy-associated hypertension and proteinuria, often with arm or facial edema. Eclampsia (seizures or coma in a patient with some indication of pregnancy-induced hypertension) before labor is antepartum; if seizures appear before 28 weeks' gestation, then it is early antepartum eclampsia. Intrapartum eclampsia is present if seizures occur after labor has started; postpartum eclampsia obtains after delivery of the fetus and placenta. Eclampsia often occurs postpartum: 44% were postpartum, 12% after the first 48 hours and 2% more than a week after delivery[64]; 48% had postpartum eclampsia after 48 hours.[65] Postpartum eclampsia has a worse prognosis, often with adult respiratory distress syndrome (ARDS) and DIC.[66]

Hypertension may be "relative": blood pressures that would not be of concern in older patients may cause cerebral ischemia, edema, hemorrhage, or vasospasm. Modest increases in blood pressure (eg, 140/70 mm Hg) may be seen with eclampsia, but more recently, absolute measurements of at least 140/90 mm Hg 6 hours apart define hypertension (American College of Obstetrics and Gynecology Bulletin).[67] Sheehan and Lynch[68] reported that about half of the patients had convulsions with systemic blood pressures between 160 and 195 mm Hg. Proteinuria is defined as a urinary protein of greater than 300 mg per 24 hours or 30 mg/dL on urine sample.[67] The pathologic edema typically affects the face and upper limbs. Severe preeclampsia is present when: blood pressure is 160 mm Hg or more systolic, or 110 mm Hg or more diastolic, twice, at least 6 hours apart during bed rest; or proteinuria is greater than 5 g per 24 hours or 3^+ to 4^+ by dipstick; or urine output is less than 400 mL per day; or there is thrombocytopenia or hemolysis; cyanosis or pulmonary edema; upper quadrant pain; or cerebral dysfunction/visual disturbances.[67]

Eclampsia occurs in 0.05% to 0.20% of pregnancies in developed countries, increasing to 1% in developing countries. It is a leading cause of maternal death.[65]

Many patients have an incomplete clinical triad either in preeclampsia or eclampsia, but a seizure or coma define eclampsia. Up to 20% of patients may lack one of the cardinal features.[69] The appearance of eclampsia may not correlate with preeclampsia severity, or the presence of the 3 features of preeclampsia.[64,70] In fact it may appear postpartum without the triad appearing before admission to an emergency room. In effect, the seizures may appear without proteinuria, edema, or known postpartum hypertension. In addition to the typical triad, there may also be pulmonary edema, oliguria, or hepatic dysfunction. Thrombocytopenia can occur with coagulopathy. Neurologic features include confusion, headache, raised intracranial pressure and cerebral edema, infarction, and hemorrhage. There may be paralysis, aphasia, blindness, psychosis, and coma. Seizures can start focally, but often generalize.

Recent mechanisms believed to underlie eclampsia include: (1) hematologic abnormalities with vascular damage activation by neutrophils, macrophages, and T-cell lymphocytes interacting with platelets, complement, and the coagulation system; (2) endothelial damage from impaired prostaglandin metabolism; and (3) arterial spasm or vasospasm.[71–73] The process may cause damage to cortical, subcortical, and brainstem areas from small, medium, and large hemorrhages. There may be bland infarcts due to vasospasm as well as exudation through vessel walls with cerebral edema. Coagulopathies with DIC and bleeding diatheses cause hemorrhage, along with the coagulopathy of HELLP syndrome.[71,74–76] There is a proclivity for the posterior rather than the anterior watershed zones.[19,46,68,77–83]

A mechanism underlying preeclampsia-eclampsia is believed to be the faulty transformation of the placental vascular system from impaired cytotrophoblastic migration through the decidua to the inner third of the myometrium. In preeclampsia, there may be incomplete transformation of the spiral arteries to a pregnant "low-pressure" system. Studies have uncovered mitochondrial defects underlying the impaired cytotrophoblastic invasion.[84] This uteroplacental arterial insufficiency leads to release of inflammatory factors and cytokine production, inducing a more generalized maternal inflammatory response, and may interfere with the normal downregulation of the immune system that moderates inflammatory reactions—part of the dynamic known as the "maternal-fetal genetic conflict."[85] The neuropeptide neurokinin B may have a marked pressor effect, and is increased in preeclampsia and pregnancy-induced hypertension.[86]

Diagnosis is largely clinical, but can be strengthened by cerebral imaging. The MRI findings are those of hypertensive encephalopathy, with posterior leukoencephalopathy. Imaging may reveal infarction, hemorrhage, edema, and even herniation or hydrocephalus. Typical imaging patterns are the serpiginous subcortical white matter edema with a predilection for the posterior watershed zone and the tips of the occipital lobe.[26] Cerebral edema is usually reversible with treatment of hypertension, occurring typically over days. Larger infarctions or hemorrhages cause permanent sequelae.[71,79,80,87–90]

Management

Management is directed at intensive treatment of hypertension, if necessary in an intensive care unit. Treatment may include labetolol, hydralazine, or nifedipine. Magnesium sulfate may stop recurrent seizures and reverse the vasospastic process without, strictly speaking, acting as an anticonvulsant. The Eclampsia Trial Collaborative Group[91] compared the recurrence rate of seizures in 1682 women with eclampsia in the developing world. One arm provided diazepam as an intravenous bolus of 10 mg over 2 minutes followed by infusion of 40 mg and 500 mL normal saline over 24 hours. Phenytoin was given intravenously as a 1-g load followed by 100 mg every 6 hours for 24 hours. This study showed a 52% lower incidence of recurrent seizures after magnesium sulfate compared with diazepam. There was a 67% decrease with magnesium sulfate compared with phenytoin. The Parkland Memorial Trial revealed that 10 of 1089 preeclamptic women treated with phenytoin had a seizure,[92] whereas none of 1049 patients on magnesium sulfate had a seizure,[93] but women included in the study largely had pregnancy-induced hypertension without other signs of preeclampsia, and phenytoin levels were in the subtherapeutic or low-therapeutic range.

Prognosis

Ten percent of untreated women with eclampsia have further seizures. The mortality is 15% to 20% after ICH in eclampsia. About 20% have recurrent eclampsia.[64,94–98]

SEIZURES AND STATUS EPILEPTICUS

Status epilepticus (SE) may have a high morbidity, so some experts advocate a shortening of the duration needed for SE, defining it as 20, 10, or even 5 minutes.[99]

Pregnancy may increase seizure frequency in women with epilepsy, but produces no effect in most women; some have fewer seizures.[100,101] Pregnancy decreases the total blood levels of most antiepileptic drugs (AEDs) by 50%, and somewhat less so for the free level. Free valproate levels may increase. Lamotrigine levels may decrease from enhanced clearance of up to 300% during pregnancy, starting within 1 to 2 weeks.[102]

The highest morbidity in SE occurs with convulsive SE. Frequent causes of SE are a low level of AEDs, new strokes, infections, abscesses, and vascular malformations. SE carries a worse prognosis with acute symptomatic causes, and a better prognosis when caused by low AED levels.

Management is directed at seizure control and investigation of possible underlying causes. Treatment includes diazepam, lorazepam, phenytoin, barbiturates, or anesthetic agents if necessary. The best outcomes are achieved with treatment in an intensive care unit, preferably with electroencephalographic monitoring. Lightly obtunded or confused patients can usually be managed without barbiturates or anesthesia.

COAGULOPATHIES DURING PREGNANCY
Hemolysis, Elevated Liver Function Tests, and Low Platelets (HELLP Syndrome)

HELLP produces coma by the volume-expanding effects of ICH, or by direct involvement of the brainstem. It is a highly morbid complication and possibly a unique variant of preeclampsia/eclampsia.[103,104] There is no universal consensus regarding the exact elements of HELLP, nor the degree of abnormality needed in the individual tests used in diagnosis of the syndrome. For thrombocytopenia, cutoff values range from 75,000/mm^3 to 279,000/mm^3. Many large series define platelet counts as being less than 100 to 150,000/mm^3; aspartate aminotransferase abnormality as being above 40 to 70 U/L; and lactate dehydrogenase exceeding 600 U/L.

HELLP may occur postpartum in up to 30%, usually within 48 hours, but can occur up to a week later. A review with decision and treatment pathways is provided by Barton and Sibai.[105]

Clinical complaints may include right upper quadrant or epigastric pain, nausea and vomiting, and malaise. HELLP usually involves older pregnant women, the multiparous, and patients with preeclampsia usually before 31 weeks of pregnancy. There is often marked weight gain and generalized edema, but not infrequently without absolute or even relative hypertension (see preeclampsia/eclampsia). HELLP may be distinguished from acute fatty liver of pregnancy (AFLP) by the absence of proteinuria, and liver function abnormalities are usually worse in HELLP.

Several disorders enter the differential diagnosis for HELLP. Laboratory investigation may include complete blood count, coagulation studies, a peripheral smear, serum electrolytes, and liver function tests.

Pathophysiology
A microangiopathic hemolytic anemia with hemolysis is characteristic of HELLP, believed to arise from fibrin deposition on a damaged intima. Peripheral smears may reflect the presence of burr cells, echinocytes, triangular cells, and spherocytes. This microangiopathic hemolytic anemia may also be seen in other disorders such as renal disease, eclampsia, hemolytic uremic syndrome, and thrombotic thrombocytopenic purpura (TTP). HELLP typically is an afebrile illness with elevated liver enzymes, whereas TTP often has fever and targets the kidney.

Management
HELLP syndrome often has great morbidity and mortality and therefore warrants urgent management. The coagulopathy is rapidly corrected if possible, along with intensive management of the hypertension, and treatment with magnesium sulfate. If the pregnancy has reached 34 weeks, the patient is often delivered. Several randomized trials suggest that improvement may be obtained with the additional use of glucocorticoids, leading to improvement in liver function and coagulopathy. Treatment may include platelet transfusions.

Several syndromes resemble each other, namely HELLP, AFLP, hemolytic uremic syndrome, and TTP, further emphasizing the need for accurate diagnosis.

Other hematologic conditions that may appear in pregnancy or the peripartum period include sickle cell disease, DIC, and TTP.[106]

Thrombotic Thrombocytopenic Purpura
TTP can cause coma by ICH and/or by cardiovascular collapse. Features include thrombocytopenia, microangiopathic hemolytic anemia, fever, renal dysfunction, and fluctuating neurologic abnormalities. TTP peaks in the second through fourth decades and occurs with pregnancy, infections, autoimmune disorders, and malignancy. Ten

percent to 25% of patients with TTP are pregnant or postpartum.[106–112] TTP is character-ized by systemic endothelial cell damage. Pregnancy is not a poor risk factor for survival, but there may be early delivery and intrauterine fetal death from placental infarction.

Treatment of TTP involves plasma exchange and fresh frozen plasma replace-ment.[113] Others have tried vincristine, corticosteroids, or other immunosuppressive medications. In refractory cases, splenectomy has been tried.[114–117]

METABOLIC CAUSES OF COMA
Glucose Dysregulation

Diabetes causing high or low blood sugar that can lead to coma occurs in pregnancy and the peripartum period. Causes specific to pregnancy include morning sickness, which may cause the mother to avoid glucose-lowering medication and facilitate hyperglycemia. Vomiting with dehydration can cause hypernatremia while diarrhea may lead to hypokalemia and cardiac dysrhythmias that may lead to coma. Other electrolytic disturbances are even less common.[118]

Treatment principles follow those of diabetic hyperglycemia or hypoglycemia.

Wernicke Encephalopathy

Wernicke encephalopathy can present with confusion, eye movement disorders and nystagmus, ataxia, and rarely, coma. Hyperemesis gravidarum may cause Wernicke encephalopathy by depleting the body thiamine stores in a well-nourished woman even in 3 to 6 weeks. It occurs more rapidly in malnourished women or alcoholics. Wernicke encephalopathy may be precipitated by intravenous glucose. Rapid correc-tion of hyponatremia may independently precipitate central pontine myelinolysis. Rapid, intravenous thiamine repletion is important, and clinical signs including eye movement abnormalities may disappear within the day. Treatment may require daily parenteral thiamine repletion for 7 to 10 days.[25,119–124]

Acute Intermittent Porphyria

Acute intermittent porphyria (AIP) is caused by an autosomal dominant inherited abnor-mality of heme biosynthesis with toxic accumulation of aminolevulinic acid and porpho-bilinogen. AIP can be precipitated in women during menarche, perimenstrually, and in pregnancy. Many drugs can precipitate crises, including antiepileptic drugs and barbitu-rates. A crisis may include an acute axonal polyneuropathy with paralysis resembling Guil-lain-Barré syndrome. There may be severe pain, autonomic dysfunction with tachycardia and constipation, cognitive and behavioral abnormalities, and psychosis, occasionally with coma. Seizures may be difficult to control because of the porphyrinogenic nature of most AEDs. Precipitants include fasting, surgery, or an acute febrile illness.[25,120,121]

Treatment is directed at decreasing fever, avoiding porphyrinogenic drugs, and administering intravenous hematin to break the crisis. During pregnancy, both hematin and glucose are used acutely in AIP, although this is not endorsed by the manufac-turers of hematin, and its effects are unknown.[122]

Safe drugs that stop seizures and can break SE include the benzodiazepines. For chronic use, AEDs that do not precipitate porphyria, such as gabapentin, levetirace-tam, or vigabatrin, are recommended.

Individual attacks remit but recurrence is typical, often with cumulative neurologic deficit.

ENDOCRINE DISTURBANCES IN PREGNANCY

Thyrotoxicosis rarely worsens to the point of coma, as may an Addisonian state. Pitu-itary apoplexy can arise from increased vascularity, and enlargement of the pituitary may result in antepartum infarction or hemorrhage. Postpartum there may be end-circulation ischemia, usually after massive maternal blood loss.

Coma arises from electrolyte or metabolic disturbance, seizures, or cerebral edema. Detailed treatment may be found in texts on endocrine disorders.

Sheehan Syndrome

With anterior pituitary necrosis after hypovolemia and hypotension in severe maternal blood loss, there may be a decrease in several circulating hormones, known as Sheehan syndrome. The pituitary, because of its pregnancy-associated hyperplasia and increased vascularity, is particularly vulnerable to hypovolemia and hypotension. Retrospective surveys suggest that 3% to 4% of pregnant women with acute shock may be affected.[125–127]

Classically there is fatigue, hypothyroidism, and diminished consciousness. Acute pituitary apoplexy with abrupt infarction, hemorrhage, or necrosis within the pituitary or in a pituitary adenoma represents an emergency with high mortality, often from compression of the hypothalamus. Consciousness is impaired and there is the danger of acute adrenal failure and further hypotension. Pituitary apoplexy is rare in women and is rarely described in pregnancy. Symptoms include severe frontal, retroorbital, or diffuse headache, meningismus, vomiting (thus resembling SAH), and coma. Other features include ophthalmoplegia, ptosis, pupillary defects, or even bilateral third nerve palsies.[128]

Treatment is aimed at acute replacement of corticosteroids intravenously. Surgery to decompress the hypothalamus or optic nerve is occasionally warranted.[128]

Pheochromocytoma

Coma rarely occurs with pheochromocytoma, but may occur because of hypertensive ICH (also caused by eclampsia/PRES). Pheochromocytoma is a tumor of chromaffin tissue in the adrenal gland, but may also arise in chromaffin tissue anywhere along the adrenal developmental pathway. The tumors secrete catecholamines, including epinephrine, norepinephrine, dopamine, and their metabolites (vanillylmandelic acid and metanephrine), leading to hemodynamic instability and acute hypertensive crises.[129,130] Pheochromocytomas comprise 0.3% to 1.9% of secondary causes of hypertension, but remains rare in pregnancy. Ten percent are malignant. Some cases have been successfully managed with epidural anesthesia, magnesium infusion, and cesarean section.[130,131] If confirmed before 24 weeks' gestation, it should be resected. After the 24th week, the pregnancy is usually continued under adrenergic blockade until the fetus is mature, with cesarean section to avoid hypertensive crises. Diagnosis is made with CT or MRI as well as metaiodobenzylguanidine (MIBG) scintigraphy scanning. An alternative to surgery is radioactive iodine-132 MIBG. Extramedullary tumors are usually malignant.

INFECTIONS AND INFESTATIONS

There is mild immunosuppression in pregnancy associated with alterations in circulating maternal steroids. There may be a slight increase in certain systemic infections and septicemia, but rarely coma.

Rarely, parasitic infestations can cause coma in pregnancy. At least 4 cases of cysticercosis with seizures or coma during pregnancy have been described.[132] Coma was produced by unilocular cysts near the third ventricle producing acute hydrocephalus. Treatment was successful with intraventricular drainage.

ORGAN FAILURE OCCASIONALLY LEADING TO COMA
Acute Renal Failure in Pregnancy

Acute renal failure (ARF) can cause coma, but rarely occurs in pregnancy.[133] ARF may be caused by hemorrhagic or septic shock, or severe preeclampsia. During pregnancy ARF may follow malignant hypertension, infections, scleroderma, vasculitis, microangiopathic hemolytic anemia transplant rejection, hemolytic uremic syndrome, malignancies, or drug toxicity. HELLP may lead to a decrease in glomerular filtration and renal failure, occasionally with acute tubular necrosis.[134,135] Most cases of ARF in HELLP syndrome resolve.[136–139] ARF may be caused by DIC. Rarer causes include mesangial proliferative glomerular nephritis, Sjögren syndrome, malaria, multicystic dysplastic kidneys, and toxins. Necrotizing fasciitis and Group A streptococcus may induce toxic shock syndrome, while in utero exposure to nonsteroidal anti-inflammatory drugs may produce neonatal renal failure.

Acute Liver Failure

Acute fulminant liver failure may occur prepartum or postpartum with eclampsia, HELLP syndrome, or acute viral hepatitis. It may arise from unrecognized peripartum cardiomyopathy. Acute fatty liver and HELLP syndrome occur most frequently in the third trimester, with jaundice, liver function enzyme increases, and coagulopathy. There may be itching, diarrhea, and jaundice. Acute-on-chronic causes include hepatic failure on chronic hepatitis B virus–related cirrhosis. If occurring after early delivery, patients with encephalopathy, coagulopathy, hypoglycemia, and other significant problems should be candidates for urgent liver transplantation.[140–144]

Acute Fatty Liver of Pregnancy

AFLP affects about 1 in 7000 to 16,000 pregnancies,[145,146] usually is seen in the third trimester of pregnancy, and presents with hepatic failure, microvesicular fatty infiltration of the liver, and encephalopathy.[147,148] Maternal mortality is almost 20% while neonatal mortality may be as high as 58%.[145–149] Frequent symptoms are nausea and vomiting (75%), jaundice, or epigastric pain. There may be DIC, acute tubular necrosis, and pulmonary edema. The illness is usually monophasic,[150,151] with clinical and laboratory findings similar to those seen in preeclampsia, HELLP, and pancreatitis. Hypoglycemia may occur in about 50% of patients. Treatment is with supportive measures until the disease regresses. On occasion, liver transplantation is recommended.[145,146,149,152]

PULMONARY DISEASE AND FAILURE IN PREGNANCY
Acute Respiratory Failure and Adult Respiratory Distress Syndrome

Acute respiratory failure and ARDS, and all of the pulmonary disorders listed herein, may cause coma from hypoxia. Acute respiratory failure in pregnancy accounts for more than 30% of maternal deaths.[153] It is usually caused by thromboembolism, AFE, venous air embolism, or ARDS. Treatment involves managing the underlying disease, hemodynamic, ventilation, and other multisystem problems, and avoiding complications[154] (see later discussion).

Clinical features of ARDS are nonspecific and include respiratory distress, tachycardia, tachypnea, and dyspnea. The patient may be cyanotic. Chest radiograph findings may range from minimal interstitial infiltrate to white-out of the lungs. Criteria for ARDS are: (1) identifiable risk factors; (2) respiratory distress; (3) exclusion of cardiogenic pulmonary edema; (4) bilateral opacification on chest radiograph; (5) PaO_2/FIO_2 ratio of less than 200. In pregnancy, the specific risk factors may be difficult to identify.[154,155]

Injury to the endothelial lining, activation of neutrophils, and consequent damage to the capillary endothelium can lead to capillary leak, increased vascular resistance, pulmonary edema, decreased lung compliance, and intrapulmonary vascular shunting. After the 30th week of pregnancy, the relative hypervolemia may worsen ARDS and outcome.[156]

Mortality in ARDS follows that of comorbid illnesses, multiorgan system failure, and duration of ventilation. It ranges from 30% to 70% even with improvements in critical care. It may be difficult to differentiate between sepsis, ARDS, and systemic inflammatory response syndrome.[157]

Treatment of sepsis, fluid overload, protecting against alveolar distention, and ensuring oxygenation are the cornerstones of management. ARDS often displays a mixed picture of abnormal and normal alveoli. Overextension of alveoli by restricting tidal volumes to 6 to 8 mL/kg, and the lowest level of positive end-expiratory pressure may help.[157]

Aspiration pneumonia may arise during decreased consciousness in labor and delivery, an increase in intragastric pressure by compression by the pregnant uterus, and delayed gastric emptying, all contributing to significant of maternal morbidity and mortality but rarely leading to coma. Most patients show early pulmonary infiltrates on chest radiograph progressing to ARDS. Prognosis ranges from mild reversible to sudden death.[158,159]

Management is directed at prevention, with use of regional anesthesia, avoiding oral feedings, use of H2 blockers; and supportive care with antibiotics, mechanical ventilation, and avoiding hypoxia.[158,159]

Venous Air Embolism

Venous air embolism can occur with abortion, delivery, labor, and other interventions, and is caused by air entry into the subplacental venous sinuses. Air travels to the heart and prevents blood flow to the lungs, frequently causing a blood-air interface, with microemboli, platelet injury, and inflammatory white cell response leading to ARDS.[153]

Typical clinical features include shortness of breath, tachypnea and tachycardia, hypotension, and sweating. Treatment includes support of blood pressure and pulmonary function, often for 2 to 3 days. Death may occur following small amounts of infused air, although women have survived amounts greater than 1.5 L.[153,160]

Toxic Pulmonary Edema

Pulmonary edema can be caused by selective and nonselective β2-adrenergic agents, with tachycardia, shortness of breath, tachypnea, chest pain, and orthopnea. Chest radiography may reflect fluid overload within 1 to 2 days of using β-adrenergic agents. Pulmonary edema may be caused by cardiac toxicity, fluid overload, a decrease in colloid osmotic pressure, and increased capillary permeability. Treatment involves stopping the drug, coupled with supportive care. Symptoms usually resolve within a day.[153]

HEAD AND ABDOMINAL TRAUMA AND COMA

Motor vehicle accidents account for up to 3900 fetal losses per year[161] making it a leading cause, with other trauma, of nonobstetric maternal coma and mortality in the United States. Most patients die of internal injuries of the abdomen, thorax, and pelvis. Obstetric consequences include premature delivery, higher rate of abruption, and low birth weight at delivery. Fetal outcome depends on gestational age rather than injury. Trauma in pregnancy may cause sepsis or miscarriage.[162]

In coma following head trauma, investigations are aimed at the anatomic and pathophysiological causes of coma. Imaging may demonstrate cranial fractures, cerebrovascular problems, intracranial shifts, hemorrhage, and the features and progression of raised intracranial pressure. Management largely follows the pathway used for nonpregnant patients, with stabilization of vital systems and CNS compromise. Attention is also directed at fetal health, with obstetric consultation on the viability of the fetus. These investigations may provide guidance regarding medications electively used in management when there is less mortality or morbidity.

REFERENCES

1. Amias AG. Cerebral vascular disease in pregnancy, II: occlusion. J Obstet Gynaecol Br Commonw 1970;77:312–25.
2. Srinavasan K. Cerebral venous and arterial thrombosis in pregnancy and puerperium: a study of 135 patients. Angiology 1983;34:731–46.
3. Huggenberg HR, Kesselring F. Postpartuale cerebrale komplikationen. Gynaecologia 1958;146:312–5 [in German].
4. Barnes JE, Abbott KH. Cerebral complications incurred during pregnancy and the puerperium. Am J Obstet Gynecol 1961;82:192–207.
5. Lorincz AB, Moore RY. Puerperal cerebral venous thrombosis. Am J Obstet Gynecol 1962;83:311–8.
6. Goldman JA, Eckerling B, Gans B. Intracranial venous sinus thrombosis in pregnancy and puerperium: report of fifteen cases. J Obstet Gynaecol Br Commonw 1964;71:791–6.
7. Carroll JD, Leak D, Lee HA. Cerebral thrombophlebitis in pregnancy and the puerperium. Q J Med 1966;35:347–68.
8. Cross JN, Castro PO, Jennett WB. Cerebral strokes associated with pregnancy and the puerperium. Br Med J 1968;3:214–8.
9. Simolke GA, Cox SM, Cunningham FG. Cerebrovascular accidents complicating pregnancy and the puerperium. Obstet Gynecol 1991;78:37–42.
10. Wiebers DO. Ischemic cerebrovascular complications of pregnancy. Arch Neurol 1985;42:1106–13.
11. Sharshar T, Lamy C, Mas JL. Incidence and causes of strokes associated with pregnancy and puerperium. Stroke 1995;26:930–6.
12. Wiebers DO, Whisnant JP. The incidence of stroke among pregnant women in Rochester, Minn, 1955 through 1979. JAMA 1979;254:3055–7.
13. Lidegaard O. Orgal contraceptives, pregnancy and the risk of cerebral thromboembolism: the influence of diabetes, hypertension, migraine and previous thrombotic disease. Br J Obstet Gynaecol 1995;102:153–9.
14. Grosset DG, Ebrahim S, Bone I, et al. Stroke in pregnancy and puerperium: what magnitude of risk? [editorial]. J Neurol Neurosurg Psychiatr 1995;58:129–31.
15. Awada A, Rajeh SA, Duarte R, et al. Stroke and pregnancy. Int J Gynaecol Obstet 1995;48:157–61.
16. Jeng J-S, Tang S-C, Yip P-K. Stroke in women of reproductive age: comparison between stroke related and unrelated to pregnancy. J Neurol Sci 2004;221:25–9.
17. Kittner SJ, Stern BJ, Feeser BR, et al. Pregnancy and the risk of stroke. N Engl J Med 1996;335(11):768–74.
18. Biller J, Adams HP. Cerebrovascular disorders associated with pregnancy. Air Force Physician 1986;33:125–32.
19. Donaldson JO. Eclampsia. In: Donaldson JO, editor. Neurology of pregnancy. 2nd edition. London: WB Saunders Co; 1989. p. 269–310.

20. Homans DC. Peripartum cardiomyopathy. N Engl J Med 1985;312:1432–7.
21. Knepper LE, Giuliani MJ. Cerebrovascular disease in women. Cardiology 1995; 86:339–48.
22. Schafer AI. The hypercoagulable states. Ann Intern Med 1985;102:814–28.
23. Finley BE. Acute coagulopathy in pregnancy. Med Clin North Am 1989;73: 723–43.
24. Bódis L, Szupera Z, Pierantozzi M, et al. Neurological complications of pregnancy. J Neurol Sci 1998;153:279–93.
25. Donaldson JO. Neurologic emergencies in pregnancy. Obstet Gynecol Clin North Am 1991;18(2):199–212.
26. Digre KB, Varner MW. Diagnosis and treatment of cerebrovascular disorders in pregnancy. In: Adams HP Jr, editor. Handbook of cerebrovascular disorders in pregnancy. New York: Marcel Dekker; 1993. p. 255–86.
27. Huong DLT, Wechsler B, Edelman P, et al. Postpartum cerebral infarction associated with aspirin withdrawal in the antiphospholipid antibody syndrome. J Rheumatol 1993;20:1229–32.
28. Elkayam U, Tummala PP, Rao K, et al. Maternal and fetal outcomes in women with peripartum cardiomyopathy. N Engl J Med 2001;344:1567–71.
29. Kozelj M, Novak-Antolic Z, Grad A, et al. Patent foramen ovale as a potential cause of paradoxical embolism in the postpartum period. Eur J Obstet Gynecol Reprod Biol 1999;84:55–7.
30. Jaigobin C, Silver FL. Stroke and pregnancy. Stroke 2000;31:2948–51.
31. Witlin AG, Mattar F, Sibai BM. Postpartum stroke: a twenty-year experience. Am J Obstet Gynecol 2000;183:83–8.
32. Veldtman GR, Connolly HM, Grogan M, et al. Outcomes of pregnancy in women with tetralogy of Fallot. J Am Coll Cardiol 2004;44:174–80.
33. Dias MS, Sekhar LN. Intracranial hemorrhage from aneurysm and arteriovenous malformations during pregnancy and the puerperium. Neurosurgery 1990;27: 855–66.
34. Biousse V, Bousser M-G. Cerebral venous thrombosis. Neurologist 1999;5: 326–49.
35. Einhaupl KM, Villringer A, Meister W. Heparin treatment in sinus venous thrombosis. Lancet 1991;338:597–600.
36. De Bruijn SF, Stam J. Randomized placebo controlled trial of anticoagulate treatment with low molecular weight heparin for cerebral sinus thrombosis. Stroke 1999;30:484–8.
37. Breteau G, Mounier-Vehier F, Godefroy O, et al. Cerebral venous thrombosis 3-year clinical outcome in 55 consecutive patients. J Neurol 2003;250(1):29–35.
38. Ferro JM, Canhão P, Stam J, et al. Prognosis of cerebral and dural sinus thrombosis. Stroke 2004;35:664–70.
39. Ameri A, Bousser MG. Cerebral venous thrombosis. Neurol Clin 1992;10: 87–111.
40. Bell DA, Davis WL, Osborn AG, et al. Bithalamic hyperintensity on T2-weighted MR: vascular causes and evaluation with MR angiography. AJNR Am J Neuroradiol 1994;15:893–9.
41. Geocadin RG, Razumovsky AY, Wityk RJ, et al. Intracerebral hemorrhage and postpartum cerebral vasculopathy. J Neurol Sci 2002;205:29–34.
42. Geraghty JJ, Hock DB, Robert ME, et al. Fatal puerperal cerebral vasospasm and stroke in a young woman. Neurology 1991;41:1145–7.
43. Singhal AB. Postpartum angiopathy with reversible posterior leukoencephalopathy. Arch Neurol 2004;61:411–6.

44. Calado S, Vale-Santos J, Lima C, et al. Postpartum cerebral angiopathy: vasospasm, vasculitis or both? Cerebrovasc Dis 2004;18:340–1.
45. Ursell MR, Marras CL, Farb R, et al. Recurrent intracranial hemorrhage due to postpartum cerebral angiopathy: implications for management. Stroke 1998; 29:1995–8.
46. Garner BF, Burns P, Bunning RD, et al. Acute blood pressure elevation can mimic arteriographic appearance of cerebral vasculitis (a postpartum case with relative hypertension). J Rheumatol 1990;17:93–7.
47. Tuffnell DJ. Amniotic fluid embolism. Curr Opin Obstet Gynecol 2003;15:119–22.
48. Muth CM, Shank ES. Primary care: gas embolism. N Engl J Med 2000;342:476–82.
49. De Wilde R, Holzgreve W, Zubke W. [Rupture of a cerebral angioma in pregnancy]. Geburtshilfe Frauenheilkd 1987;47(9):654–5 [in German].
50. Velut S, Vinikoff L, Destrieux C, et al. Cerebro-meningeal hemorrhage secondary to ruptured vascular-malformation during pregnancy and post-partum. Neurochirurgie 2000;46(2):95–104.
51. Barno A, Freeman DW. Maternal death due to spontaneous subarachnoid hemorrhage. Am J Obstet Gynecol 1976;125(3):384–92.
52. Wiebers DO. Subarachnoid haemorrhage in pregnancy. Semin Neurol 1988;8: 226–9.
53. Robinson JL, Hall CS, Sedzimir CB. Arteriovenous malformations, aneurysms, and pregnancy. J Neurosurg 1974;41:63–70.
54. Selo-Ojeme DO, Marshman LA, Ikomi A, et al. Aneurysmal subarachnoid haemorrhage in pregnancy. Eur J Obstet Gynaecol Reprod Biol 2004;116:131–43.
55. Mosiewicz A, Jakiel G, Janusz W, et al. Treatment of intracranial aneurysms during pregnancy. Ginekol Pol 2001;72(2):86–92.
56. Weir B, MacDonald N, Mielke B. Intracranial vascular complications of choriocarcinoma. Neurosurgery 1978;2:138–42.
57. Fox MW, Harms RW, Davis DH. Selected neurologic complications of pregnancy. Mayo Clin Proc 1990;65:1595–618.
58. Wityk RJ, Hillis A, Beauchamp N, et al. Perfusion-weighted magnetic resonance imaging in adult moyamoya syndrome: characteristic patterns and change after surgical intervention: case report. Neurosurgery 2002;51:1499–505.
59. Komiyama M, Yasui T, Kaitano S, et al. Moyamoya disease in pregnancy: case report and review of the literature. Neurosurgery 1998;43:360–9.
60. Williams DL, Martin IL, Gully RM. Intracerebral hemorrhage and moyamoya disease in pregnancy. Can J Anaesth 2000;47:996–1000.
61. Schwartz RB. Neuroradiographic imaging techniques and safety considerations. Adv Neurol 2002;90:1–8.
62. Tyndall DA, Sulik KK. Effects of magnetic resonance imaging on eye development in the C57BL/6J mouse. Teratology 1991;43:263–75.
63. Mas JL, Lamy C. Stroke in pregnancy and the puerperium. J Neurol 1998;245: 305–13.
64. Douglas K, Redman CW. Eclampsia in the United Kingdom. BMJ 1994;309: 1395–400.
65. Sibai BM. Preeclampsia-eclampsia. In: Sciarra JJ, editor. Gynecology and obstetrics, vol. 2. Philadelphia: JB Lippincott; 1989. p. 1–12.
66. Phelan JP. Pulmonary edema in obstetrics. Obstet Gynecol Clin North Am 1991; 18:319–31.
67. American College of Obstetrics and Gynecology. Diagnosis and management of preeclampsia and eclampsia. ACOG practice bulletin no. 33. Obstet Gynecol 2002;99:159–67.

68. Sheehan HL, Lynch JB. In: Pathology of toxaemia of pregnancy. Baltimore: Williams & Wilkins; 1973.

69. Porapakkam S. An epidemiologic study of eclampsia. Obstet Gynecol 1983;54: 26–30.

70. Cunningham FG, MacDonald PC, Gant NF, et al. Hypertensive disorders in pregnancy. In: Cunningham FG, MacDonald PC, Gant NF, editors. Williams obstetric. 19th edition. Norwalk (CT): Appleton & Lange; 1993. p. 763–817.

71. Sibai BM, Ramadan MK, Chari RS, et al. Pregnancies complicated by HELLP syndrome (hemolysis, elevated liver enzymes, and low platelets): subsequent pregnancy outcome and long-term prognosis. Am J Obstet Gynecol 1995;172: 125–9.

72. Roberts JM, Redman CW. Preeclampsia: more than pregnancy-induced hypertension. Lancet 1993;341:1447–51.

73. Easton JD, Mas JL, Lamy C, et al. Severe preeclampsia/eclampsia: hypertensive encephalopathy of pregnancy? Cerebrovasc Dis 1998;8:53–8.

74. Barton JR, Sibai BM. Hepatic imaging in HELLP syndrome (hemolysis, elevated liver enzymes, and low platelet count). Am J Obstet Gynecol 1996;174:1820–5 [discussion: 1825–7].

75. Sullivan CA, Magann EF, Perry KG Jr, et al. The recurrence risk of the syndrome of hemolysis, elevated liver enzymes, and low platelets (HELLP) in subsequent gestations. Am J Obstet Gynecol 1994;171:940–3.

76. Isler CM, Rinehart BK, Terrone DA, et al. Maternal mortality associated with HELLP (hemolysis, elevated liver enzymes, and low platelets) syndrome. Am J Obstet Gynecol 1994;181:924–8.

77. Zunker P, Happe S, Georgiadis AC, et al. Maternal cerebral hemodynamic changes in pregnancy-related hypertension: a prospective transcranial Doppler study. Ultrasound Obstet Gynecol 2000;16:179–87.

78. Williams KP, Wilson S. Persistence of cerebral hemodynamic changes in patients with eclamspsia. Am J Obstet Gynecol 1999;181:1162–5.

79. Qureshi AI, Frankel MR, Ottenlips JR, et al. Cerebral hemodynamics in preeclampsia and eclampsia. Arch Neurol 1996;53:1226–31.

80. Naidu K, Moodley J, Coor P, et al. Single photon emission and cerebral computerized tomographic scan and transcranial Doppler sonographic findings in eclampsia. Br J Obstet Gynaecol 1997;104:1165–72.

81. Call GK, Fleming MC, Sealfon S, et al. Reversible cerebral segmental vasoconstriction. Stroke 1988;19:1159–70.

82. Will AD, Lewis KL, Hinshaw DB Jr, et al. Cerebral vasoconstriction in toxemia. Neurology 1987;37:1555–7.

83. Schobel HP, Fischer T, Heuszer K, et al. Preeclampsia—a state of sympathetic overactivity. N Engl J Med 1996;335:1480–5.

84. Widschwendter M, Schrocksnadel H, Mortl MG. Opinion: pre-eclampsia: a disorder of placental mitochondria? Mol Med Today 1998;4:286–91.

85. Haig D. Genetic conflicts in human pregnancy. Q Rev Biol 1993;68:495–532.

86. Page NM, Woods RJ, Gardiner SM, et al. Excessive placental secretion of neurokinin β during the third trimester causes pre-eclampsia. Nature 2000;405: 797–800.

87. Schwartz RB, Jones KM, Kalina P, et al. Hypertensive encephalopathy: findings on CT, MR imaging, and SPECT imaging in 14 cases. AJR Am J Roentgenol 1991;159:379–83.

88. Crawford S, Varner MW, Digre KB, et al. Cranial magnetic resonance imaging in eclampsia. Obstet Gynecol 1985;70:474–7.

89. Raroque HG, Orrison WW, Rosenberg GA. Neurologic involvement in toxemia of pregnancy: reversible MRI lesions. Neurology 1980;40:167–9.
90. Sibai BM. Eclampsia. In: Goldstein PJ, Stern BJ, editors. Neurological disorders of pregnancy. 2nd edition. Mount Kisco (NY): Futura Publishing Co; 1992. p. 1–24.
91. Eclampsia Trial Collaborative Group. Which anticonvulsant for women with eclampsia? Lancet 1995;45:1455–63.
92. Pritchard JA, Cunningham FG, Pritchard SA. The Parkland Hospital protocol for treatment of eclampsia: evaluation of 245 cases. Am J Obstet Gynecol 1984; 148:951–63.
93. Lucas L, Leveno K, Cunningham G. A comparison of magnesium sulfate with phenytoin for the prevention of eclampsia. N Engl J Med 1995;333:201–5.
94. Sibai B, el-Nazer A, Gonzalez-Ruis A. Severe preeclampsia-eclampsia in young primigravid women: subsequent-related hypertension: a prospective transcranial Doppler study. Ultrasound Obstet Gynecol 1986;16:179–87.
95. Lanska DJ, Kryscio RJ. Stroke and intracranial venous thrombosis during pregnancy and puerperium. Neurology 1998;51:1622–8.
96. Sibai BM, Spinnato JA, Watson DL, et al. Eclampsia: IV. Neurologic findings and future outcome. Am J Obstet Gynecol 1985;152:184–92.
97. Chesley LC, Annitto JE, Cosgrove RA. The remote prognosis of eclamptic women. Am J Obstet Gynecol 1976;124:446–59.
98. Lamy C, Sharshar T, Mas J-L. Prognosis of cerebrovascular pathology associated with pregnancy and the postpartum period. Rev Neurol (Paris) 1996;152:422–40.
99. Lowenstein DH, Bleck T, Macdonald RL. It's time to revise the definition of status epilepticus. Epilepsia 1999;40(1):120–2.
100. Schmidt D. The effect of pregnancy on the natural history of epilepsy: review of the literature. In: Jan D, Dam M, Richens A, et al, editors. Epilepsy, pregnancy and the child. New York: Raven Press; 1982. p. 3–14.
101. Schmidt D, Canger R, Avanzini G, et al. Changes of seizure frequency in pregnant epileptic women. J Neurol Neurosurg Psychiatr 1983;46:751–5.
102. Pennell PB. Antiepileptic drug pharmacokinetics during pregnancy and lactation. Neurology 2003;61:S35–42.
103. MacKenna J, Dover NL, Brame RG. Preeclampsia associated with hemolysis, elevated liver enzymes, and low platelets: an obstetric emergency? Obstet Gynecol 1983;62:751–4.
104. Weinstein L. Syndrome of hemolysis, elevated liver enzymes, and low platelet count: a severe consequence of hypertension in pregnancy. Am J Obstet Gynecol 1982;142:159–67.
105. Barton JR, Sibai BM. Diagnosis and management of hemolysis, elevated liver enzymes, and low platelets syndrome. Clin Perinatol 2004;31:807–33.
106. Pinewte MG, Vinttziloes AM, Ingardia CJ. Thrombotic thrombocytopenic puerperal as a cause of thrombocytopenia in pregnancy: literature review. Am J Perinatol 1989;6:55.
107. Gasser C, Gautier E, Steck A, et al. Hämolytischurämische syndrome: bilaterale Nierenrindennekrosen bei akuten erworbenen hämolytischen Anämien. Schweiz Med Wochenschr 1955;85:905–9 [in German].
108. Lämmle B, Kremer Hvinga JA, Alberio L. Thrombotic thrombocytopenic purpura. J Thromb Haemost 2005;3(8):1663.
109. Ezra Y, Michaelson-Cohen R, Abramov Y, et al. Prelabor rupture of the membranes at term: when to induce labor? Eur J Obstet Gynecol Reprod Biol 2004;115(1):23–7.

110. Ezra Y, Rose M, Eldor A. Therapy and prevention of thrombotic thrombocyto-penic purpura during pregnancy. A clinical study of 16 pregnancies. Am J Hematol 1996;51:1–6.

111. Egerman RS, Witlin AG, Friedman SA, et al. Thrombotic thrombocytopenic purpura and hemolytic uremic syndrome in pregnancy. Review of 11 cases. Am J Obstet Gynecol 1996;175:950–6.

112. Proia A, Paesano R, Torcia F, et al. Thrombotic thrombocytopenic purpura and pregnancy: a case report and a review of the literature. Ann Hematol 2002;81: 210–4.

113. Byrnes JJ, Khurana M. Treatment of thrombotic thrombocytopenic purpura with plasma. N Engl J Med 1977;297:1386–9.

114. Ruggenenti P, Remuzzi G. The pathophysiology and management of thrombotic thrombocytopenic purpura. Eur J Haematol 1996;56:191–207.

115. George JN. How I treat patients with thrombotic thrombocytopenic purpura-hemolytic uremic syndrome. Blood 2000;96:1223–39.

116. Moalke JL, Chow TW. Thrombotic thrombocytopenic purpura: understanding a disease no longer rare. Am J Med Sci 1998;316:105–19.

117. Rock GA. Management of thrombotic thrombocytopenic purpura. Br J Haematol 2000;109:496–507.

118. Evers IM, Ter Braak EW, De Valk HW, et al. Risk indicators predictive for severe hypoglycemia during the first trimester of Type * diabetic pregnancy. Diabetes Care 2002;25:554–9.

119. Fraser D. Central pontine myelinolysis as a result of treatment of hyperemesis gravidarum. Br J Obstet Gynaecol 1988;95:621.

120. Kanaan C, Veille JC, Lakin M. Pregnancy and acute intermittent porphyria. Obstet Gynecol Surv 1989;44:244.

121. Kaplan PW, Lesser RP, Fisher RS, et al. No, magnesium sulfate should not be used in treating eclamptic seizures. Arch Neurol 1988;45:1361.

122. Lamon JM, Frykholm BC, Hess RA, et al. Hematin therapy for acute porphyria. Medicine 1979;58(3):252–69.

123. Mumford CJ. Papilloedema delaying diagnosis of Wernicke's encephalopathy in a coma patient. Postgrad Med J 1989;65:371.

124. Reuler JB, Girard DE, Cooney TG. Current concepts. Wernicke's encephalop-athy. N Engl J Med 1985;312:1035–9.

125. Sheehan HL. Post-partum necrosis of the anterior pituitary. J Pathol Bacteriol 1937;45:189–214.

126. Hall MR. The incidence of anterior pituitary deficiency following post-partum haemorrhage: cases reviewed from the Oxfordshire and Buckinghamshire area. Proc R Soc Med 1962;55:468–70.

127. Moszkowski EF. Postpartum pituitary insufficiency. Report of five unusual cases with long-term followup. South Med J 1973;66:878–82.

128. Grimes HG, Brooks MH. Pregnancy in Sheehan's syndrome. Report of a case and review. Obstet Gynecol Surv 1980;35:481–8.

129. Bullough AS, Karadia S, Watters M. Phaeochromocytoma: an unusual cause of hypertension in pregnancy. Anaesthesia 2001;56:1365–2044.

130. Pomares FJ, Canas R, Rodriguez JM, et al. Differences between sporadic and multiple endocrine neoplasia type 2A phaeochromocytoma. Clin Endocrinol 1998;48:195–200.

131. Harper MA, Murnaghan GA, Kennedy L, et al. Phaeochromocytoma in preg-nancy. Five cases and a review of the literature. Br J Obstet Gynaecol 1989; 96:594–606.

132. Suarez VR, Iannucci TA. Neurocysticercosis in pregnancy: a case initially diagnosed as eclampsia. Obstet Gynecol 1999;93(5 Pt 2):816–8.

133. Pertuiset N, Grunfeld JP. Acute renal failure in pregnancy. Baillieres Clin Obstet Gynaecol 1994;8:333–51.

134. Lakkis FG, Campbell OC, Badr KF. Microvascular diseases of the kidney. In: Brenner BM, editor. The kidney. 5th edition. Philadelphia: W.B. Saunders Co; 1996. p. 1713–30. Chapter 35.

135. Thadhani R, Pascaul M, Bonventre JV. Acute renal failure. N Engl J Med 1996; 334:1448–60.

136. Sibai BM, Ramadan MK, Usta I, et al. Maternal morbidity and mortality in 442 pregnancies with hemolysis, elevated liver enzymes, and low platelets (HELLP syndrome). Am J Obstet Gynecol 1993;169:1000–6.

137. Selcuk NY, Odabas AR, Centikaya R, et al. Outcome of pregnancies with HELLP syndrome complicated by acute renal failure (1989-1999). Ren Fail 2000;22: 319–27.

138. Abraham KA, Connolly G, Farrell J, et al. The HELLP syndrome, a prospective study. Ren Fail 2001;23:705–13.

139. Abraham KA, Kennelly M, Dorman AM, et al. Pathogenesis of acute renal failure associated with the HELLP syndrome: a case report and review of the literature. Eur J Obstet Gynecol Reprod Biol 2003;108:99–102.

140. Riely CA. Hepatic disease in pregnancy. Am J Med 1994;96(1A):18s–22s.

141. Locarnini SA, Cunningham AL. Clinical treatment of viral hepatitis. In: Jeffries DJ, De Clerq E, editors. Antiviral chemotherapy. Chichester (UK): Wiley; 1995. p. 441–530.

142. Castro MA, Fassett MJ, Reynolds TB, et al. Reversible peripartum liver failure: a new perspective on the diagnosis, treatment, and cause of acute fatty liver of pregnancy, based on 28 consecutive cases. Am J Obstet Gynecol 1999; 181:389–95.

143. Sheikh RA, Yasmeen S, Pauly MP, et al. Spontaneous intrahepatic hemorrhage and hepatic rupture in HELLP syndrome. J Clin Gastroenterol 1999;28:323–8.

144. Paternoster DM, Gerace PF, Manganelli F, et al. Acute hepatic failure in pregnancy. Eur J Obstet Gynecol Reprod Biol 2004;112:230–2.

145. Castro MA, Fasset MJ, Reynolds TB, et al. Reversible peripartum liver failure: a new perspective on the diagnosis, treatment, and cause of acute fatty liver of pregnancy based on 28 cases. Am J Obstet Gynecol 2000;181:389–95.

146. Reyes H, Sandoval L, Wainstein A, et al. Acute fatty liver of pregnancy: a clinical study of 12 episodes in 11 patients. Gut 1994;35(1):101–6.

147. Mabie WC. Acute fatty liver of pregnancy. Crit Care Clin 1991;7:799–808.

148. Sibai BM, Kustermann L, Velasco J. Current understanding of severe preeclampsia, pregnancy associated hemolytic uremic syndrome, thrombotic thrombocytopenic purpura, hemolysis, elevated liver enzymes, and low platelet syndrome, and postpartum acute renal failure: different clinical syndromes or just different names? Curr Opin Nephrol Hypertens 1994;3:436–45.

149. Usta IM, Barton JR, Amon EA, et al. Acute fatty liver of pregnancy: an experience in the diagnosis and management of fourteen cases. Am J Obstet Gynecol 1994;171:1342–7.

150. Fesenmeier MF, Coppage KH, Lambers DS, et al. Acute fatty liver of pregnancy in 3 tertiary care centers. Am J Obstet Gynecol 2004;192:1416–9.

151. Fett JD. Peripartum cardiomyopathy: insights from Haiti regarding a disease of unknown etiology. Minn Med 2002;85:46–8.

152. Rolfes DB, Ishak KG. Acute fatty liver of pregnancy: a clinicopathologic study of 35 cases. Hepatology 1985;5:1149–58.

153. Hollingsworth HM, Irwin RS. Acute respiratory failure in pregnancy. Clin Chest Med 1992;13:723–40.
154. Deblieuz P, Summer WR. Acute respiratory failure in pregnancy: pulmonary diseases in pregnancy. Clin Obstet Gynecol 1996;39(1):143–59.
155. Gurman G, Schlaeffer F, Kopernic G. Adult respiratory distress syndrome as a complication of acute pyelonephritis during pregnancy. Eur J Obstet Gynecol Reprod Biol 1990;36:75–80.
156. Collop NA, Sahn SA. Critical illness in pregnancy: an analysis of 20 patients admitted to a medical intensive care unit. Chest 1993;103:1548–52.
157. Gattinoni L, Pelosi P, Pesenti A, et al. CT scan in ARDS: clinical and physiopathological insights. Acta Anaesthesiol Scand 1991;35S:87–96.
158. Rodrigues J, Niederman MS. Pneumonia complicating pregnancy. Clin Chest Med 1992;13:679–92.
159. Clinton MJ, Niederman MS. Noninfectious respiratory disease in pregnancy. Cleve Clin J Med 1993;60:233–44.
160. Lowenwirt IP, Chi DS, Handwerker SM. Nonfatal venous air embolism during cesarean section: a case report and review of the literature. Obstet Gynecol Surv 1994;49:72–6.
161. Dobo SM, Johnson VS. Evaluation and care of the pregnant patient with minor trauma. Emergenza 2001;1–24.
162. Weiss HB, Lawrence B, Miller T. Prevalence and risk of hospitalized pregnant occupants in car crashes. Annu Proc Assoc Adv Automot Med 2002;46:355–66.

Psychogenic Unresponsiveness

Trevor A. Hurwitz, MBChB, MRCP(UK), FRCP(C)[a,b,*]

KEYWORDS

• Stupor • Coma • Catatonia • Psychogenic

PSYCHOGENIC UNRESPONSIVENESS

Psychiatric illness most commonly presents as a disturbance in the form and content of consciousness. Psychiatric illness may, however, present to the neurologist as an unresponsive state suggesting a disturbance in the level of consciousness, thereby creating diagnostic challenges with specific implications for treatment.

From a neurologic perspective, stupor and coma are organic impairments in the level of consciousness during which the patient has a complete or partial absence of awareness of self and the environment.[1] Organic stupors (OSs) and comas are caused by a variety of biological insults to the integrity and/or electrochemical functioning of the neural structures that support wakefulness: the ascending reticular activating system (ARAS) and its thalamic connections or widely distributed cortical and subcortical networks.[2–4] Stupor and coma are part of a continuum in the pathology of wakefulness. At the normal end is the awake and alert patient. With escalating severity of disruption, the patient passes through the stages of drowsiness (obtundation), then stupor, and finally coma. These and other terminologies in use have, however, created confusion with uncertain boundaries between the categories of implied severity. Pathologic degradations in the level of consciousness are better defined by observable and elicitable behaviors at the bedside, which have been operationalized in the most commonly used assessment tool, the Glasgow Coma Scale (GCS) (**Table 1**).

Psychiatric illness may also present cross-sectionally as an unresponsive state and may additionally feature characteristic and specific motor disturbances. These motor disturbances include catalepsy/waxy flexibility (in which the patient allows a body part to be placed into fixed even bizarre positions by the examiner), posturing (the patient holds self-initiated persistent positions), and rigidity (a motiveless maintenance of

This work was supported by the ERIN Fund, BC Neuropsychiatry Program.
The author has nothing to disclose.
[a] Division of Neurology, Department of Psychiatry and Medicine, University of British Columbia, Canada
[b] BC Neuropsychiatry Program, British Columbia, Canada
* UBC Hospital, 2255 Wesbrook Mall, Vancouver, British Columbia, Canada V6T 2A1.
E-mail address: t.hurwitz@ubc.ca

Table 1 The GCS					
Eye Opening		**Best Verbal Response**		**Best Motor Response**	
Observation	Score	Observation	Score	Observation	Score
Spontaneous	4	Orientated	5	Obeying	6
To speech	3	Confused	4	Localizing to pain	5
To pain	2	Inappropriate words	3	Withdrawal response	4
None	1	Incomprehensible sounds	2	Flexor decorticate response	3
—		None	1	Extensor decerebrate response	2
—				None	1

From Teasdale G, Jennett B. Assessment of coma and impaired consciousness: a practical scale. Lancet 1974;2(7872):81–4; with permission.

a rigid position despite efforts to be moved).[5,6] Unlike the mechanisms in OSs and coma, the unresponsive component of these psychiatric states is caused by varying degrees of muteness and immobility linked to the underlying primary psychiatric condition. At its extreme, a psychiatrically mute and immobile patient may be easily mistaken for an organically comatose patient with no verbal output and no motor responses, both patients scoring 1 on each of the relevant GCS subscales. Here, however, the resemblance with typical stupor and coma ends, although, rarely, such patients do present with flaccid coma.[7–9] Most patients with psychiatrically linked hyporesponsive states do not appear drowsy or asleep.[10] They typically display eyes open staring[5,10] (a form of oculomotor posturing[6]). If closed, the eyes resist being pried open. To an external observer, this resistance to passive movement, similar to the patient's failure to initiate movement on command, appears motiveless, a phenomenon known as negativism. Negativism must be distinguished from an identifiably angry, defiant, and uncooperative patient. Such consciously motivated behavior is labeled as oppositional and is not part of the catatonic syndrome. Negativism is also reflected in gegenhalten (a seemingly motiveless resistance to passive movement, which is proportional to the strength of the stimulus) and rigidity (a seemingly motiveless maintenance of a rigid position) when attempting to move a patient's limbs. By contrast, unless there is underlying intrinsic central nervous system (CNS) injury, decorticate, and decerebrate posturing, spasticity and extensor plantar responses are not seen. Some of these psychogenically driven motor abnormalities, such as gegenhalten and rigidity, may also be seen in various organic brain pathologic conditions and can only then be correctly attributed by the company they keep.

The most common diagnostic label applied to such psychiatrically based presentations is catatonia or the catatonic syndrome, with mutism and immobility as its most consistent features.[5,11] This term is, however, confusing because it is used to describe unresponsiveness alone, unresponsiveness with typical motor disturbances, or motor disturbances alone.[7,9,11,12]

Catatonia can be separated into 2 factors: one that identifies mutism, negativism, and stupor and correlates to the syndrome of negativistic stupor and the other identifying stereotypy, catalepsy, and automatic obedience.[13,14] The separation of catatonic inhibition, that is, mutism, motor inhibition, rigidity, gegenhalten, and parakinesias (bizarre awkward or disconnected voluntary movements), from other catatonic motor symptoms was also found in another more recent factor analysis of patients presenting with a catatonic syndrome.[15] Catatonia is thus best reserved as a specifier of the characteristic motor disturbances but using existing neurologic terminology and established criteria, such as those embodied in the GCS, to capture unresponsiveness. This separation of unresponsiveness from catatonic motor abnormalities aligns modern psychiatric and neurologic views of an unresponsive patient and avoids conceptual confusion such as comatoid catatonia to describe a state of psychogenic flaccid unresponsiveness.[9] In both disciplines, unresponsiveness is operationalized as failing verbal and motor output and termed stupor. This usage is a resurrection of older views of stupor in psychiatry. Stupor was seen as distinct from catatonia and defined as a temporary reduction or obliteration of reactive and spontaneous relational functions (ie, action and speech).[16]

Terminology aside, a fundamental understanding about these patients is that the underlying disturbance is a functional major primary psychiatric illness, usually a mood disorder or psychosis, in which the underlying brain disturbance lies in one or more neurotransmitter systems.[17–19] These patients are correctly described as having a psychogenically driven unresponsiveness to distinguish their apparent alteration in level of consciousness from those caused by organic pathologies. Psychogenic used in this context indicates that the pathogenetic mechanisms are caused by a primary functional psychiatric disturbance and in no way implies that the state is self-induced and under volitional control.[7]

A final complexity is the well-described tendency of a variety of nonpsychiatric organic brain insults to present as a catatonic syndrome diagnosed in the past as secondary catatonia or, using *Diagnostic and Statistical Manual of Mental Disorders* (Fourth Edition) nomenclature, as a catatonic disorder due to a general medical condition.[20] In these patients, there is a clear and unequivocal organic brain disturbance due to intrinsic neurologic diseases, such as CNS infections, systemic metabolic disorders, or exogenous substances. The organic brain disturbance is presumably affecting those neural structures or systems that are disturbed in primary functional psychiatric disorders, giving rise to similar psychobehavioral manifestations, which in these cases is a catatonic syndrome—varying degrees of muteness and immobility coupled with the characteristic catatonic motor displays. The fact that the catatonic symptoms of these organic conditions respond to the same interventions as the catatonic symptoms of primary psychiatric disorders lends support to the hypothesis of overlapping mechanisms responsible for the psychobehavioral inhibition and motor symptoms.[5,11] Treatment must still be directed at the underlying organic condition, which also determines the ultimate prognosis.[20] These patients, owing to their presentation, are vulnerable to psychiatric misattribution and may not receive the full attention and diagnostic energies of the consultant neurologist to the detriment of both.

When faced with an unresponsive patient, the neurologist must thus address 4 broad diagnostic categories:

1. Organic stupor (OS)
   An organic condition causing varying degrees of unresponsiveness
2. Organic catatonic stupor (OCS)
   An organic condition causing varying degrees of unresponsiveness and accompanied by catatonic motor signs
3. Psychogenic stupor (PS)
   A primary functional psychiatric disorder causing varying degrees of unresponsiveness
4. Psychogenic catatonic stupor (PCS)
   A primary functional psychiatric disorder causing varying degrees of unresponsiveness and accompanied by catatonic motor signs.

The term stupor used earlier and hereafter follows clinical custom with due regard for the controversy around terminology and simply refers to varying degrees of unresponsiveness due to an apparent decreased level of consciousness. The diagnosis of coma applies when the patient is totally unresponsive, although such patients may still have preserved brainstem reflexes. In each instance, the diagnostic category should be accompanied by a recorded GCS evaluation. The specifier catatonic refers to the presence of the characteristic catatonic motor phenomena (**Box 1**).

Organic Stupor

Organic stupors (OSs) are more fully addressed in this volume and so the discussion in this article is focused on the essentials of diagnosis. Anatomically, organic causes of decreased level of consciousness are ultimately due to 1 of 3 intracranial pathologies: damage to the ARAS and its projection to the thalamus, especially the intralaminar nuclei; unilateral hemispheric lesions that by mass effect compromise the rostral ARAS and thalamus; or diffuse bilateral hemispheric insults.[1-4] This knowledge guides investigations. Regardless of how convincing the premorbid and cross-sectional psychiatric aspects are, each and every patient with an apparent decreased level of consciousness requires structural imaging, which at a minimum is a cranial computed tomographic scan and, if indicated, magnetic resonance imaging. Imaging visualizes the contents of the posterior fossa in addition to the hemispheres and addresses their structural integrity. Unless these imaging procedures demonstrate an unequivocal noninfectious or hemorrhagic cause, a lumbar puncture is required to rule out such pathologies as meningitis, encephalitis, and subarachnoid hemorrhage with cerebrospinal fluid sent for the appropriate studies. Electroencephalography (EEG) is also mandatory to rule out nonconvulsive status epilepticus[21] or to confirm a generalized disturbance of hemispheric function indicated by the presence of generalized slowing.[22] Appropriate laboratory investigations are also performed and include analysis of blood gases; a complete blood cell count; determination of electrolytes, calcium, magnesium, thyrotropin, inflammatory markers, serum glucose, and serum iron levels; renal and liver chemistries; vasculitis screen; serological tests for human immunodeficiency virus (HIV) and syphilis; serum alcohol level and urine drug screen. Additional diagnostic tests may be required based on the clinical picture and the outcome of this initial test battery and could include determining drug, carboxyhemoglobin, and serum ammonia levels. Treatment and prognosis follow diagnostic clarification.

Organic Catatonic Stupor

Patients with organic catatonic stupors (OCS) present with a typical catatonic syndrome, displaying mutism, withdrawal (refusal to eat and drink), immobility, and negativism combined with other typical catatonic motor disturbances.[20] OCS is caused by intrinsic CNS diseases, such as infections (HIV infection, syphilis, and others), multiple sclerosis and epilepsy, systemic metabolic disorders such as uremia and hypercalcemia, and neurotoxic states from ingested substances that include phencyclidine, disulfiram, and neuroleptics.[20,23] OCS may also be caused by withdrawal from benzodiazepines.[24] In general psychiatric wards, between 16% and 21.4% of patients admitted with a diagnosis of catatonia are shown to have the condition secondary to a variety of nonpsychiatric medical or neurologic causes.[5,10] In a given instance, the specific cause is identified by the history and investigations, which also determine treatment and prognosis. Treatment of OCS is less well studied and is based mostly on case reports or small numbers of patients in case series. OCS often, but not always, responds to same interventions used for motor symptoms and unresponsiveness in PCS and are described later.[5,11,25]

Box 1
Catatonic motor signs

Negativism

    Seemingly motiveless resistance to passive movement or examination by an examiner or failure to follow instructions to move

Gegenhalten

    Motiveless resistance to passive movement, which is proportional to strength of the stimulus. Gegenhalten is a specific form of negativism

Rigidity

    Motiveless maintenance of a rigid position despite efforts to be moved. Rigidity is also a specific form of negativism

Posturing

    Spontaneous self-initiated active maintenance of a posture without reacting and includes conventional everyday positions such as sitting and standing or odd, bizarre, and socially inappropriate postures. Posturing includes staring (maintaining a fixed gaze with decreased blinking) or head held off the bed (psychic pillow)

Waxy flexibility/catalepsy

    Allowing the examiner to place a body part into persistent bizarre positions comparable to that of bending a candle

Grimacing

    Maintenance of odd facial expressions. These may be hyperkinetic (short, simple, and rapid) or dystonic (slow and sustained) and involve a single or several facial muscles

Stereotypy

    Repetitive non–goal-directed motor activity (eg, finger play, repeatedly touching, patting, or rubbing self)

Mannerisms

    Odd purposeful movements that are either exaggerated caricatures of conventional movements or bizarre idiosyncratic movements

Echopraxia/echolalia

    Mimicking the examiner's movements/speech, for example, the examiner scratches his/her head in an exaggerated manner

Automatic obedience

    Exaggerated cooperation with examiner's request even if these are senseless or dangerous. Patient obligingly follows requests such as "stick out your tongue I want to stick a pin in it." Mitmachen and mitgehen are special instances of automatic obedience. In mitmachen (to take part), the patient's body can be put into any posture, despite instructions given that the patient resists. Mitgehen (to go along with) is an extreme form of mitmachen in which very slight pressure leads to movement in any direction. This is done despite instructions that the patient resists, such as "Do not let me move your arm."

Ambitendency

    Patient shows conflicting or opposing emotions or thoughts reflected in actions. Patient appears stuck in indecisive hesitant movement

Data from Refs.[6,37,52,53]

One of the more commonly encountered neurotoxic states causing OCS and deserving special attention in the clinical setting of a patient with a known psychiatric condition and on psychoactive medication is the neuroleptic malignant syndrome (NMS). The NMS is an idiosyncratic complication of treatment with both typical (eg, haloperidol) and atypical (eg, olanzapine) antipsychotic drugs. Dopamine receptor blockade lies at the heart of this potentially life-threatening disturbance. NMS presents with mental status changes, fever, severe muscle rigidity and autonomic disturbances, and, mostly but not always, catatonic motor signs.[26–28] These clinical features bear a striking similarity with cases of severe PCS, also known as malignant (lethal) catatonia. In malignant catatonia, psychogenic unresponsiveness is combined with catatonic motor signs, fever, and autonomic instability (tachycardia, tachypnea, and hypertension).[23,29,30] Some investigators have suggested that NMS is simply a variant of malignant catatonia.[23,30,31]

The diagnosis of NMS is made on the basis of a history of exposure to antipsychotic medication or other dopamine antagonists, such as metoclopramide, and the typical clinical features. Laboratory investigations that are helpful are elevations in serum creatine phosphokinase levels due to rhabdomyolysis (keeping in mind that mild creatine phosphokinase elevations may be caused by prior intramuscular [IM] injections), leukocytosis, and an EEG result that shows generalized slowing consistent with a metabolic encephalopathy. NMS is self-limited and may respond to supportive measures such as rehydration and stopping the offending antipsychotic medication. Lorazepam, 1 to 2 mg IM or intravenously (IV), every 4 to 6 hours is usually effective but may not help in NMS that lacks catatonic motor signs.[27,28] Other medications that may be useful are amantadine, bromocriptine, and dantrolene. Electroconvulsive therapy (ECT; 6–10 treatments using a bilateral electrode placement) is invariably effective in medically refractory or moderate to severe cases.[26]

Another important diagnostic consideration is serotonin toxicity (ST), also known as the serotonin syndrome. ST is caused by an excess of serotonin in the brain and presumed to be mediated via the $5\text{-}HT_{2A}$ receptor. ST presents as a febrile agitated delirium with spontaneous or inducible clonus and hyperreflexia maximal in the lower extremities, myoclonus, opsoclonus, and shivering. Rigidity and tremor may occur. Catatonic motor symptoms are not, however, part of this syndrome.[32,33] Most cases of ST relate to drug interactions most commonly seen when a selective serotonin reuptake inhibitor is combined with a monoamine oxidase inhibitor, but many other serotonergic agents have been associated with ST.[33] Treatment centers on supportive care and stopping of any serotonergic medications. There may be a role for specific serotonin antagonists such as cyproheptadine.[33]

PSYCHOGENIC STUPOR AND PSYCHOGENIC CATATONIC STUPOR

Psychiatric illness may present as acute onset, sustained and profound muteness, and immobility that on examination is indistinguishable from a flaccid coma with a GCS score of 3.[7–9] There are no systematic studies concerning the prevalence of psychogenic coma. The published literature consists of isolated case reports suggesting that such presentations are uncommon. PS is much more common. In general psychiatric wards, 9% to 15% of acute admissions meet diagnostic criteria for catatonia. The predominant presentation is with varying degrees of immobility and muteness.[5,34] In the psychiatric literature, such presentations are diagnosed as the retarded-stuporous variety of catatonia.[11,34] These patients are diagnosed as having either PS or PCS depending on the absence or presence of catatonic motor signs and after the diagnostic workup identifies no organic explanation. The qualifier malignant PS or PCS is applied when unresponsiveness is associated with fever and autonomic instability (tachycardia, tachypnea, and hypertension). The psychiatric disorders associated with these presentations are most commonly mood disorders (46%–50%), especially mania, schizophrenia (7%–20%), and schizoaffective disorder (3.6%–6.0%).[5,10,11]

Patients with PS and PCS receive the same investigations as any patient presenting in an unresponsive state. In PS and PCS, all structural imaging and laboratory investigations have negative results. The EEG result is normal in more than 90% of patients with a catatonic syndrome secondary to a psychiatric illness.[25] In one prospective case series, one schizophrenic patient with a catatonic syndrome demonstrated diffuse nonspecific slowing.[35] Mild EEG changes such as theta slowing may also be seen in PS and PCS[36] and may be caused by psychotropic medication, such as neuroleptics, which the patient may already be taking. EEG abnormalities must raise doubt about a primary psychiatric cause, and the search for organic causes such as epilepsy, a systemic metabolic disturbance, or a toxidrome, such as NMS, should be energetically pursued.

PATHOPHYSIOLOGY

Psychogenic unresponsiveness with catatonic motor signs is now best understood as a nonspecific syndrome due to multiple causes but with final common pathways.[37] The underlying pathophysiology, however, remains a matter of speculation. The major psychiatric disorders associated with a catatonic syndrome persist for years after the catatonic symptoms have resolved, and identical symptoms are seen in a variety of intrinsic neurologic diseases and neurotoxic states. Moreover, regardless of the underlying cause, acute but not chronic catatonic symptoms respond to the same interventions: lorazepam and ECT.[5,25,38] These observations have given rise to 2 chief hypotheses concerning catatonic symptom production.

The first is based on neurobiology and suggests that both the associated psychiatric disorders and the medical/neurologic conditions disrupt similar neurobiology, with data mostly supporting alterations and abnormal reactivity of γ-aminobutyric acid (GABA) class A receptors with possible involvement of the glutamatergic N-methyl-D-aspartate (NMDA) receptors.[6] This hypothesis may explain the response to lorazepam, a GABA receptor modulator, and amantadine and memantine, both glutamatergic NMDA receptor antagonists.

The second hypothesis is psychological and psychodynamic. Retrospective interviews of psychiatric patients have revealed severe anxiety (a state of fright) seemingly in response to paranoid delusions, depressive mood, or traumatic experiences.[6] In Rosebush and Mazurek's series of 180 episodes of catatonia in 148 individuals, more than 75% of catatonic patients across diagnostic groups reported having psychotic symptoms during the episode. The anxiety identified by these patients is considered as reactive to the psychosis, depression, or trauma and mobilizes an evolutionary fear response resulting in massive psychobehavioral inhibition, producing a condition of tonic immobility, a state of being "scared stiff" akin to fear-induced freezing studied in experimental animals.[39] The implication is that the neurologic and medical conditions associated with the catatonic syndrome do so indirectly by first provoking severe anxiety. Here the anxiety arises as an understandable but pathologic psychological reaction to the neurologically or medically threatening illness. Anxiety may also stem from activation of anxiogenic neurobiology, such as anxiety provoked by amygdala activation in temporal lobe epilepsy,[40] or in response to psychosis or mood dysregulation caused directly by the specific neurologic and medical condition. Such a formulation, with anxiety as the central psychodynamic, also accounts for the dramatic response to lorazepam, which has its customary and primary use in clinical practice as an anxiolytic. Indeed the response to lorazepam is dramatic and swift with the expectation that up to 85% of patients will have complete resolution of catatonic features within 3 hours of receiving 1 to 3 mg of IM or sublingual lorazepam.[25] The response to IV lorazepam is even more dramatic, with patients responding within minutes.[5] After 2 mg lorazepam IV, there is a 60% reduction in symptoms within 10 minutes.[5,41]

TREATMENT

Although no double-blind placebo-controlled trials have been performed, treatment begins with 1 to 2 mg lorazepam administered sublingually, IM, or IV and repeated in 3 hours and then again in 3 hours if the first 2 doses are ineffective (**Box 2**). This regimen constitutes an adequate trial for most patients who have been symptomatic with PS or PCS for less than 3 weeks.[10] Some patients may, however, require higher doses ranging from 12 to 16 mg per day.[41] Initial treatment is often by the parenteral route because many patients are not capable of taking orally administered medication. Lower initial doses should be considered in the elderly patient. The same lorazepam regimen is used to treat catatonic syndromes from organic causes. Remarkably, patients with acute catatonic syndromes seem to tolerate such high doses of benzodiazepines with little sedation or ataxia.

The dose of lorazepam that is effective in resolving the catatonic syndrome is continued until the underlying primary psychiatric or neurologic/medical condition is effectively controlled. Catatonic symptoms may resurface if the lorazepam is discontinued prematurely.[10]

ECT should be given to all patients who fail to respond to lorazepam. The duration of a trial of lorazepam before moving on to ECT is unclear. Carroll and colleagues[42] suggest 1 to 3 days during which time the workup for the safe administration of

---

Box 2
Standard treatment algorithm for catatonic syndrome

Nonmalignant catatonic syndrome (no fever or autonomic instability)

    Antipsychotic medication should be avoided until catatonic symptoms remit

    Day 1

        Lorazepam 1 to 2 mg every 3 hours for 3 doses by any route (by mouth, IM, or IV)

    Days 2 and 3

        Lorazepam 6 mg/d in 3 divided doses; higher doses (12–16 mg/d) may be needed if response is suboptimal

    Day 4

        Lorazepam responders: continue with the effective dose of lorazepam until the underlying primary psychiatric or neurologic/medical condition is effectively controlled

        Lorazepam nonresponders: 12 to 15 ECT using a bilateral electrode placement. ECT is administered 3 times a week

Malignant catatonic syndrome (with fever and/or autonomic instability)

    Antipsychotic medication should be avoided until catatonic symptoms remit

    Bilateral ECT given daily until autonomic dysfunction resolves

Data from Refs.[10,41–44]

ECT is completed. Specific guidelines for ECT in the treatment of catatonic syndromes are also not available, but patients typically receive an average of 12 to 15 treatments using a bilateral electrode placement.[43,44] ECT should also be considered a first-line intervention for patients who present with malignant catatonic syndromes (fever and autonomic instability). For such very ill patients, daily, rather than the customary thrice weekly, treatments should be given until autonomic dysfunction resolves.[44] Antipsychotic medication should be avoided until catatonic symptoms remit because neuroleptics may provoke NMS in patients while they are still catatonic. These medications can be safely introduced if indicated by the underlying primary psychiatric disorder once the catatonic syndrome is over.[10]

A trial with an antipsychotic medication is also appropriate if the patient fails to respond to lorazepam and ECT, given that most patients with the catatonic syndrome are psychotic and bearing in mind the higher risk of provoking NMS when using this class of medication while the patient still has catatonic symptoms.[10] Other agents that the have been shown in small case series or case reports to have a role in the treatment of the catatonic syndrome include zolpidem (a nonbenzodiazepine $GABA_A$ agonist[45]); amantadine and memantine (both glutamatergic NMDA antagonists)[42]; carbamazepine, possibly via its anticonvulsant effect[46]; topiramate, possibly via an indirect NMDA antagonism[47]; and valproic acid.[48]

The response to lorazepam for acute PS and PCS is generally good to very good and depends on the underlying primary psychiatric illness. Overall response rates vary between 69% and 80%.[5,25,49] Patients with affective disorders do best (greater than 80% responders), whereas those with schizophrenia do poorest (response rates of 40%–50%).[25] Lorazepam does not improve the chronic catatonic motor signs found in schizophrenia. These patients typically present with mannerisms, stereotypes, and perseverative behavior, which have been present for many years. These patients do not have full-blown stupor or persistent and complete mutism.[50] This lack of response to lorazepam suggests that the catatonic motor signs in this population reflect a different underlying neurobiology or mediating psychopathology.

For lorazepam failures, the response to ECT is excellent. Complete resolution of the catatonic syndrome can be expected in more than 80% of patients.[5,44,51] Poorer response to ECT (59%) may result if ECT is delayed.[44]

SUMMARY

Unresponsive patients with or without catatonic motor signs are etiologically heterogeneous, and all require a comprehensive neurodiagnostic assessment to rule out organic causes. Most cases prove to be caused by primary psychiatric disorders, mostly mood disorders, especially mania, rather than schizophrenia. These patients respond to lorazepam administered by any route and, failing this, ECT. Those patients with associated fever and autonomic instability are medical emergencies and need urgent treatment.

ACKNOWLEDGMENTS

The author would like to thank Robert Stowe, MD, for his helpful review and feedback of the draft manuscript.

REFERENCES

1. Posner JB, Saper CB, Schiff ND, et al. Plum and Posner's diagnosis of stupor and coma. 4th edition. Oxford (UK): Oxford University Press; 2007.

2. Bateman DE. Neurological assessment of coma. J Neurol Neurosurg Psychiatry 2001;71(Suppl 1):i13–i7.
3. Young GB. Coma. Ann N Y Acad Sci 2009;1157(1):32–47.
4. Wijdicks EFM. The bare essentials: coma. Pract Neurol 2010;10(1):51–60.
5. Bush G, Fink M, Petrides G, et al. Catatonia II. Treatment with lorazepam and electroconvulsive therapy. Acta Psychiatr Scand 1996;93(2):137–43.
6. Northoff G. What catatonia can tell us about "top down modulation": a neuropsychiatric hypothesis. Behav Brain Sci 2002;25(5):555–604.
7. Freudenreich O, McEvoy JP, Goff DC, et al. Catatonic coma with profound bradycardia. Psychosomatics 2007;48(1):74–8.
8. Baxter CL, White WD. Psychogenic coma: case report. Int J Psychiatry Med 2003;33(3):317–22.
9. Bender KG, Feutrill J. Comatoid catatonia. Aust N Z J Psychiatry 2000;34(1):169–70.
10. Rosebush PI, Mazurek MF. Catatonia and its treatment. Schizophr Bull 2010; 36(2):239–42.
11. Taylor MA, Fink M. Catatonia in psychiatric classification: a home of its own. Am J Psychiatry 2003;160(7):1233–41.
12. Benegal V, Hingorani S, Khanna S, et al. Is stupor by itself a catatonic symptom? Psychopathology 1992;25(5):229–31.
13. Abrams R, Taylor MA, Coleman Stolurow KA. Catatonia and mania: patterns of cerebral dysfunction. Biol Psychiatry 1979;14(1):111–7.
14. Taylor MA. Catatonia: a review of a behavioral neurologic syndrome. Neuropsychiatry Neuropsychol Behav Neurol 1990;3(1):48–72.
15. Krüger S, Bagby RM, Höffler J, et al. Factor analysis of the catatonia rating scale and catatonic symptom distribution across four diagnostic groups. Compr Psychiatry 2001;44(6):472–82.
16. Berrios GE. Stupor revisited. Compr Psychiatry 1981;22(5):466–78.
17. Lee S, Jeong J, Kwak Y, et al. Depression research: where are we now? Mol Brain 2010;3(8):1–10.
18. Moncrieff J. A critique of the dopamine hypothesis of schizophrenia and psychosis. Harv Rev Psychiatry 2009;17(3):214–25.
19. Howes OD, Kapur S. The dopamine hypothesis of schizophrenia: version III—the final common pathway. Schizophr Bull 2009;35(3):549–62.
20. Carroll B, Anfinson T, Kennedy J, et al. Catatonic disorder due to general medical conditions. J Neuropsychiatry Clin Neurosci 1994;6(2):122–33.
21. Meierkord H, Holtkamp M. Non-convulsive status epilepticus in adults: clinical forms and treatment. Lancet Neurol 2007;6(4):329–39.
22. Fisch BJ, Spehlmann R. Fisch and Spehlmann's EEG primer: basic principles of digital and analog EEG. 3rd edition. Amsterdam: Elsevier; 1999.
23. Philbrick K, Rummans T. Malignant catatonia. J Neuropsychiatry Clin Neurosci 1994;6(1):1–13.
24. Rosebush PI, Mazurek MF. Catatonia after benzodiazepine withdrawal. J Clin Psychopharmacol 1996;16(4):315–9.
25. Rosebush PI, Mazurek MF. Catatonia: re-awakening to a forgotten disorder. Mov Disord 1999;14(3):395–7.
26. Strawn JR, Keck PE, Caroff SN. Neuroleptic malignant syndrome. Am J Psychiatry 2007;164(6):870–6.
27. Lee JW. Catatonic variants, hyperthermic extrapyramidal reactions, and subtypes of neuroleptic malignant syndrome. Ann Clin Psychiatry 2007;19(1):9–16.
28. Lee JW. In response to the letter to the editor by Dr. Andrew Francis and Dr. Adeeb Yacoub. Ann Clin Psychiatry 2008;20(4):232–3.

29. Detweiler M, Mehra A, Rowell T, et al. Delirious mania and malignant catatonia: a report of 3 cases and review. Psychiatr Q 2009;80(1):23–40.
30. Fink M, Taylor MA. The many varieties of catatonia. Eur Arch Psychiatry Clin Neurosci 2001;251(Suppl 1):i8–i13.
31. Carroll BT, Taylor RE. The nondichotomy between lethal catatonia and neuroleptic malignant syndrome. J Clin Psychopharmacol 1997;17(3):235–6.
32. Dunkley EJC, Isbister GK, Sibbritt D, et al. The Hunter serotonin toxicity criteria: simple and accurate diagnostic decision rules for serotonin toxicity. QJM 2003; 96(9):635–42.
33. Isbister GK, Buckley NA, Whyte IM. Serotonin toxicity: a practical approach to diagnosis and treatment. Med J Aust 2007;187(6):361–5.
34. Rosebush PI, Hildebrand AM, Furlong BG, et al. Catatonic syndrome in a general psychiatric inpatient population: frequency, clinical presentation, and response to lorazepam. J Clin Psychiatry 1990;51(9):357–62.
35. Carroll BT, Goforth HW, Boutros NN, et al. Electroencephalograph in catatonic disorders due to general medical conditions and psychiatric disorders. CNS Spectr 1998;3(2):57–61.
36. Louis ED, Pflaster NL. Catatonia mimicking nonconvulsive status epilepticus. Epilepsia 1995;36(9):943–5.
37. Fink M, Taylor MA. Catatonia: subtype or syndrome in DSM? Am J Psychiatry 2006;163(11):1875–6.
38. Ungvari GS, Caroff SN, Gerevich J. The catatonia conundrum: evidence of psychomotor phenomena as a symptom dimension in psychotic disorders. Schizophr Bull 2010;36(2):231–8.
39. Moskowitz AK. "Scared stiff": catatonia as an evolutionary-based fear response. Psychol Rev 2004;111(4):984–1002.
40. Cendes F, Andermann F, Gloor P, et al. Relationship between atrophy of the amygdala and ictal fear in temporal lobe epilepsy. Brain 1994;117:739–46.
41. Francis A. Catatonia: diagnosis, classification, and treatment. Curr Psychiatry Rep 2010;12(3):180–5.
42. Carroll BT, Goforth HW, Thomas C, et al. Review of adjunctive glutamate antagonist therapy in the treatment of catatonic syndromes. J Neuropsychiatry Clin Neurosci 2007;19(4):406–12.
43. Rohland BM, Carroll BT, Jacoby RG. ECT in the treatment of the catatonic syndrome. J Affect Disord 1993;29(4):255–61.
44. van Waarde JA, Tuerlings JH, Verwey B, et al. Electroconvulsive therapy for catatonia: treatment characteristics and outcomes in 27 patients. J ECT 2010;26(4): 248–52.
45. Thomas P, Rascle C, Mastain B, et al. Test for catatonia with zolpidem. Lancet 1997;349(9053):702.
46. Kritzinger PR, Jordaan GP. Catatonia: an open prospective series with carbamazepine. Int J Neuropsychopharmacol 2001;4(03):251–7.
47. McDaniel WW, Spiegel DR, Sahota AK. Topiramate effect in catatonia: a case series. J Neuropsychiatry Clin Neurosci 2006;18(2):234–8.
48. Krüger S, Bräunig P. Intravenous valproic acid in the treatment of severe catatonia. J Neuropsychiatry Clin Neurosci 2001;13(2):303–4.
49. Northoff G, Wenke J, Demisch L, et al. Catatonia: short-term response to lorazepam and dopaminergic metabolism. Psychopharmacology 1995;122(2):182–6.
50. Ungvari GS, Chiu HFK, Chow LY, et al. Lorazepam for chronic catatonia: a randomized, double-blind, placebo-controlled cross-over study. Psychopharmacology 1999;142(4):393–8.

51. McCall WV. The response to an amobarbital interview as a predictor of therapeutic outcome in patients with catatonic mutism. Convuls Ther 1992;8(3):174–8.
52. Northoff G, Koch A, Wenke J, et al. Catatonia as a psychomotor syndrome: a rating scale and extrapyramidal motor symptoms. Mov Disord 1999;14(3): 404–16.
53. Bush G, Fink M, Petrides G, et al. Catatonia. I. Rating scale and standardized examination. Acta Psychiatr Scand 1996;93(2):129–36.

Nontraumatic Coma in Children and Adolescents: Diagnosis and Management

Shashi S. Seshia, MD (Bombay), FRCPC&E[a],*,
William T. Bingham, MD, FRCPC[b], Fenella J. Kirkham, MD, FRCPCH[c,d],
Venkatraman Sadanand, PhD, MD, FRCSC[e]

KEYWORDS

- Nontraumatic • Coma • Children • Adolescents • Causes
- Management • Increased intracranial pressure

Coma, defined as an impairment of arousal, is an important clinical emergency in pediatric practice. Despite the advances in diagnostic techniques since one of us wrote on this subject in 1977,[1] clinical acumen is still central to diagnosis, management, and prognostication, and the approach of Plum and Posner[2] remains relevant.

The focus of our review is nontraumatic coma (NTC) in children (the term includes adolescents, ie, those <20 years of age). Nonaccidental head injury (NAHI) is addressed in so far as it enters into the differential diagnosis of NTC. Coma of less than 1 hour in duration is excluded from discussion.

DIFFERENTIAL DIAGNOSIS

The assessment of consciousness is dependent on motor responses. Hence, a child with total generalized loss of motor function, as may happen with severe myasthenia

Disclosures/conflict of interest (all authors): None.
[a] Division of Pediatric Neurology, Department of Pediatrics, Royal University Hospital, University of Saskatchewan, 103 Hospital Drive, Saskatoon, Saskatchewan, S7N 0W8, Canada
[b] Department of Pediatrics, Royal University Hospital, University of Saskatchewan, 103 Hospital Drive, Saskatoon, Saskatchewan, S7N 0W8, Canada
[c] Neurosciences Unit, UCL Institute of Child Health, 30 Guilford Street, London, WC1N 1EH, UK
[d] Department of Child Health, Southampton General hospital NHS Trust, Tremona Road, Southampton, SO16 6YD, UK
[e] Department of Neurosurgery, Loma Linda University Medical Center, 11234 Anderson Street, Loma Linda, CA 92354, USA
* Corresponding author.
E-mail address: sseshia@yahoo.ca

Neurol Clin 29 (2011) 1007–1043
doi:10.1016/j.ncl.2011.07.011
0733-8619/11/$ – see front matter © 2011 Elsevier Inc. All rights reserved.

gravis, botulinum poisoning, or Guillain Barré syndrome, may be erroneously labeled as comatose; the pupils are normally reactive in these situations despite presumed deep coma and absent oculomotor reflexes.

Apparent coma may be presentations of conversion or factitious disorders and malingering: resistance to eyelid opening with a normal Bell phenomenon, normal responses to cold caloric testing (including nystagmus), and otherwise normal neurologic examination should make one suspect these possibilities.

The electroencephalogram (EEG) is normal for age and reactive to stimuli in these situations.

EPIDEMIOLOGY

Relative incidences vary by country, region, season, especially for infective causes, and period of data collection.[3] Ethnicity is relevant for several inborn errors of metabolism (IEM) that produce coma.[4,5] The age-specific incidence of NTC was 160 per 100,000 children per year for those less than 1 year of age, and less than 40 per 100,000 children in those aged 2 years to 16 years for the period July 1994 to December 1995, in a population-based study in England.[6] NTC has also been commoner in children less than 6 years than in older children in hospital-based studies.[1,7–9] The higher incidence in early childhood is likely because of greater susceptibility to infective causes. Anemia, malnutrition, and adverse socioeconomic factors predispose to infectious encephalopathy, children being most vulnerable.

GENETIC SUSCEPTIBILITY?

Kobayashi and colleagues'[10] data suggest that polymorphisms in the sodium channel $\alpha 1$ subunit may predispose to some acute encephalopathies. Variations in the carnitine palmitoyl transferase II (CPT II) gene, apparently common in East Asians (eg, Japanese), may be a risk factor for a variety of acute encephalopathies among them.[11–13]

CAUSES

We have used the concepts of Plum and Posner[2] to classify the causes of NTC in children[3]; the distinction between (1) conditions associated with structural changes in the brain and (2) those in which metabolic or toxic disturbances predominate (often with no or little structural change), and between those with focal signs and diffuse signs may still have practical merit (**Box 1**). However, the differentiation is often indistinct in clinical practice. Clinical features may evolve from focal to diffuse, and conditions listed under the structural category may produce metabolic dysfunction, and vice versa. Clinical, laboratory, EEG, and neuroimaging data should be considered collectively when attempting to arrive at a specific diagnosis. Some causes are discussed in further detail. Because of travel and migration, physicians, especially in Western countries, should be familiar with important global causes, particularly infective and genetic.

Infective Causes

A variety of organisms (bacterial, viral, protozoal, and fungal) can cause sepsis or invade the nervous system (meningoencephalitis) and produce coma. Many occur exclusively or more frequently in some geographic regions than others, and several are seasonal.

The incidence of bacterial meningoencephalitis has been greatly reduced in many advanced economies with the introduction of conjugate vaccines, but vaccines are not available everywhere, and in some countries, bacterial strains different from those in the vaccines are emerging. Immunization programs have markedly reduced if not eliminated encephalitis secondary to communicable childhood infectious disease like chickenpox, measles, mumps, and rubella.

Mycoplasma pneumoniae is becoming recognized as the most frequent cause of infection-related encephalopathy in many countries; several factors, including direct infection and immune-mediated reactions may be responsible for coma and neurologic dysfunction.[14–16]

Tuberculous meningoencephalitis (TBM) still occurs in many parts of the world, those with human immunodeficiency virus and possibly diabetes mellitus (DM) being at high risk. The diagnosis is challenging and often delayed because current tests are insensitive; central nervous system (CNS) TB was identified in 20 cases between June 1998 and October 2005 in the California encephalitis project.[17]

The minimum incidence of childhood acute encephalitis syndromes was 10.5 per 100,000 cases in Western industrialized countries, the specific incidence for children in tropical countries being unknown; cause could not be established in a high percentage, likely because of inadequate diagnostic techniques; the incidence of herpes simplex virus (HSV) encephalitis was uniform across the globe.[18] Japanese encephalitis (JE) is decreasing in the Far East, likely because of immunization programs, but increasing in South Asian countries where vaccines are not yet universally available.[18]

Seasonal outbreaks of West Nile virus encephalitis have occurred in several parts of the world, including Canada and the United States, children also being affected.[19,20] Chikunguya infection has also become a global risk, and can associate with encephalitis.[21,22] The recent pandemic of H1N1 was associated with cases of encephalitis in children.[23,24]

Infective Causes in Advanced Economies

Encephalitides from arboviruses like western equine, eastern equine, Venezuelan equine, and West Nile are seasonal (related to mosquito vectors) and have often occurred in epidemics (or outbreaks) in certain parts of North America. *M pneumoniae* can also be associated with outbreaks, with encephalitis being a complication.[25] *M pneumoniae* was the most common responsible agent in the California Encephalitis Project (June 1998–2006), children being more affected than adults[16]; of the 34 children in coma, 12 (35%) had *M pneumoniae* encephalitis, 13 (38%) had a variety of bacterial (meningoencephalitic) or rickettsial infections, 7 (20%) had HSV1, and 2 had enterovirus encephalitis. Precise pediatric data could not be teased out from a French study.[26] In a population-based study from England, HSV accounted for 16% of 76 children diagnosed with encephalitis, almost all being less than 2 years of age; a diagnosis could not be established in 42%.[27] Arbovirus encephalitides were uncommon in the European studies. Neuroborreliosis occurs in parts of North America and Europe but coma is an uncommon presentation.

Infective Causes in (Mainly Tropical) Emerging Economies

The causes are likely to be different in rural and urban populations. Socioeconomic status and access to health care are major influencing variables, as they are in developed countries. In recent series, infection (eg, sepsis, bacterial meningoencephalitides, cerebral malaria, viral encephalitides, gastroenteritis) has accounted for 28% to 78%, and toxic/metabolic causes for 13% to 38% of children with NTC.[8,9,28–33] Cases of malaria can be seen throughout the year in endemic areas. JE and cerebral malaria occur in clusters/epidemics, especially during the monsoon, when mosquito populations are high.[28,32,34–41] TBM remains a frequent and important cause of

---

Box 1
Cause of childhood coma. The history, physical examination, electroencephalographic, laboratory, and neuroradiologic findings should be considered in determining the presence or absence of 'structural/anatomic abnormality,' metabolic or toxic disturbance, and diffuse or focal features

1. Those with predominant structural lesions
   a. Focal (focal or localizing features present)
      i. Head injury, accidental or nonaccidental (NAHI is most common <1 year of age)
      ii. Vascular (age of presentation is cause dependent)
         1. Arteriovenous malformation or aneurysm
         2. Migraine
         3. Embolism
         4. Hypertensive encephalopathy
         5. Intracranial arterial vasculopathy
         6. Carotid or vertebral arterial dissection
         7. Venous thrombosis
         8. Hypercoagulable or hypocoagulable states
      iii. Mass
         1. Hematoma (often associated with i, ii1, ii3, ii4, ii7, ii8 under point 1)
         2. Abscess (association with congenital cyanotic heart disease, sinusitis)
         3. Others (eg, tumor, tuberculoma; coma is a late presentation)
      iv. Intracranial infection (presentation at any age; specific cause is country/region/season specific; common and important)
         1. Meningitis (often meningoencephalitis; focal signs in bacterial or TB meningoencephalitis usually caused by vasculitis)
         2. Encephalitis
      v. Immune-mediated: ADEM (diagnosis by MRI) and immune-mediated encephalitides
   b. Diffuse (ie, clinical features are not localizing)
      i. Accidental/NAHI
      ii. Vascular (age of presentation is cause dependent)
         1. Migraine
         2. Venous thrombosis (eg, dehydration, sepsis, hypercoagulable states)
         3. Diffuse arteriopathy
         4. Hypertensive encephalopathy
         5. Diffuse intracranial bleeding (bleeding disorder)
      iii. Intracranial infection (presentation at any age; specific cause is country/region/season specific; common and important)
         1. Meningoencephalitis
         2. Encephalitis
      iv. Immune-mediated: ADEM and immune-mediated encephalitides
      v. Hypoxia-ischemia (presentation at any age; several potential triggers)

        1. Cardiorespiratory arrest (eg, acute life-threatening event, near drowning, choking)

        2. Shock/hypotension (eg, dehydration, sepsis, bleeding)

   vi. ANE of childhood[a]

  vii. HSE syndrome

 viii. Complications of malignancy (disease or treatment)

   ix. IEM affecting the brain primarily (eg, mitochondrial cytopathies; usually present in infancy or early childhood)

    x. Hydrocephalus/shunt dysfunction

2. Those with predominant metabolic (or toxic) disturbance (anatomic abnormalities if present are usually potentially reversible; CNS features are usually diffuse but may rarely be asymmetric or focal)

  a. Fluid-electrolyte acid-base disturbance (infants are at highest risk but can occur at any age)

     i. Hypernatremia

    ii. Hyponatremia

   iii. Acidosis

   iv. Alkalosis

    v. Water intoxication

   vi. Inappropriate antidiuretic hormone (often complicates bacterial or TB meningitis or severe head injury)

  vii. Diabetes insipidus

 viii. Rapid correction of dehydration, electrolyte or acid-base imbalance (*Note*: risk of central pontine myelinosis)

  b. Infection-septicemia (encephalopathy of sepsis)

  c. Poisoning (numerous agents; bimodal age distribution: 1–5 years and 13–20 years)

  d. Hepatic failure

  e. Renal failure

  f. Respiratory failure

  g. Endocrine

     i. Hypoglycemia (ketotic and nonketotic)

    ii. DM (an important and increasingly common disorder)

   iii. Hypothyroidism

   iv. Other, including adrenal insufficiency (in which hypoglycemia may be the cause of coma and a prominent metabolic abnormality)

  h. IEM (primarily systemic; presentation is typically in the neonatal period, infancy and early childhood but can be during adolescence and later). Some examples:

     i. Urea cycle

    ii. Congenital lactic acid syndromes

   iii. Intermittent maple syrup urine disease

   iv. Mitochondrial cytopathies

    v. Carnitine palmitoyltransferase deficiency

(*continued on next page*)

Box 1
(continued)

   i. Hypothermia/hyperthermia

   j. Nutritional deficiencies

   k. Iatrogenic

      i. Parenteral nutrition

      ii. Pediatric phosphate enema

   l. Toxic

      i. Shigella infection

      ii. Burns

      iii. Intussusception

   m. Iatrogenic

3. Not readily classifiable as above

   a. Idiopathic SE (particularly nonconvulsive); acute epileptic encephalopathies (FIRES[a]; AERRPS[a], AESD[a])

   b. Associated with congenital heart disease, especially postoperative complications

   c. Central pontine myelinosis

Abbreviations: ADEM, acute disseminated encephalomyelitis; AERRPS, acute encephalitis with refractory repetitive partial seizures; AESD, acute encephalopathy with biphasic seizures and late reduced diffusion; ANE, acute necrotizing encephalopathy; CNS, central nervous system; DM, diabetes mellitus; FIRES, fever-induced refractory epileptic encephalopathy in school-aged children; HSE, hemorrhagic shock and encephalopathy; IEM, inborn errors of metabolism; MRI, magnetic resonance imaging; NAHI, non-accidental head injury; SE, status epilepticus; TB, tuberculous.

[a] Genetic susceptibility and immune-mediated responses may have a role in causation.

From Seshia SS, Bingham WT, Griebel RW. Coma in childhood. Handb Clin Neurol 2008;90:329–50; with permission.

---

coma and morbidity.[28,41,42] Encephalitis from childhood communicable diseases, rabies, and shigella gastroenteritis still occur; seizures and coma are important features with shigellosis.[43]

Chronic ear infections predispose to brain abscess and intracranial venous sinus thrombosis. Gastroenteritis and sepsis often associate with metabolic dysfunction that includes fluid, electrolyte and acid-base disturbances, hypoglycemia, and hypovolemia. Endotoxins, inflammatory, and immunologic reactions produced by the infective agents also contribute to the encephalopathy in these situations.

Immune-mediated Encephalitides (Excluding Acute Disseminated Encephalomyelitis)

Immune-mediated encephalitides are being increasingly recognized in children, *N*-methyl-D-aspartate receptor (NMDAR) antibodies related, being the best example.[27,44,45] Girls are mainly affected in this disorder. Psychiatric symptoms and sleep disturbance are prominent at the outset, seizures occur, coma is common, and dyskinesia often a striking feature. Associations with acute *M pneumoniae* infection and teratomas, especially ovarian, have been reported.[44,45]

Acute encephalitis with refractory repetitive partial seizures (AERRPS), reported from Japan, has been associated with GluRε2 antibodies in serum or cerebrospinal fluid (CSF) in some cases[46]; the condition is characterized by fever, and refractory repetitive partial seizures consisting primarily of eye deviation and facial twitching. The prognosis is often unfavorable.

Hemorrhagic Shock and Encephalopathy Syndrome

Infants and young children seem most affected. The presenting features include seizures, coma, fever, shock, and often multiorgan failure. Neuroimaging and autopsy show hemorrhagic cortical lesions. Clustering during winter was reported in 1 series.[47] The relative incidence of hemorrhagic shock and encephalopathy (HSE) in the causes of coma is unknown. The cause is likely to be multifactorial, including genetic predisposition, immune mediated, and IEM, with infection being a possible trigger rather than the primary cause.

Acute Demyelinating Encephalomyelitis

Acute demyelinating encephalomyelitis (ADEM) is a diagnosis being made increasingly with the advent of magnetic resonance imaging (MRI).[27,48,49] ADEM is often post-infectious or after immunization.[50] *M pneumoniae* is an important cause.[14] Most cases have a monophasic course, although some may have relapses, not dissimilar to those seen with demyelinating diseases such as multiple sclerosis.[51]

Acute Necrotizing Encephalopathy

This condition first reported by Mizuguchi from Japan, has also been described from other countries.[52–56] Infants and young children are typically affected. Onset is with symptoms of upper respiratory viral illness and vomiting, followed by high fever, coma, and seizures. Associated features include hepatomegaly and impaired liver functions. The prognosis is poor, with significant residual neurodevelopmental dysfunction in most patients. The hallmark of acute necrotizing encephalopathy (ANE) is the presence of multiple, symmetric, necrotic lesions in the thalamus, cerebral white matter, brainstem, and cerebellum on computed tomography (CT), MRI, and at autopsy. The differential diagnosis includes Leigh mitochondrial cytopathy. Missense mutations in RANBP2 may be responsible for familial or recurrent cases.[56] Variations in the CPT II gene may be a risk factor for developing ANE after infections[13]; such genetic traits may explain the high incidence of these disorders in East Asia.

Other Acute Encephalopathies of Uncertain Origin

Fever-induced refractory epileptic encephalopathy in school-aged children (FIRES) often occurs about 1 to 6 days after a nonspecific febrile illness or vaccination.[57–61] Subjects develop partial seizures involving perisylvian areas, and impairment of consciousness; seizures become continuous and refractory; some respond well to the ketogenic diet. Tests for infective agents and autoimmune antibodies have been negative, and MRI unremarkable. The possibility of genetic susceptibility, immune-mediated reaction (eg, voltage-gated potassium channel complex antibodies), or IEM should be considered. FIRES is not dissimilar to AERRPS.

Acute encephalopathy with biphasic seizures and late reduced diffusion (AESD),[62] described from Japan, is characterized by fever, prolonged initial seizure, impairment of consciousness, and a flurry of seizures around days 4 to 6. MRI is often normal initially, but shows reduced diffusion in the frontal or frontoparietal subcortical white matter around days 3 to 9. MR spectroscopy (MRS) is characteristic, apparently suggesting excitotoxic injury. Outcome is variable. Polymorphisms in the CPT II gene may predispose to AESD.[13]

Stroke (Arterial and Venous)

Arterial and venous strokes complicate bacterial meningitides, dehydration, and sepsis. With the advent of MRI (including MR venography [MRV] and MR angiography [MRA]), arterial and venous strokes are becoming increasingly recognized as a cause of coma.[63,64] Large arterial strokes are usually seen on neuroimaging but venous sinus thrombosis may not be accompanied by infarction and should be specifically sought. Hematologic conditions such as iron deficiency anemia, sickle cell disease, and β-thalassemia predispose to stroke. The latter 2 conditions are relatively more common in ethnic groups such as African, Southeast Asian, South Asian, Chinese, Mediterranean, and Middle Eastern. Preventive measures in these populations, and a high index of suspicion for stroke when they present with neurologic symptoms, are important in management.[65]

Cerebral aneurysms (and arteriovenous malformations) can present in childhood, usually adolescence, with subarachnoid hemorrhage and hemorrhagic stroke.[66]

Hypertensive Encephalopathy and Posterior Reversible Encephalopathy Syndrome

Hypertensive encephalopathy is uncommon in children compared with adults. However, it can occur with renal and connective tissue diseases (such as systemic lupus erythematosus), and may be the presenting feature in them. Coarctation of the aorta as a cause of hypertension is now rare, as most cases are detected in the newborn period or early infancy during routine physical examinations. In addition to hypertensive encephalopathy, other important associations with posterior reversible encephalopathy syndrome (PRES) include renal diseases and immunosuppressive therapy.[67]

Simple Metabolic Disorders

Hypoglycemia and hypernatremia are important causes, often complicating illnesses, particularly in infants. Hypoglycemia may also be secondary to poor feeding, alcohol poisoning, several IEM or endocrinopathy, especially adrenal insufficiency. Anticipation, early recognition, and prompt treatment are key to better outcome.

Diabetes Mellitus and Hyperglycemic Hyperosmolar Syndrome

There has been a dramatic increase in the global incidence of DM. The clinical distinction between type 1 and type 2 is often blurred. Coma caused by diabetic ketoacidosis was the first presentation of DM in 7 of 8 diabetic children in the study of Wong and colleagues.[6] Nonketotic hyperglycemic hyperosmolar coma may also be a presentation in DM[68–72]; timely recognition and treatment are important to minimize morbidity and mortality.

Inborn Errors of Metabolism

Coma is an important and sometimes a presenting feature of several Inborn Errors of Metabolism (IEM). These IEM include maple syrup urine disease, urea cycle enzyme defects, disorders of fatty acid oxidation, nonketotic hyperglycinemia, congenital lactic acidosis, mitochondrial cytopathies, and certain leukodystrophies (leukoencephalopathies), especially Cree and adrenoleukodystrophy.[73–75] Minor illness may trigger coma in IEM. Reye-like syndrome may be a presenting feature. Detailed discussion of these conditions is beyond the scope of this review, and readers are advised to consult current references.

Poisoning

Organophosphate insecticides are readily available in tropical/developing countries; they are an important cause of coma in those regions.[76–78] Accidental (young children), intentional or suicidal (older children) poisoning with opiates or amitriptyline in infants/children, whose caregivers may be taking these drugs, is not uncommon.[79–81]

Accidental and Other Causes

Near drowning (in warm or cold water) is a universal risk, hypoxic-ischemic encephalopathy (HIE) often being the consequence. HIE can also result from aspiration or acute life-threatening events of unknown cause. HIE is an important clinical entity in neonates but is not discussed here. Hypothermic coma is a winter risk in many countries. Coma can be a presentation of acute abdomen, especially intussusception.[82] Coma may be a feature or presenting symptom of autoimmune conditions like Hashimoto thyroiditis and systemic lupus erythematosus.

Postcardiac Surgery

Cardiac surgery, especially for correction of congenital heart defects, is occurring with increasing frequency. Neurologic complications in the postoperative period include coma, seizures, dyskinesia, and focal deficits.[83,84] The causes are multifactorial.

Non-accidental Head Injury

Young children less than the age of 3 years are the most vulnerable, those less than 1 year especially so.[85] The presentation is often of a nonspecific acute encephalopathy with impairment of consciousness. Recurrent alleged impairment of consciousness (encephalopathy) may be a rare presentation. Often, the first clue may be findings on CT of the head, including scalp injury, subgaleal or cephalhematoma, skull fracture, subdural and other intracranial hemorrhagic lesions. A systematic clinical and radiologic examination for evidence of abuse, including other injuries, should be performed.

The Neonate

Important causes include maternal drug use or administration (especially narcotics), IEM (eg, urea cycle defects; see earlier discussion), bacterial meningoencephalitis, sepsis, viral encephalitis (especially HSV), HIE, intracranial hemorrhage (from a variety of causes), and fluid or electrolyte disturbance from gastroenteritis or poor intake.

ASSESSMENT

The approach to the comatose child has been discussed by several investigators.[1,3,41,86-89] The examination is still based on that suggested by Plum and Posner.[2] The Pediatric Accident and Emergency Research Group in the United Kingdom (UK) used a Delphi process to develop national guidelines for the management of children with decreased level of consciousness.[89]

Core Principles and Immediate Measures

Staff in the front line, especially in remote communities, should have basic knowledge about the management of comatose children. Telephone and telehealth links are now available in many parts of the world; hence, early management can be optimized through consultation with a pediatric center. Emerging economies are developing specific strategies to deal with their critically ill children.

Initial steps that also have to be continued throughout the acute stage are generally multipronged (**Box 2**), particularly when coma is complicated by cardiorespiratory insufficiency, shock or status epilepticus (SE), all of which should be treated with minimal delay. Blood gases need to be checked, adequate ventilation and circulation ensured, temperature normalized, and hypoglycemia and electrolyte abnormalities excluded or if present treated. Arterial blood pressure, heart rate, electrocardiograms, central venous pressure (CVP), urinary output, and core body temperature (rectal or esophageal) must

---

Box 2
Initial and core management of nontraumatic coma and increased ICP

ABC (airway, blood pressure, circulation) or CAB (circulation, airway, blood pressure) as appropriate

Rule out and treat: hypoglycemia and electrolyte disturbance

Evaluate for clinical features of increased ICP/herniation syndromes

Investigate for cause and complications

CSF examination is an important investigation if meningitis, encephalitis, or certain IEM are under consideration but please consider if any contraindications to LP

Neuroradiologic investigations (especially MRI) high on the list

EEG (high on the list); may need continuous EEG monitoring

Treat seizures (do not mistake nonepileptic phenomena for seizures)

Specific treatment of underlying cause (eg, infective)

Maintain age-appropriate CPP

Maintain normothermia

Maintain normoxia and normocarbia

Head in the midline and avoid obstruction to venous outflow (neck)

Elevate head end of the bed to 20° to 30° if increased ICP suspected

Repeat investigations as clinically necessary; however, avoid unnecessary radiographs (including CT scans) because of the cumulative radiation dosing for children

Abbreviations: CPP, cerebral perfusion pressure; CSF, cerebrospinal fluid; CT, computed tomography; EEG, electroencephalogram or electroencephalographic; ICP, intracranial pressure; IEM, inborn error/s of metabolism; LP, lumbar puncture; MRI, magnetic resonance imaging.

Data from Tatman A, Warren A, Williams, A, et al. Development of a modified pediatric coma scale in intensive care clinical practice. Arch Dis Child 1997; 77:519–21.

---

be monitored from the outset, as may intracranial pressure (ICP). The cervical spine must be immobilized without obstructing venous return, if there is suspicion of trauma.

Evidence of brain displacement (herniation) should be sought. Decerebration, often asymmetrical, strongly suggests increased ICP with brain shift; other features include abrupt pupillary change (unilateral or bilateral), impaired upward gaze, sudden deterioration of respiration, and apnea.[3,86,90] These are indications for emergent management of increased ICP.

Once the child is stable, a detailed history should be taken and the child should be examined. These can be completed by one individual within 15 minutes, and are essential for planning investigations and further management.

General Examination

The skin should be checked for bruising, rash, and evidence of neurocutaneous syndromes. In infants, the head circumference should be measured and compared with previous values, the anterior fontanelle (AF) checked for fullness, and sutures assessed for separation. Transillumination can be performed in infants. The head should be auscultated for bruits. The length and weight should be taken, and ideally plotted with earlier measurements. Signs of meningeal irritation (neck stiffness; Kernig sign) should be sought. The spine, including the sacral area, should be inspected for sinuses. The chest and abdomen should be examined.

Comments on Some General Clinical Clues

History and general examination invariably provide clues to cause. The following is a brief list:

1. Fever suggests an infective cause. Infants with sepsis may be hypothermic or body temperature may decrease during transportation; hence, infection should also be considered in those who are hypothermic.[1,3] Fever may trigger metabolic decompensation in those with IEM.[3]
2. The absence of neck stiffness in comatose children does not exclude (bacterial) meningitis.
3. Failure to thrive and neurodevelopmental dysfunction before onset of coma may suggest IEM.[3]
4. Parental consanguinity, family history of similar disorder, and particular ethnicity of the child may suggest an IEM, or in the event of a stroke, β-thalassemia or sickle cell disease. Those of East Asian ancestry are susceptible to a variety of unique acute encephalopathies (discussed earlier).
5. Recurrent coma may suggest epilepsy with recurrent nonconvulsive SE (NCSE), IEM, or nonaccidental poisoning.[3,91]
6. A comatose child with a previously established diagnosis of epilepsy may be in NCSE. However, NCSE may be the first presentation of a seizure disorder.
7. Multifocal/myoclonic seizures favor an IEM if HIE is excluded.
8. Focal seizures or focal deficit typically suggest a structural lesion as outlined in **Box 1**. However, focal seizures or deficit can occur with hypoglycemia, and hemiparesis can be postictal.
9. A full AF suggests increased ICP; a sunken AF may point to dehydration.
10. Meningococcal and rickettsial infections often have a characteristic rash, as may Lyme infection.
11. Presence of bruising (especially thumb marks), frenular tears, or cigarette burns suggest nonaccidental injury (NAI). Bruising alone may be secondary to hematologic derangement, which should be excluded.
12. Leigh's mitochondrial cytopathy and central pontine myelinosis should be considered in those with symptoms and signs of brainstem dysfunction.
13. Poisoning with opioid substances should be excluded in those with miotic pupils[80]; intravenous (IV) naloxone is diagnostic and therapeutic in this situation.
14. Evidence of cardiac lesion may point to a stroke.
15. Hepatomegaly/splenomegaly may suggest an IEM. Splenomegaly may be present in malaria.
16. Abdominal pain and watery bloody stools (not necessarily currant jelly), suggest infective gastroenteritis or intussusception.
17. Chronic suppurative ear infection may suggest brain abscess or cerebral sinus venous thrombosis.

Grading of Coma and Coma Scales

The Glasgow coma scale (GCS) is widely used in adults.[92] There are several modifications of the scale for use in children; these have been studied for interobserver agreement and reviewed critically.[3,86,93,94] One modification of the GCS was found to have good interrater agreement, and has been endorsed by the British Pediatric Neurology Association.[86,95] A slightly revised version of the scale is shown in **Table 1**. Scales modeled on the GCS have some limitations:

1. Swollen eyelids confound eye opening.
2. Aphasia, intubation, and deafness can affect responses to verbal stimuli.

Table 1 Modified Glasgow coma scale for children		
Item	>5 y	<5 y
Eye opening		
E4	Spontaneous	As older child
E3	To verbal stimulus	As older child
E2	To pain	As older child
E1	No response to pain	As older child
ET	Unable to test response (state reason)	
Verbal (not used in intubated children: use Grimace instead)		
V5	Orientated	Alert, babbles, coos, words or sentences to usual ability
V4	Confused	Less than usual ability or spontaneous Irritable cry
V3	Inappropriate words	Cries to pain
V2	Incomprehensible sounds	Moans to pain
V1	No response to pain	No response to pain
VT (go to Grimace)	Intubated	Intubated
Grimace (use in intubated children regardless of age or in those considered to be aphasic)		
G5	Spontaneous normal facial oromotor activity (eg, sucks tube, coughs, sounds)	
G4	Less than usual spontaneous ability or only responds to touch	
G3	Vigorous grimace to pain	
G2	Mild grimace or some change in facial expression to pain	
G1	No response to pain	
GT	Unable to test response (state reason)	
Motor		
M6	Obeys commands	Normal spontaneous movements or withdraws to touch
M5	Localizes to pain stimulus	As older child or vigorous motor response to painful stimulus
M4	Withdraws from pain	As older child or less than vigorous response to painful stimulus or needs more intense/sustained painful stimulus
M3	Abnormal flexion to pain	As older child
M2	Abnormal extension to pain	As older child
M1	No response to pain	As older child
MT	Unable to test motor response	

ET, VT, GT, MT represent minor additions to the original.

Data from Tatman A, Warren A, Williams A, et al. Development of a modified pediatric coma scale in intensive care clinical practice. Arch Dis Child 1997;77:519–21.

3. Limb injury can influence motor response.
4. Although it is commonplace to describe a patient by the summed score, this must only be done with a description of each component and a complete physical and neurologic examination.[3,96]

Neurologic Examination

Interobserver agreement was fair to almost perfect for 12 items used in the assessment of comatose children, although the sample size was limited to 15 and observers to 2.[97]

Fundal examination

Multilayered retinal hemorrhage is considered characteristic of NAHI or shaken baby syndrome.[85] Papilledema is rare early in acute coma.[1] Venous pulsations are often difficult to assess; their presence makes increased ICP unlikely; their absence is unhelpful.

Extraocular assessment

Observation Repetitive horizontal eye movements with rapid saccades with or without quivering of the eyelids suggest NCSE. Ophthalmoplegia, ocular bobbing, convergent or divergent spasms, spontaneous blinking, or episodes of lid retraction usually imply brainstem dysfunction.[1] Noticeable nystagmus is seen in barbiturate or phenytoin overdose/poisoning.

Ocular movements Ocular movements are tested by the doll's eye maneuver and ice water caloric test. The former should not be performed if cervical spine injury is suspected. Impaired upward gaze strongly suggests central herniation, a finding that calls for urgent intervention to reduce ICP and investigation for the cause. Impaired lateral gaze and partial or complete ophthalmoplegia generally result from brainstem structural lesions. However, these symptoms may be seen with myasthenia gravis, botulinum poisoning, and the Fisher variant of the Guillain Barré syndrome, or as an effect of neuromuscular blocking agents; pupillary reaction is generally preserved in these situations but may be affected in botulinum poisoning and the Fisher variant of the Guillain Barré syndrome.

Corneal reflexes

Corneal reflexes tend to be abolished in deep coma. Weak eye closure on 1 side (with good closure on the other) can occur contralateral to a hemispheric lesion or ipsilateral to a pontine/brainstem one.

Pupillary responses

The size of the pupils in the resting state and reaction to light (direct, consensual, and ciliospinal) should be noted. Normal or relatively normal pupillary responses despite other evidence of brainstem/pontine dysfunction may suggest a toxic or metabolic cause for coma. A unilateral fixed dilated pupil or the sudden occurrence of bilateral fixed dilated pupils suggests transtentorial or central herniation respectively. Fixed dilated pupils with relative preservation of ocular movements may be caused by administration of topical pupil dilating agents. Otherwise, they may occur secondary to poisoning with barbiturates, sympathomimetics, or anticholinergics. Small pupils are usually caused by poisoning with narcotics (opiates), phenothiazines, ethanol, valproic acid, or anticholinesterases.

Motor system Muscle tone should be checked, and response to a supraorbital painful stimulus assessed. Limb withdrawal to pressure over the fingertips or the sternum may be reflex. Decorticate and decerebrate patterns are often asymmetric and intermittent, and should not be mistaken for seizures. They may be provoked by stimulation.[1,3,90] Decerebrate and decorticate posturing may be seen in coma associated with structural damage or toxic/metabolic causes. Dystonia or dyskinesia in a comatose child strongly suggests poisoning with drugs such as phenothiazines or phenytoin. However, these may also be seen in IEM (eg, glutaric aciduria type 1, mitochondrial cytopathies), and anti-NMDAR encephalitis. Flaccidity and areflexia are serious signs in coma; however, the effect of neuromuscular blocking agents, high levels of depressant drugs, and disorders of the lower motor neurone or neuromuscular junction should be excluded.

Respiration
Plum and Posner[2] suggested that the pattern of breathing was helpful in localizing site of dysfunction and assessing rostral-caudal progression of supratentorial lesions (normal; Cheyne-Stokes: deep in the cerebral hemisphere or diencephalon; central neurogenic hyperventilation: brainstem or tegmentum; apneustic: pontine; ataxic: medulla; apnea: lower medulla). In one study, abnormalities of breathing were not found useful in assessing clinical course; ataxic respiration and apnea often occurred with little warning.[1] Examples of Leigh's mitochondrial cytopathy have been associated with central neurogenic hyperventilation, apneustic, and ataxic respiration.

Blood pressure
Hypertension can be secondary to intracranial lesions or increased ICP, the latter often associated with Cushing triad. Without previous history, the differentiation from primary hypertension can be difficult; clinical, neuroradiologic, and ICP data may be helpful. Neuroradiologic features of PRES may favor hypertensive encephalopathy.

Temperature and temperature regulation
Infections are usually responsible for fever. Fever can occur with anticholinergic poisoning. Central causes for fever are uncommon. Temperature and blood pressure regulation are lost in severe hypothermia or brain death.

INVESTIGATIONS

Some investigations are generic. Many others have to be case-specific and problem-specific, based on clinical symptoms and diagnostic considerations. Bowker and colleagues[98] have discussed the UK recommendations.

Generic

A comatose child is generally a critically ill one. Initial tests even before detailed history and examination include complete blood count, blood gases, acid-base status, urine examination, and blood-based biochemical tests such as electrolytes, glucose, creatinine, calcium, magnesium, phosphate, lactate, ammonia, and alanine aminotransferase. These tests should be supplemented by additional ones based on the diagnostic considerations.

Tests for Infectious and Immune-mediated Causes

Investigations have to be specific for the clinical presentation, and organisms prevalent in the geographic region and season. We involve our pediatric infectious disease expert from the outset. Polymerase chain reaction is becoming the gold standard for diagnosis of several infective agents, and molecular studies can also be useful. Further detailing of tests is beyond the scope of this review.

Tests for immune-mediated encephalitides should be undertaken, when these are clinically suspected or if the cause is not apparent.

CSF Examination: to Lumbar Puncture or not to Lumbar Puncture?

Intracranial infection is a common cause of NTC. However, because brain edema often complicates most infective causes of NTC,[99,100] there is fear of lumbar puncture (LP) precipitating dangerous brain shifts in the acute phase. On the other hand, Kneen and colleagues[101,102] found that many children who should have had LPs did not even have a deferred procedure. CSF examination contributes to the choice of the appropriate antimicrobial agent, minimizing risk of antibiotic resistance. The UK Pediatric Accident and Emergency Research Group suggests that LP be deferred under the following situations[89]: (1) shock, (2) pulse rate more than 60 beats per minute, (3) hypertension, (4) clinical evidence of systemic meningococcal disease, (5) GCS summed score ≤ 8, (6) deteriorating GCS, (7) focal neurologic signs, (8) seizure lasting more than 10 minutes and GCS ≤ 12, and (9) clinical features to suggest increased ICP or brain shift.[89] Two of us (SSS; WTB) have reservations about situations 5, 6, 7 and 8 being absolute individual (evidence-based) contraindications. A normal CT scan does not exclude increased ICP.[3,89,95,103]

The decision to perform an LP or not, immediately on admission, is a clinical one and should always be made by an experienced clinician. If the LP is deferred, the decision should be reviewed within 4 hours (when cultures are still likely to be positive despite antibiotics), then every 12 hours, and the LP should be performed as soon as it is considered safe. The decision on timing is especially important in countries where bacterial and tuberculous meningoencephalitides still occur; early specific diagnosis and knowledge about organism sensitivity are crucial determinants of outcome. Like the United Kingdom, other countries (or regions) should develop local guidelines.

The pressure must always be measured when LP is performed. If the pressure is increased, then the minimum quantity of CSF should be removed, and mannitol (0.25–0.5 g/kg) should be administered promptly, and the patient monitored,[3,86] a practice for which there is no evidence. If LP is considered to be contraindicated then the most appropriate therapeutic agent/s should be started. CSF samples should be obtained for all potential infectious and noninfectious possibilities, ideally before antimicrobial treatment is started. The blood glucose level should be checked near simultaneously with the LP. CSF analyses are often incomplete in many who have LPs; hence, it is helpful for each hospital/region to develop guidelines for sample collection and testing. When the cause of coma is uncertain, CSF lactate should be assayed, and a sample of CSF saved to test for IEM and immune-mediated encephalitides.

Toxicology Screen

A toxicology screen (typically in the urine but a blood sample may be required in some situations) should be performed, particularly in teenagers and toddlers, if the cause of coma is not apparent from the history or examination. Toxicology screens are standardized for regions; hence, it may be necessary to discuss the suspected agents with the clinical chemist to ensure these are tested.

Tests for Inborn Errors of Metabolism

Given their complexity, in consultation with an expert in metabolic diseases, the possible tests could include: plasma ammonia (disorders of the urea cycle), venous or capillary lactate and lactate:pyruvate ratio (congenital lactic acidosis syndromes and mitochondrial cytopathies), plasma carnitine and acylcarnitine, plasma and urine amino acids and urine organic acids, CSF assay for lactate, amino acids, MRS, and specific enzyme assay or molecular genetic studies to confirm the specific cause.

Electroencephalography

An EEG is essential in most comatose patients for the following reasons: (1) EEG patterns can provide a clue to the cause (example: HSV encephalitis: **Fig. 1**), (2) a high percentage of children with coma have clinical and electrographic seizures,[1,3,86,104,105] and (3) serial EEGs can help with prognostication.[3,86,106,107] Continuous EEG monitoring is mandatory under the following situations: refractory seizures; and patients who are heavily sedated, receiving neuromuscular blocking agents, or being treated with barbiturates for increased ICP. Clinical and electrographic seizures can increase ICP.[108]

Neuroimaging

Causes determine the imaging modality and protocol that should be used for any given clinical situation. Hence, consultation with a pediatric neuroradiologist is essential to obtain the maximum diagnostic yield.

Ultrasonography of the brain

Ultrasonography (US) is a simple cost-effective screening bedside test for those with an open AF, especially neonates, but its diagnostic value in coma is limited.

Computed tomographic scanning

CT scanning is readily available on an emergent basis in many centers, and is often the first imaging modality of choice. The diagnostic considerations determine if the procedure should include bone windows, contrast enhancement, and CT angiography/venography. Radiation dose should be minimized by performing only those studies considered essential. The CT scan is ideal for showing acute hemorrhage and skull fractures.

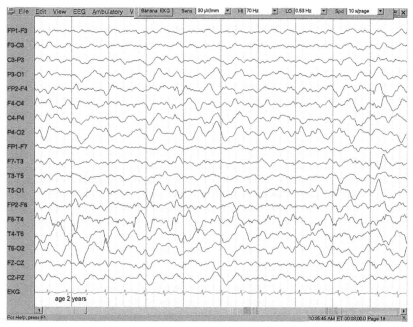

Fig. 1. Focal (regional) slowing over the right posterior temporal region with generalized increase in slow in the background, in a 2-year-old presenting with fever, left focal status epilepticus, and left hemiparesis. Final diagnosis: herpes simplex (type 1) encephalitis.

Magnetic resonance imaging

In the absence of known or suspected acute trauma, MRI is rapidly becoming the investigation of choice for several reasons: (1) there is no radiation dose; (2) depending on the techniques used, one can obtain a wide range of information; (3) MRI is especially superior for assessing change in the deeper parts of the cerebral hemispheres, brainstem, and spinal cord; (4) stroke, IEM, and ADEM can be diagnosed more readily; (5) MRA and MRV can be diagnostic in arterial or venous strokes; (6) MRI is superior for detecting traumatic lesions of different ages, as can occur with NAHI; and (7) MRI is superior for detecting diffuse axonal injury.

Figs. 2–6 illustrate the value of CT and MRI in diagnosis and management.

Magnetic resonance spectroscopy

MRS of brain and muscle can be diagnostic in some IEM, in HIE, and AESD.

Ultrasonography of the optic nerve sheath

US of the optic nerve sheath, a noninvasive procedure, may help to determine if the ICP is increased or not.[109,110] Further studies are needed to establish its role.

Evoked potentials Visual, auditory, and somatosensory evoked potentials (SEPs) may provide information about the site of dysfunction and complement assessment in those who are on large doses of depressant drugs.

Serum biomarkers Serum biomarkers such as serum neuron-specific enolase, S100B, and myelin basic protein were increased in most of those with accidental HI (AHI) and

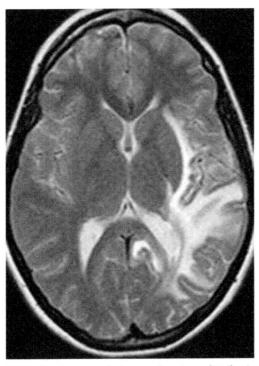

Fig. 2. T1-weighted MRI showing signal abnormality, in a distribution characteristic for herpes simplex type 1 encephalitis (different child from **Fig. 1**).

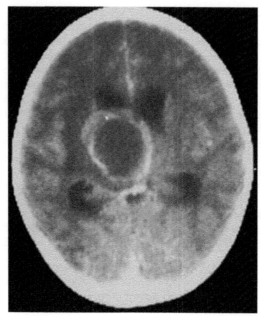

Fig. 3. CT scan showing intracranial abscess in a toddler with sickle cell anemia. Note obliteration of extra-axial space and dilatation of ventricles.

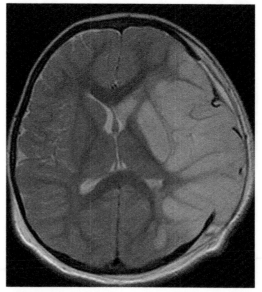

Fig. 4. T2-weighted MRI showed hemispheric infarction secondary to internal carotid occlusion in a toddler. The child survived with moderate handicap after surgical decompression.

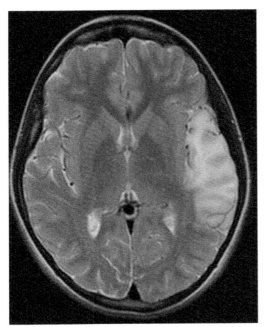

Fig. 5. T1-weighted MRI showing signal change in a nonvascular distribution, suggestive of mitochondrial encephalopathy with lactic acidosis and strokelike episodes.

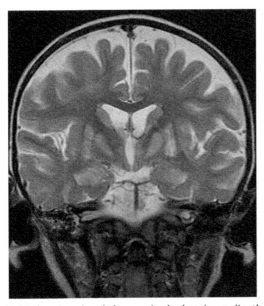

Fig. 6. T2-weighted MRI showing signal changes in the basal ganglia, thalamus, and brainstem. Child became unconscious in the course of H1N1 influenza. Radiologic findings consistent with Leigh's mitochondrial cytopathy.

NAHI, "including well appearing children in whom the diagnosis might be missed."[111] However, these biomarkers may also be increased in NTC. Hence, further studies are needed to determine their diagnostic value in NAHI, and in prognosticating outcome.

Other tests Some of the other investigations that may be needed are cardiac assessment if a cardiac disorder is suspected, skeletal survey if NAI is suspected, hematological studies in those with hemorrhagic or ischemic stroke, tests for connective tissue or autoimmune diseases, and abdominal US (or other tests as advised by the pediatrician or radiologist) for conditions such as intussusception.

The investigations of a previously well afebrile comatose child often include tests for IEM, immune-mediated encephalitides or ADEM, stroke, connective tissue/autoimmune diseases, poisoning, and NAHI in young children.

MANAGEMENT

The general (core) management of the comatose child is outlined earlier (see **Box 2**). Many aspects of management are based on best clinical practice and consensus rather than high levels of evidence.

Specific Management

Specific treatment should be directed to the (suspected) underlying cause (eg, infective, metabolic). Antimicrobial or antiviral agents are not specified; the sensitivity of organisms to, and the availability of, specific agents varies from country to country. The rapid development of resistance to therapeutic agents creates additional challenges. Treatment of HSV encephalitis and neuroborreliosis should be started promptly even if these are remote possibilities.

IV methylprednisolone[48] and IV immune globulin or plasmapheresis (first-line immunotherapy) should be considered in those with ADEM and immune-mediated encephalitides; cyclophosphamide and azathioprine may be required in some cases. Antibiotics with good penetration of the CNS are also advised when *M pneumoniae* is the responsible agent.[14,112] Treatment of an underlying tumor if present (usually teratoma), and first-line immunotherapy should be offered early for those with anti-NMDAR encephalitis; second-line immunotherapy with cyclophosphamide and rituximab may be needed in some.[45]

Thrombolysis may occasionally be indicated for arterial stroke, especially for basilar occlusion in which the evidence suggests a limit of 12 hours compared with 4.5 hours for anterior circulation stroke. Anticoagulation should be considered in arterial dissection or venous thrombosis, ideally in consultation with a pediatric hematologist.[65,113]

Seizures

Seizures occur frequently in comatose children, often heralding the onset of coma: in an older study, seizures occurred more often with intracranial infection (84%) than with other causes; repetitive seizures and SE are also common.[1,7] Several recent publications have discussed the management of recurrent seizures and SE.[89,114–121] Guidelines should be tailored for specific populations/countries/regions and clinical situations.

Children who are comatose often have a variety of systemic derangements: circulatory, hepatic, renal, and hematologic. They may be on other medications. All these elements, together with the cause of the comatose state and pharmacogenetic issues, have to be factored in the choice and dose of specific antiepileptic agents (AEDs). The complexity of the situation often requires input from a pediatric clinical pharmacist. A few key points are summarized:

1. Metabolic derangements can contribute to seizures; hence, these must be identified and treated. In turn, convulsive seizures contribute to metabolic derangement such as hypoglycemia and metabolic acidosis.
2. Although effective for acute seizures and SE, inappropriate or more than one dose of benzodiazepines can cause or contribute to respiratory depression.[122] Cardiorespiratory function is often compromised in comatose children. In this situation, the administration of benzodiazepines (especially diazepam, in the views of SSS and WTB), to those who may also have received phenobarbital, may provoke cardiorespiratory arrest.[1] We recommend their avoidance in unventilated patients with a GCS of less than 12.
3. Seizures, both clinical and electrographic, can increase ICP and provoke brain shifts.[108]
4. Nonepileptic motor phenomena, especially decerebration, should not be mistaken for seizures. Mobile phones, now with built-in cameras, are now commonplace, even in rural areas. A videoclip of the patient can be transmitted from remote areas to specialty hospitals for opinion and guidance regarding management.
5. As discussed earlier, continuous (video-) EEG monitoring is often essential in some cases.
6. The longer a seizure lasts the more difficult it is to control.
7. The intranasal (lorazepam or midazolam),[115,123] buccal (midazolam), or sublingual (sublingual lorazepam tablets where available) routes can be used if it is not possible to insert an IV line. Buccal or intranasal (midazolam) and rectal (diazepam or paraldehyde) routes are preferred in the United Kingdom (FJK). In Saskatoon (WTB, SSS), we advocate the intraosseous route for administration in this situation, because bioavailability is superior, especially if circulation is impaired.
8. A Cochrane review on the drug management of acute tonic-clonic seizures and SE in children suggested[116]: (1) IV lorazepam was at least as effective as IV diazepam and had fewer adverse effects; (2) when IV access is not available, buccal midazolam may be the treatment of choice, and superior to rectal diazepam; and (3) there is moderate evidence for the superiority of intranasal lorazepam over intramuscular paraldehyde; those treated with lorazepam were less likely to require further AEDs.
9. Clinicians should be cognizant of the potential toxicity of excipients in IV AEDs, especially for neonates and infants.[124,125]

Lorazepam is our first choice. If there is a risk of repetitive seizures, then a loading dose of phenobarbital or phenytoin (fosphenytoin is now preferred to phenytoin for children; cost and availability may be a limiting factor in some countries; phenytoin and fosphenytoin are used interchangeably in this article) should be administered. Phenytoin may not be effective in febrile seizures.[126] Phenobarbital and phenytoin have significant drug-to-drug interactions. The former is predictable in its pharmacokinetic behavior. The zero order kinetics and unpredictable half-life of phenytoin in infants makes it a challenging drug for maintenance treatment. Phenobarbital should be avoided if the child has already received two doses of a benzodiazepine and has poor cardiorespiratory status, phenytoin being preferred. It may be necessary to use both in controlled settings, if seizures persist. Their levels can guide maintenance dosing: free phenytoin levels may be important if the child is protein deficient. IV levetiracetam is a promising option for the treatment of repetitive seizures and SE because of the absence of drug interactions.[114,119] Valproic acid can be used intravenously for treating recurrent seizures/SE; however, it should be avoided if an IEM is suspected, when there is evidence of hepatic or hematologic dysfunction, and if the child is already on other drugs (polytherapy increases the risk of hepatotoxicity).

If seizures are refractory to initial management with 2 or 3 conventional agents (benzodiazepine + phenytoin or fosphenytoin or phenobarbital or levetiracetam), then further steps include: (1) confirm the epileptic nature of the events with an EEG; continuous EEG monitoring may now become necessary; (2) exclude/investigate for an underlying metabolic cause, including IEM; perform or repeat MRI scan if not already done so; MR study must be tailored to the possible differential diagnoses being entertained; (3) in young children, administer pyridoxine (ideally pyridoxal phosphate) 100 mg intravenously: response occurs within 15 minutes in most of those with an IE of pyridoxine metabolism; (4) in neonates and young infants, consider possibility of biotinidase deficiency and folinic acid responsive seizures: the latter often respond to pyridoxine.

Refractory seizures may require management with infusion of midazolam or pentobarbital. Faulty compliance in a known epileptic patient, intracranial infections, certain IEM, and abnormalities of brain development are the usual causes of refractory seizures and SE.

INTRACRANIAL PRESSURE
General

Relatively young age and genetic predisposition may be factors that determine the occurrence and severity of brain edema in traumatic and NTC. Infants and young children may experience significant brain swelling secondary to even minor head injury compared with adults,[127,128] although precise comparisons are not possible. Severe potentially fatal brain swelling has been reported after apparently trivial head injury in those who have the S218L mutation in the CACNA1A gene, which is also associated with familial hemiplegic migraine.[129,130]

ICP is increased because of brain edema in children not only after AHI or NAHI but also in those suffering NTC from a variety of causes that include intracranial infection, hepatic encephalopathy, diabetic ketoacidosis, stroke, and IEM.[3,40,86,99,100,131–137] Subdural effusions and hydrocephalus can complicate bacterial (including tubercular) and other meningoencephalitides, and contribute to increased ICP, as can intracranial hematoma and hydrocephalus in those with NAHI. We are not aware of any evidenced-based studies that have clarified the role for ICP monitoring or the treatment of increased ICP in NTC in children,[138] a factor that may explain the considerable intercenter and intracenter variability in practice, at least earlier in this decade.[139]

However, there are compelling clinical reasons to monitor ICP in selected children with NTC: (1) the high risk and incidence of brain edema in these situations, as outlined earlier; (2) the consequent compromise of cerebral blood flow and (CPP); and (3) risk of herniation, all of which increase the odds of death and severity of handicap.

Recently, we suggested that the general guidelines for the management of increased ICP after severe traumatic brain injury (TBI) in children[103] be adapted for NTC.[3]

ICP should be monitored in the following situations: (1) summed GCS of less than 8, (2) those who show clinical or radiologic features of brain swelling/shifts even if the summed GCS is greater than 8; (3) those at risk for increased ICP, and (4) those heavily sedated or treated with neuromuscular blocking agents, in whom reliable clinical assessment is not possible.

The presence of an open AF or sutures does not preclude the development of increased ICP, and a normal CT scan does not exclude clinically significant increased ICP.

The management of increased ICP has been discussed recently,[3,136,137,140] and there is a relative uniformity of approach. Some of the specific methods do not apply to neonates.

Intracranial Pressure and Cerebral Perfusion Pressure

ICP varies with age. ICP of 20 mm Hg is the upper threshold (regardless of age) for considering treatment. However, treatment should be started at lower pressures if there is evidence of brain shift. In TBI, Chambers and colleagues[141] suggested that CPPs of 53, 63, and 66 mm Hg should be the minimum to aim for in those aged 2 to 6 years, 7 to 10 years, and 11 to 16 years, respectively. There is little information on the effective CPP in those less than 2 years of age. The range is probably between 30 and 40 mm Hg in preterm infants, around 40 mm Hg in the term newborn, increasing to 53 mm Hg in the 2-year-old.[3] Maintenance of an adequate CPP may improve outcome.[142] Transcutaneous and transcranial near-infrared spectroscopy are being evaluated to assess ICP and CPP noninvasively; it may also be possible to monitor brain tissue oxygenation, oxygen delivery, and lactate/pyruvate to assess for brain ischemia.[140]

How to Measure Intracranial Pressure

A ventricular catheter connected to an external strain gauge is the most accurate, low-cost, reliable method of monitoring ICP; it also allows for therapeutic CSF drainage.[3,103] Other methods include the use of epidural, subdural and intraparenchymal devices. The Camino intraparenchymal device (Camino Laboratories, San Diego, CA, USA) is the first choice in the United Kingdom, a ventricular catheter being used if the ICP is difficult to manage.

Procedures to Treat Increased Intracranial Pressure

The core principles of management have not changed since Lundberg discussed ICP monitoring and increased ICP 50 years ago.[143] Opinions regarding the relative roles for mannitol, hypertonic saline (HS), and decompression craniectomy (DC) have swung over the past 5 to 6 decades. The information that follows has been summarized from several recent sources.[3,103,136,137,140] A critically ill comatose child, especially one with seizures, increased ICP, or multisystem derangement is best managed by a multidisciplinary team in a pediatric intensive care unit. The management of increased ICP in NTC is summarized in flow diagrams (**Figs. 7** and **8**). The distinction between first-tier and second-tier therapy is artificial, and one may have to proceed to second-tier therapy emergently in some cases.

General steps

General steps include treating shock and maintaining blood pressure but avoiding overhydration (hence, monitoring CPP is important). It may be necessary to give fluid boluses and inotropic agents to maintain age-appropriate CPPs[3,142]; head end of the bed elevated to 30°; head in the midline; avoid mechanical obstruction to venous outflow from the head (tight cervical collars are major culprits); minimize unnecessary stimulation. The Pao_2 should be maintained at 100 mm Hg.

Body temperature

Hyperthermia has several deleterious effects,[3] and a target core body temperature of 32°C to 33°C for those with severe or refractory ICP has been suggested.[3] Mild hypothermia (33.5°C–35°C) may improve outcome in acute childhood encephalopathies and encephalitis if instituted within 12 hours but worsen outcome if attempted later[144]; randomized control trials are required.

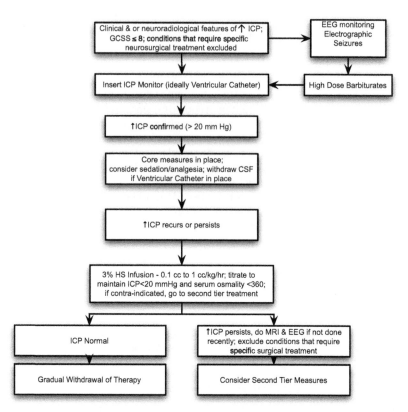

Fig. 7. First-tier treatment of increased intracranial pressure (ICP) in nontraumatic coma (NTC). CSF, cerebrospinal fluid; EEG, electroencephalogram; GCSS, Glasgow coma summed score; HS, hypertonic saline; MRI, magnetic resonance imaging. Note: GCSS often of limited value (see page 11).

Sedation and neuromuscular blockade

Sedation and neuromuscular blockade should be used judiciously. Mechanical ventilation can be facilitated and episodes of potentially dangerous ICP increases minimized. Neuromuscular blockade prevents the shivering that occurs with hypothermia. We do not advocate infusion of propofol. Midazolam can be used for its sedative and antiepileptic effects. Continuous EEG monitoring is mandatory if a child is heavily sedated or paralyzed.

Hyperventilation

The $Paco_2$ should be maintained around 35 mm Hg. However, vigorous hyperventilation may be necessary for a brief period for acute increases of ICP or occurrence of brain shift. $Paco_2$ should not be allowed to decrease less than 30 mm Hg. $Paco_2$ values may have to be corrected for body temperature and altitude.[145]

Ventricular catheter drainage

If a ventricular catheter is used for monitoring, then drainage of CSF is the simplest, quickest, and safest method for reducing ICP promptly.

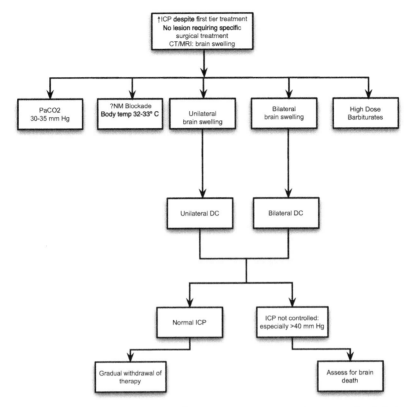

Fig. 8. Second-tier treatment of increased ICP in NTC. CT, computed tomography; DC, decompression craniectomy; EEG, electroencephalogram; ICP, intracranial pressure; MRI, magnetic resonance imaging; NM blockade, neuromuscular blockade; NTC, nontraumatic coma.

Hyperosmolar therapy

A systematic review supported the use of oral glycerol in acute bacterial meningitis and IV HS (3% being the commonest strength used) over mannitol, in traumatic and NTC; improvements in ICP and CPP were sustained for longer when HS was given as an infusion.[133] Hematologic derangements and the osmotic demyelinating syndrome are potential risks of treatment with HS.[146] Both HS and mannitol can be associated with rebound. HS should not be used if there is hypernatremia. Mannitol should be avoided if the child is dehydrated or hypotensive. Both should be avoided in hyperosmolar states; in that case barbiturate coma, hypothermia, and DC are alternatives.

Furosemide

Furosemide may be of benefit in those who are overhydrated or in cardiac failure.

Barbiturates

High-dose barbiturates (pentobarbital or thiopental) may be considered if frequent doses or continuous infusion of hyperosmolar agents are required, if side effects complicate their use, or hypothermia is ineffective. Such barbiturates are often the treatment of choice if intractable seizures also occur. The infusion has to be titrated to the ICP and CPP, under continuous EEG monitoring. It is not always necessary to aim for burst suppression on the EEG if objectives of treatment are achieved at lower doses. The hypotensive effects of barbiturates may limit dosing and duration of treatment. Hence, for the management of increased ICP, IV barbiturates are often used short-term while exploring options such as hypothermia or DC. The use of pentobarbital or thiopental often confounds and delays assessment for brain death.

Steroids

Steroids may have a role in some forms of bacterial meningoencephalitis, immune-mediated encephalitides, and ADEM. They do not have a specific role in ICP management.

Decompression craniectomy

DC should be considered relatively early in a potentially salvageable patient who has refractory increased ICP from NTC or NAHI.[3,64,147,148]

Withdrawal of treatment of increased intracranial pressure

We suggest that treatment of increased ICP be withdrawn gradually (1) when the ICP has been less than 20 mm Hg for 24 hours and (2) is not increased by suctioning, handling, or changes of position.[3] Conversely, failure to control ICP less than 40 mm Hg even after second-tier therapy is a grave sign and associated with poor outcome, particularly if the CPP cannot be maintained greater than 30 mm Hg; a decision to withdraw such care after an adequate trial period may have to be made.

Nutritional state

There is increased recognition of the importance of nutritional support, maintaining normal plasma proteins, and treating anemia in comatose children. A pediatric nutritionist should ideally be involved.

OUTCOME

Clinical variables are generally scaled from best (normal) to worst, and when used in a composite fashion, together with investigative data, can guide prognostication (see **Table 2** for outcome categories).[6,7,28,42,87,97,104,149] Some key points (not necessarily evidenced-based) are listed:

1. Prognostication (like diagnosis of cause) is generally based on statistical probabilities rather than certainties. The odds of being incorrect are greater when one attempts to prognosticate early in the patient's comatose state. Because substantial improvement can occur over the first year, earlier predictions about quality of outcome can only be tentative. Conversely, even after a 2-year follow-up, adverse outcomes like attention deficit, learning dysfunction, behavior dysfunction, and late-onset seizures cannot be predicted in young children. Factors such as adequate stimulation and access to rehabilitative services also influence outcome.
2. The mortality and morbidity are higher in infants and young children but it is uncertain if age is independent of cause and severity of illness as a predictor.
3. Adverse socioeconomic factors are associated with a poor outcome.[31,150] The reasons for the association are likely to be multifactorial, timely access to pediatric care being one of them.
4. Anemia and malnutrition, which often associate with poor socioeconomic status, are associated with a poor prognosis (death, deficits) from infective causes of coma, including malaria.[31,151]

Table 2
Outcome categories

Outcome Groups	Neurologic Status	Developmental Status/Behavior
1. Normal	Normal Seizures if present well (100%) controlled	Normal
2. Mild handicap	Minimal alterations of tone Isolated cranial nerve palsy Minimal weakness (grade 4) Minimal ataxia Seizures if present fairly well (99%–75%) controlled	Mild handicap
3. Moderate handicap	Moderate weakness (grade 3) Multiple cranial nerve palsies Moderate ataxia Seizures if present moderately (74%–50%) controlled	Moderate handicap
4. Severe handicap	Severe weakness (>grade 3) or ataxia Feeding/swallowing difficulties Uncontrolled seizures	Severe handicap (MCS)
5. Profound handicap	Profound motor handicap Uncontrolled seizures	Vegetative (UWS)
6. Dead		

Abbreviations: MCS, minimally conscious state; UWS, unresponsive wakefulness syndrome.
From Seshia SS, Johnston B, Kasian G. Non-traumatic coma in childhood: clinical variables in prediction of outcome. Dev Med Child Neurol 1983;25(4):493–501 (update of table 1); with permission from MacKeith Press gratefully acknowledged.

5. The more critically ill a child (based on physiologic indices, abnormalities of respiration, circulation, and multiorgan dysfunction), the greater the odds of death or handicap.
6. Cause has a strong statistical association with outcome, regardless of severity of clinical findings. However, outcome is influenced by promptness and appropriateness of treatment. Outcome is generally favorable in those with toxic or simple metabolic encephalopathies. Outcome in IEM is dependent on the specific cause. Diabetic coma can be associated with high mortality if treatment is delayed or inappropriate.[68] HIE usually has a poor prognosis, but HIE secondary to hypothermic exposure or immersion in cold water can have a favorable outcome. The risk of death or significant handicap is still high with bacterial (including TB) meningitis, cerebral malaria, JE, and perhaps *M pneumoniae* encephalitis.[14,31,34,42,104,152,153]
7. In the absence of depressant drugs several neurologic variables have predictive value. These variables include the depth and duration of coma, extraocular muscles, pupillary reactions, motor responses, central control of temperature, blood pressure, and respiration. The odds of a good outcome are greater when the responses are normal and worsen with increasing abnormality.
8. Multifocal /myoclonic seizures and SE increase the odds of an adverse outcome.
9. EEG patterns, especially on serial records, can be helpful in prognostication provided the effects of metabolic derangement, hypothermia, and depressant drugs can be excluded. Burst suppression, α-like activity, very low background

amplitude for age, unresponsive background, and electrocerebral silence are clearly of adverse significance.[104,106,107]

10. The presence or absence of SEPs has predictive value. However, Carrai and colleagues[154] caution against using SEPs to determine withdrawal of treatment; studies comparing the predictive role of SEPs with that of clinical variables are needed.

11. ICP greater than 40 mm Hg refractory to second-tier treatment is an adverse sign, especially if the CPP has been allowed to decrease less than 30 mm Hg.

12. CT and MRI scans, MRS, near-infrared spectroscopy, and serum biomarkers have all been considered (in various articles) to provide information of prognostic value, but their specific contribution to prognostication (over and above that of clinical variables) has not been studied.

DISORDERS OF AWARENESS

Children emerging from coma may evolve through states of altered awareness, remain in them indefinitely, or recover awareness to varying degrees, usually based on underlying cause. Children in the vegetative state (VS; the term unresponsive wakefulness syndrome [UWS], has been proposed as a substitute for VS[155]) show sleep-wake cycles but are unaware. The emergence of this state within a few days of the onset of NTC suggests a high probability of clinically significant long-term disability.[156,157] The prefix persistent is discouraged. Awareness may return even after 19 months in those initially vegetative after HIE, although the probability of continuing severe disability remains high.[158] Children in the minimally conscious state (MCS) are minimally aware, have sleep-wake cycles, and experience discomfort but are otherwise severely handicapped.[159] The level of awareness is substantially greater in the locked-in syndrome and may even be normal, but motor function is essentially absent and the patient may be able to communicate only with slight eye movements.[87] Neuropsychological testing or functional imaging may be needed to determine if the child is in a VS (UWS), MCS, or locked-in syndrome.[155] Drugs like amantidine may improve awareness in these situations.[160] Zolpidem likely has no effect.[161]

BRAIN DEATH

Age-dependent criteria for brain death (brain arrest) have been updated in some countries, but there is need for global consensus.[162–164] Joffe and colleagues[165] remind us that even with these criteria, brain death especially in infants is not always equivalent to death.

REHABILITATION

Children who have recovered from coma should be rehabilitated and followed up regularly until they are into their school years and referred for therapy, depending on the nature of their deficits. A multidisciplinary team should ideally be involved from the outset.

PREVENTION AND SUMMARY

Many infective causes of NTC are preventable with vaccines,[153] and controlled or prevented by eliminating malnutrition/anemia. Other essential public health measures include safe water supply, sewage disposal, mosquito control, education on personal hygiene, and timely access to child health care, both preventive and illness related. Education may also minimize poisoning and NAHI, as it has the incidence of pediatric head injuries in Western countries. Other steps include being aware of and identifying populations at high risk for IEM, strokes, and certain encephalopathies. The systematic clinical approach proposed by Plum and Posner remains the cornerstone of diagnosis and management.

NOTE

Readers are advised to consult current pediatric drug formulary and dosage guidelines for their region. We have not addressed history taking in the comatose child. It is an art that is best learnt at the bedside.

ACKNOWLEDGMENTS

We thank Gregg Parchomchuk for the flow diagrams in **Figs. 7** and **8**, Molly Seshia for reviewing the manuscript, and Bryan Young for helpful suggestions. SSS is grateful to the Department of Pediatrics and the Faculty of Medicine, University of Saskatchewan, for continuing support. FJK was funded by the Wellcome Trust.

REFERENCES

1. Seshia SS, Seshia MM, Sachdeva RK. Coma in childhood. Dev Med Child Neurol 1977;19(5):614–28.
2. Plum F, Posner JB. The diagnosis of stupor and coma. Philadelphia: F.A. Davis; 1966. 1972, 1980. Note: all three editions have been cited for their seminal contributions.
3. Seshia SS, Bingham WT, Griebel RW. Coma in childhood. Handb Clin Neurol 2008;90:329–50.
4. Haworth JC, Dilling LA, Seargeant LE. Increased prevalence of hereditary metabolic diseases among native Indians in Manitoba and northwestern Ontario. CMAJ 1991;145(2):123–9.
5. Prasad C, Johnson JP, Bonnefont JP, et al. Hepatic carnitine palmitoyl transferase 1 (CPT1 A) deficiency in North American Hutterites (Canadian and American): evidence for a founder effect and results of a pilot study on a DNA-based newborn screening program. Mol Genet Metab 2001;73(1):55–63.
6. Wong CP, Forsyth RJ, Kelly TP, et al. Incidence, aetiology, and outcome of non-traumatic coma: a population based study. Arch Dis Child 2001;84(3): 193–9.
7. Seshia SS, Johnston B, Kasian G. Non-traumatic coma in childhood: clinical variables in prediction of outcome. Dev Med Child Neurol 1983;25(4):493–501.
8. Balaka B, Balogou K, Bakonde B, et al. Childhood non-traumatic coma in the University of Lome. Arch Pediatr 2005;12(4):475–6.
9. Khodapanahandeh F, Najarkalayee NG. Etiology and outcome of non-traumatic coma in children admitted to pediatric intensive care unit. Iran J Pediatr 2009; 19(4):393–8.
10. Kobayashi K, Ouchida M, Okumura A, et al. Genetic seizure susceptibility underlying acute encephalopathies in childhood. Epilepsy Res 2010;91(2/3):143–52.
11. Chen Y, Mizuguchi H, Yao D, et al. Thermolabile phenotype of carnitine palmitoyltransferase II variations as a predisposing factor for influenza-associated encephalopathy. FEBS Lett 2005;579(10):2040–4.
12. Kubota M, Chida J, Hoshino H, et al. Thermolabile CPT II variants and low blood ATP levels are closely related to severity of acute encephalopathy in Japanese children. Brain Dev 2011. [EPub ahead of print]. PMID: 21277129.
13. Shinohara M, Saitoh M, Takanashi J, et al. Carnitine palmitoyl transferase II polymorphism is associated with multiple syndromes of acute encephalopathy with various infectious diseases. Brain Dev 2011;33(6):512–7.
14. Bitnun A, Ford-Jones E, Blaser S, et al. *Mycoplasma pneumoniae* ecephalitis. Semin Pediatr Infect Dis 2003;14(2):96–107.

15. Domenech C, Leveque N, Lina B, et al. Role of *Mycoplasma pneumoniae* in pediatric encephalitis. Eur J Clin Microbiol Infect Dis 2009;28(1):91–4.
16. Christie LJ, Honarmand S, Talkington DF, et al. Pediatric encephalitis: what is the role of *Mycoplasma pneumoniae*? Pediatrics 2007;120(2):305–13.
17. Christie LJ, Loeffler AM, Honarmand S, et al. Diagnostic challenges of central nervous system tuberculosis. Emerg Infect Dis 2008;14(9):1473–5.
18. Jmor F, Emsley HC, Fischer M, et al. The incidence of acute encephalitis syndrome in Western industrialised and tropical countries. Virol J 2008;5:134.
19. Guyon G, Ladet S, Maestracci M, et al. West Nile virus infections in children. Arch Pediatr 2009;16(Suppl 2):S85–8.
20. Lindsey NP, Hayes EB, Staples JE, et al. West Nile virus disease in children, United States, 1999–2007. Pediatrics 2009;123(6):e1084–9.
21. Das T, Jaffar-Bandjee MC, Hoarau JJ, et al. Chikungunya fever: CNS infection and pathologies of a re-emerging arbovirus. Prog Neurobiol 2010;91(2):121–9.
22. Jaffar-Bandjee MC, Ramful D, Gauzere BA, et al. Emergence and clinical insights into the pathology of Chikungunya virus infection. Expert Rev Anti Infect Ther 2010;8(9):987–96.
23. Centers for Disease Control and Prevention (CDC). Neurologic complications associated with novel influenza A (H1N1) virus infection in children–Dallas, Texas, May 2009. MMWR Morb Mortal Wkly Rep 2009;58(28):773–8.
24. Ekstrand JJ, Herbener A, Rawlings J, et al. Heightened neurologic complications in children with pandemic H1N1 influenza. Ann Neurol 2010;68(5):762–6.
25. Walter ND, Grant GB, Bandy U, et al. Community outbreak of *Mycoplasma pneumoniae* infection: school-based cluster of neurologic disease associated with household transmission of respiratory illness. J Infect Dis 2008;198(9):1365–74.
26. Mailles A, Stahl JP, Steering Committee and Investigators Group. Infectious encephalitis in France in 2007: a national prospective study. Clin Infect Dis 2009;49(12):1838–47.
27. Granerod J, Ambrose HE, Davies NW, et al. Causes of encephalitis and differences in their clinical presentations in England: a multicentre, population-based prospective study. Lancet Infect Dis 2010;10(12):835–44.
28. Bansal A, Singhi SC, Singhi PD, et al. Non traumatic coma. Indian J Pediatr 2005;72(6):467–73.
29. Ali AM, Al-Abdulgader A, Kamal HK, et al. Traumatic and non-traumatic coma in children in the referral hospital, Al-Hasa, Saudi Arabia. East Mediterr Health J 2007;13(3):608–14.
30. Fouad H, Haron M, Halawa EF, et al. Nontraumatic coma in a tertiary pediatric emergency department in Egypt: etiology and outcome. J Child Neurol 2011; 26(2):136–41.
31. Bondi FS. Childhood coma in Ibadan. Relationship to socio-economic factors. Trop Geogr Med 1991;43(3):288–92.
32. Sofiah A, Hussain IH. Childhood non-traumatic coma in Kuala Lumpur, Malaysia. Ann Trop Paediatr 1997;17(4):327–31.
33. Ibekwe RC, Ibekwe MU, Onwe OE, et al. Non-traumatic childhood coma in Ebonyi State University Teaching Hospital, Abakaliki, South Eastern Nigeria. Niger J Clin Pract 2011;14(1):43–6.
34. Baruah HC, Biswas D, Patgiri D, et al. Clinical outcome and neurological sequelae in serologically confirmed cases of Japanese encephalitis patients in Assam, India. Indian Pediatr 2002;39(12):1143–8.
35. Bejon P, Berkley JA, Mwangi T, et al. Defining childhood severe falciparum malaria for intervention studies. PLoS Med 2007;4(8):e251.

36. Bell DJ, Molyneux ME. Treatment of childhood *Plasmodium falciparum* malaria: current challenges. Expert Rev Anti Infect Ther 2007;5(1):141–52.
37. Crawley J, Smith S, Kirkham F, et al. Seizures and status epilepticus in childhood cerebral malaria. QJM 1996;89(8):591–7.
38. Idro R. Severe anaemia in childhood cerebral malaria is associated with profound coma. Afr Health Sci 2003;3(1):15–8.
39. Idro R, Marsh K, John CC, et al. Cerebral malaria: mechanisms of brain injury and strategies for improved neurocognitive outcome. Pediatr Res 2010;68(4):267–74.
40. Solomon T, Dung NM, Kneen R, et al. Seizures and raised intracranial pressure in Vietnamese patients with Japanese encephalitis. Brain 2002;125(Pt 5):1084–93.
41. Sharma S, Kochar GS, Sankhyan N, et al. Approach to the child with coma. Indian J Pediatr 2010;77(11):1279–87.
42. Garg RK. Tuberculous meningitis. Acta Neurol Scand 2010;122(2):75–90.
43. Khan WA, Dhar U, Salam MA, et al. Central nervous system manifestations of childhood shigellosis: prevalence, risk factors, and outcome. Pediatrics 1999; 103(2):E18.
44. Gable MS, Gavali S, Radner A, et al. Anti-NMDA receptor encephalitis: report of ten cases and comparison with viral encephalitis. Eur J Clin Microbiol Infect Dis 2009;28(12):1421–9.
45. Dalmau J, Lancaster E, Martinez-Hernandez E, et al. Clinical experience and laboratory investigations in patients with anti-NMDAR encephalitis. Lancet Neurol 2011;10(1):63–74.
46. Sakuma H, Awaya Y, Shiomi M, et al. Acute encephalitis with refractory, repetitive partial seizures (AERRPS): a peculiar form of childhood encephalitis. Acta Neurol Scand 2010;121(4):251–6.
47. Thebaud B, Husson B, Navelet Y, et al. Haemorrhagic shock and encephalopathy syndrome: neurological course and predictors of outcome. Intensive Care Med 1999;25(3):293–9.
48. Singhi PD, Ray M, Singhi S, et al. Acute disseminated encephalomyelitis in North Indian children: clinical profile and follow-up. J Child Neurol 2006; 21(10):851–7.
49. Sztajnbok J, Lignani L Jr, Bresolin AU, et al. Acute disseminated encephalomyelitis: an unusual cause of encephalitic syndrome in childhood. Pediatr Emerg Care 1998;14(1):36–8.
50. Tenembaum S, Chamoles N, Fejerman N. Acute disseminated encephalomyelitis: a long-term follow-up study of 84 pediatric patients. Neurology 2002; 59(8):1224–31.
51. Dale RC, de Sousa C, Chong WK, et al. Acute disseminated encephalomyelitis, multiphasic disseminated encephalomyelitis and multiple sclerosis in children. Brain 2000;123(Pt 12):2407–22.
52. Bassuk AG, Burrowes DM, McRae W. Acute necrotizing encephalopathy of childhood with radiographic progression over 10 hours. Neurology 2003; 60(9):1552–3.
53. Huang SM, Chen CC, Chiu PC, et al. Acute necrotizing encephalopathy of childhood associated with influenza type B virus infection in a 3-year-old girl. J Child Neurol 2004;19(1):64–7.
54. Mizuguchi M, Abe J, Mikkaichi K, et al. Acute necrotising encephalopathy of childhood: a new syndrome presenting with multifocal, symmetric brain lesions. J Neurol Neurosurg Psychiatry 1995;58(5):555–61.
55. Mizuguchi M. Acute necrotizing encephalopathy of childhood: a novel form of acute encephalopathy prevalent in Japan and Taiwan. Brain Dev 1997;19(2):81–92.

56. Neilson DE, Adams MD, Orr CM, et al. Infection-triggered familial or recurrent cases of acute necrotizing encephalopathy caused by mutations in a component of the nuclear pore, RANBP2. Am J Hum Genet 2009;84(1):44–51.

57. Nabbout R, Mazzuca M, Hubert P, et al. Efficacy of ketogenic diet in severe refractory status epilepticus initiating fever induced refractory epileptic encephalopathy in school age children (FIRES). Epilepsia 2010;51(10):2033–7.

58. Nabbout R, Vezzani A, Dulac O, et al. Acute encephalopathy with inflammation-mediated status epilepticus. Lancet Neurol 2011;10(1):99–108.

59. Specchio N, Fusco L, Claps D, et al. Epileptic encephalopathy in children possibly related to immune-mediated pathogenesis. Brain Dev 2010;32(1): 51–6.

60. Mikaeloff Y, Jambaque I, Hertz-Pannier L, et al. Devastating epileptic encephalopathy in school-aged children (DESC): a pseudo encephalitis. Epilepsy Res 2006;69(1):67–79.

61. van Baalen A, Hausler M, Boor R, et al. Febrile infection-related epilepsy syndrome (FIRES): a nonencephalitic encephalopathy in childhood. Epilepsia 2010;51(7):1323–8.

62. Takanashi J. Two newly proposed infectious encephalitis/encephalopathy syndromes. Brain Dev 2009;31(7):521–8.

63. Sebire G, Tabarki B, Saunders DE, et al. Cerebral venous sinus thrombosis in children: risk factors, presentation, diagnosis and outcome. Brain 2005;128(Pt 3): 477–89.

64. Smith SE, Kirkham FJ, Deveber G, et al. Outcome following decompressive craniectomy for malignant middle cerebral artery infarction in children. Dev Med Child Neurol 2011;53(1):29–33.

65. Roach ES, Golomb MR, Adams R, et al. Management of stroke in infants and children: a scientific statement from a Special Writing Group of the American Heart Association Stroke Council and the Council on Cardiovascular Disease in the Young. Stroke 2008;39(9):2644–91.

66. Jordan LC, Johnston SC, Wu YW, et al. The importance of cerebral aneurysms in childhood hemorrhagic stroke: a population-based study. Stroke 2009;40(2): 400–5.

67. Ishikura K, Hamasaki Y, Sakai T, et al. Posterior reversible encephalopathy syndrome in children with kidney diseases. Pediatr Nephrol 2011. [Epub ahead of print].

68. Cochran JB, Walters S, Losek JD. Pediatric hyperglycemic hyperosmolar syndrome: diagnostic difficulties and high mortality rate. Am J Emerg Med 2006;24(3):297–301.

69. Fourtner SH, Weinzimer SA, Levitt Katz LE. Hyperglycemic hyperosmolar nonketotic syndrome in children with type 2 diabetes*. Pediatr Diabetes 2005; 6(3):129–35.

70. Rother KI, Schwenk WF 2nd. An unusual case of the nonketotic hyperglycemic syndrome during childhood. Mayo Clin Proc 1995;70(1):62–5.

71. Singhi SC. Hyperglycemic hyperosmolar state and type 2 diabetes mellitus: yet another danger of childhood obesity. Pediatr Crit Care Med 2005;6(1):86–7.

72. Venkatraman R, Singhi SC. Hyperglycemic hyperosmolar nonketotic syndrome. Indian J Pediatr 2006;73(1):55–60.

73. Fogli A, Wong K, Eymard-Pierre E, et al. Cree leukoencephalopathy and CACH/VWM disease are allelic at the EIF2B5 locus. Ann Neurol 2002;52(4):506–10.

74. Stephenson DJ, Bezman L, Raymond GV. Acute presentation of childhood adrenoleukodystrophy. Neuropediatrics 2000;31(6):293–7.

75. van der Knaap MS, Pronk JC, Scheper GC. Vanishing white matter disease. Lancet Neurol 2006;5(5):413–23.

76. Sofer S, Tal A, Shahak E. Carbamate and organophosphate poisoning in early childhood. Pediatr Emerg Care 1989;5(4):222–5.

77. Verhulst L, Waggie Z, Hatherill M, et al. Presentation and outcome of severe anti-cholinesterase insecticide poisoning. Arch Dis Child 2002;86(5):352–5.

78. Budhathoki S, Poudel P, Shah D, et al. Clinical profile and outcome of children presenting with poisoning or intoxication: a hospital based study. Nepal Med Coll J 2009;11(3):170–5.

79. Glatstein M, Finkelstein Y, Scolnik D. Accidental methadone ingestion in an infant: case report and review of the literature. Pediatr Emerg Care 2009;25(2):109–11.

80. Zamani N, Sanaei-Zadeh H, Mostafazadeh B. Hallmarks of opium poisoning in infants and toddlers. Trop Doct 2010;40(4):220–2.

81. Olgun H, Yildirim ZK, Karacan M, et al. Clinical, electrocardiographic, and laboratory findings in children with amitriptyline intoxication. Pediatr Emerg Care 2009;25(3):170–3.

82. Shaoul R, Gazit A, Weller B, et al. Neurological manifestations of an acute abdomen in children. Pediatr Emerg Care 2005;21(9):594–7.

83. Kirkham FJ. Recognition and prevention of neurological complications in pediatric cardiac surgery. Pediatr Cardiol 1998;19(4):331–45.

84. Domi T, Edgell DS, McCrindle BW, et al. Frequency, predictors, and neurologic outcomes of vaso-occlusive strokes associated with cardiac surgery in children. Pediatrics 2008;122(6):1292–8.

85. Minns RA, Brown JK. Neurological perspectives of non-accidental head injury and whiplash/shaken baby syndrome: an overview. In: Minns RA, Brown JK, editors. Shaking and other non-accidental head injuries in children. London: MacKeith Press; 2005. p. 1–105.

86. Kirkham FJ. Non-traumatic coma in children. Arch Dis Child 2001;85(4):303–12.

87. Michelson DJ, Ashwal S. Evaluation of coma and brain death. Semin Pediatr Neurol 2004;11(2):105–18.

88. Wagner BP. The comatose child. Ther Umsch 2005;62(8):519–24.

89. The Paediatric Accident and Emergency Research Group. The management of a child (aged 0–18 years) with a decreased conscious level. Review date January 2008. Available at: http://www.nottingham.ac.uk/paediatric-guideline. Accessed May 25, 2011.

90. Brown JK, Ingram TT, Seshia SS. Patterns of decerebration in infants and children: defects in homeostasis and sequelae. J Neurol Neurosurg Psychiatry 1973;36(3):431–44.

91. Dine MS, McGovern ME. Intentional poisoning of children–an overlooked category of child abuse: report of seven cases and review of the literature. Pediatrics 1982;70(1):32–5.

92. Teasdale G, Jennett B. Assessment of coma and impaired consciousness. A practical scale. Lancet 1974;2(7872):81–4.

93. Yager JY, Johnston B, Seshia SS. Coma scales in pediatric practice. Am J Dis Child 1990;144(10):1088–91.

94. Kirkham FJ, Newton CR, Whitehouse W. Paediatric coma scales. Dev Med Child Neurol 2008;50(4):267–74.

95. Tatman A, Warren A, Williams A, et al. Development of a modified paediatric coma scale in intensive care clinical practice. Arch Dis Child 1997;77(6):519–21.

96. Teasdale G, Jennett B, Murray L, et al. Glasgow coma scale: to sum or not to sum. Lancet 1983;2(8351):678.

97. Seshia SS, Yager JY, Johnston B, et al. Inter-observer agreement in assessing comatose children. Can J Neurol Sci 1991;18(4):472–5.

98. Bowker R, Green A, Bonham JR. Guidelines for the investigation and management of a reduced level of consciousness in children: implications for clinical biochemistry laboratories. Ann Clin Biochem 2007;44(Pt 6): 506–11.

99. Minns RA, Engleman HM, Stirling H. Cerebrospinal fluid pressure in pyogenic meningitis. Arch Dis Child 1989;64(6):814–20.

100. Rebaud P, Berthier JC, Hartemann E, et al. Intracranial pressure in childhood central nervous system infections. Intensive Care Med 1988;14(5):522–5.

101. Kneen R, Solomon T, Appleton R. The role of lumbar puncture in children with suspected central nervous system infection. BMC Pediatr 2002;2:8.

102. Kneen R, Solomon T, Appleton R. The role of lumbar puncture in suspected CNS infection–a disappearing skill? Arch Dis Child 2002;87(3):181–3.

103. Society of Critical Medicine. The World Federation of Pediatric Intensive and Critical Care Societies and the Paediatric Intensive Care Society UK. Guidelines for the acute medical management of severe traumatic brain injury in infants, children, and adolescents. Pediatr Crit Care Med 2003;4(Suppl 3): S1–75.

104. Johnston B, Seshia SS. Prediction of outcome in non-traumatic coma in childhood. Acta Neurol Scand 1984;69(6):417–27.

105. Saengpattrachai M, Sharma R, Hunjan A, et al. Nonconvulsive seizures in the pediatric intensive care unit: etiology, EEG, and brain imaging findings. Epilepsia 2006;47(9):1510–8.

106. Singhi PD, Bansal A, Ramesh S, et al. Predictive value of electroencephalography and computed tomography in childhood non-traumatic coma. Indian J Pediatr 2005;72(6):475–9.

107. Tasker RC, Boyd S, Harden A, et al. Monitoring in non-traumatic coma. Part II: electroencephalography. Arch Dis Child 1988;63(8):895–9.

108. Minns RA, Brown JK. Intracranial pressure changes associated with childhood seizures. Dev Med Child Neurol 1978;20(5):561–9.

109. Geeraerts T, Merceron S, Benhamou D, et al. Non-invasive assessment of intracranial pressure using ocular sonography in neurocritical care patients. Intensive Care Med 2008;34(11):2062–7.

110. Soldatos T, Chatzimichail K, Papathanasiou M, et al. Optic nerve sonography: a new window for the non-invasive evaluation of intracranial pressure in brain injury. Emerg Med J 2009;26(9):630–4.

111. Berger RP, Adelson PD, Pierce MC, et al. Serum neuron-specific enolase, S100B, and myelin basic protein concentrations after inflicted and noninflicted traumatic brain injury in children. J Neurosurg 2005;103(Suppl 1):61–8.

112. Chambert-Loir C, Ouachee M, Collins K, et al. Immediate relief of *Mycoplasma pneumoniae* encephalitis symptoms after intravenous immunoglobulin. Pediatr Neurol 2009;41(5):375–7.

113. Dlamini N, Billinghurst L, Kirkham FJ. Cerebral venous sinus (sinovenous) thrombosis in children. Neurosurg Clin N Am 2010;21(3):511–27.

114. Abend NS, Monk HM, Licht DJ, et al. Intravenous levetiracetam in critically ill children with status epilepticus or acute repetitive seizures. Pediatr Crit Care Med 2009;10(4):505–10.

115. Ahmad S, Ellis JC, Kamwendo H, et al. Efficacy and safety of intranasal lorazepam versus intramuscular paraldehyde for protracted convulsions in children: an open randomised trial. Lancet 2006;367(9522):1591–7.

116. Appleton R, Macleod S, Martland T. Drug management for acute tonic-clonic convulsions including convulsive status epilepticus in children. Cochrane Database Syst Rev 2008;3:CD001905.

117. Babl FE, Sheriff N, Borland M, et al. Emergency management of paediatric status epilepticus in Australia and New Zealand: practice patterns in the context of clinical practice guidelines. J Paediatr Child Health 2009;45(9):541–6.

118. Expert Committee on Pediatric Epilepsy, Indian Academy of Pediatrics. Guidelines for diagnosis and management of childhood epilepsy. Indian Pediatr 2009; 46(8):681–98.

119. Kirmani BF, Crisp ED, Kayani S, et al. Role of intravenous levetiracetam in acute seizure management of children. Pediatr Neurol 2009;41(1):37–9.

120. Prasad AN, Seshia SS. Status epilepticus in pediatric practice: neonate to adolescent. In: Blume WT, editor, Intractable epilepsies. Advances in neurology, 97. Philadelphia: Lippincott Williams & Wilkins; 2006. p. 229–43.

121. Sofou K, Kristjansdottir R, Papachatzakis NE, et al. Management of prolonged seizures and status epilepticus in childhood: a systematic review. J Child Neurol 2009;24(8):918–26.

122. Chin RF, Verhulst L, Neville BG, et al. Inappropriate emergency management of status epilepticus in children contributes to need for intensive care. J Neurol Neurosurg Psychiatry 2004;75(11):1584–8.

123. Wermeling DP. Intranasal delivery of antiepileptic medications for treatment of seizures. Neurotherapeutics 2009;6(2):352–8.

124. Shehab N, Lewis CL, Streetman DD, et al. Exposure to the pharmaceutical excipients benzyl alcohol and propylene glycol among critically ill neonates. Pediatr Crit Care Med 2009;10(2):256–9.

125. Federman MD, Kelly R, Harrison RE. Refractory metabolic acidosis as a complication of high-dose midazolam infusion for pediatric status epilepticus. Clin Neuropharmacol 2009;32(6):340–1.

126. Melchior JC, Buchthal F, Lennox-Buchthal M. The ineffectiveness of diphenylhydantoin in preventing febrile convulsions in the age of greatest risk, under three years. Epilepsia 1971;12(1):55–62.

127. Bruce DA, Alavi A, Bilaniuk L, et al. Diffuse cerebral swelling following head injuries in children: the syndrome of "malignant brain edema". J Neurosurg 1981;54(2):170–8.

128. Zimmerman RA, Bilaniuk LT, Bruce D, et al. Computed tomography of pediatric head trauma: acute general cerebral swelling. Radiology 1978;126(2):403–8.

129. Kors EE, Terwindt GM, Vermeulen FL, et al. Delayed cerebral edema and fatal coma after minor head trauma: role of the CACNA1A calcium channel subunit gene and relationship with familial hemiplegic migraine. Ann Neurol 2001; 49(6):753–60.

130. Stam AH, Luijckx GJ, Poll-The BT, et al. Early seizures and cerebral oedema after trivial head trauma associated with the CACNA1A S218L mutation. J Neurol Neurosurg Psychiatry 2009;80(10):1125–9.

131. Brown JK, Habel AH. Toxic encephalopathy and acute brain-swelling in children. Dev Med Child Neurol 1975;17(5):659–79.

132. Goitein KJ, Tamir I. Cerebral perfusion pressure in central nervous system infections of infancy and childhood. J Pediatr 1983;103(1):40–3.

133. Gwer S, Gatakaa H, Mwai L, et al. The role for osmotic agents in children with acute encephalopathies: a systematic review. BMC Pediatr 2010;10:23.

134. Minns RA. Problems of intracranial pressure in childhood. Clin Dev Med 113/114. London: MacKeith Press; 1991.

135. Tasker RC, Matthew DJ, Helms P, et al. Monitoring in non-traumatic coma. Part I: invasive intracranial measurements. Arch Dis Child 1988;63(8):888–94.
136. Singhi SC, Tiwari L. Management of intracranial hypertension. Indian J Pediatr 2009;76(5):519–29.
137. Sankhyan N, Vykunta Raju KN, Sharma S, et al. Management of raised intracranial pressure. Indian J Pediatr 2010;77(12):1409–16.
138. Forsyth RJ, Wolny S, Rodrigues B. Routine intracranial pressure monitoring in acute coma. Cochrane Database Syst Rev 2010;2:CD002043.
139. Segal S, Gallagher AC, Shefler AG, et al. Survey of the use of intracranial pressure monitoring in children in the United Kingdom. Intensive Care Med 2001; 27(1):236–9.
140. Pediatric care online. Increased Intracranial Pressure. Available at: http://www.pediatriccareonline.org/pco/ub/pview/Point-of-Care-Quick%20Reference/397260/2/increased%20intracranial%20pressure. Last updated March 3, 2010. American Academy of Pediatrics. Accessed May 24, 2011.
141. Chambers IR, Jones PA, Lo TY, et al. Critical thresholds of intracranial pressure and cerebral perfusion pressure related to age in paediatric head injury. J Neurol Neurosurg Psychiatry 2006;77(2):234–40.
142. Shetty R, Singhi S, Singhi P, et al. Cerebral perfusion pressure–targeted approach in children with central nervous system infections and raised intracranial pressure: is it feasible? J Child Neurol 2008;23(2):192–8.
143. Lundberg N. Continuous recording and control of ventricular fluid pressure in neurosurgical practice. Acta Psychiatr Scand Suppl 1960;36(149):1–193.
144. Kawano G, Iwata O, Iwata S, et al. Determinants of outcomes following acute child encephalopathy and encephalitis: pivotal effect of early and delayed cooling. Arch Dis Child 2010. [Epub ahead of print].
145. Stocchetti N, Maas AI, Chieregato A, et al. Hyperventilation in head injury: a review. Chest 2005;127(5):1812–27.
146. Doyle JA, Davis DP, Hoyt DB. The use of hypertonic saline in the treatment of traumatic brain injury. J Trauma 2001;50(2):367–83.
147. Aghakhani N, Durand P, Chevret L, et al. Decompressive craniectomy in children with nontraumatic refractory high intracranial pressure. Clinical article. J Neurosurg Pediatr 2009;3(1):66–9.
148. Kirkham FJ, Neville BG. Successful management of severe intracranial hypertension by surgical decompression. Dev Med Child Neurol 1986;28(4):506–9.
149. Trubel HK, Novotny E, Lister G. Outcome of coma in children. Curr Opin Pediatr 2003;15(3):283–7.
150. Obiako OR, Ogunniyi A, Anyebe E. Prognosis of non traumatic coma: the role of some socio-economic factors on its outcome in Ibadan, Nigeria. Ann Afr Med 2009;8(2):115–21.
151. Roine I, Weisstaub G, Peltola H, et al. Influence of malnutrition on the course of childhood bacterial meningitis. Pediatr Infect Dis J 2010;29(2):122–5.
152. Njuguna P, Newton C. Management of severe falciparum malaria. J Postgrad Med 2004;50(1):45–50.
153. Ramakrishnan M, Ulland AJ, Steinhardt LC, et al. Sequelae due to bacterial meningitis among African children: a systematic literature review. BMC Med 2009;7:47.
154. Carrai R, Grippo A, Lori S, et al. Prognostic value of somatosensory evoked potentials in comatose children: a systematic literature review. Intensive Care Med 2010;36(7):1112–26.

155. Bruno MA, Gosseries O, Ledoux D, et al. Assessment of consciousness with electrophysiological and neurological imaging techniques. Curr Opin Crit Care 2011;17(2):146–51.
156. Gillies JD, Seshia SS. Vegetative state following coma in childhood: evolution and outcome. Dev Med Child Neurol 1980;22(5):642–8.
157. Ashwal S. Pediatric vegetative state: epidemiological and clinical issues. Neuro-Rehabilitation 2004;19(4):349–60.
158. Heindl UT, Laub MC. Outcome of persistent vegetative state following hypoxic or traumatic brain injury in children and adolescents. Neuropediatrics 1996;27(2):94–100.
159. Ashwal S. Medical aspects of the minimally conscious state in children. Brain Dev 2003;25(8):535–45.
160. McMahon MA, Vargus-Adams JN, Michaud LJ, et al. Effects of amantadine in children with impaired consciousness caused by acquired brain injury: a pilot study. Am J Phys Med Rehabil 2009;88(7):525–32.
161. Snyman N, Egan JR, London K, et al. Zolpidem for persistent vegetative state–a placebo-controlled trial in pediatrics. Neuropediatrics 2010;41(5):223–7.
162. Shemie SD, Doig C, Dickens B, et al. Severe brain injury to neurological determination of death: Canadian forum recommendations. CMAJ 2006;174(6):S1–13.
163. Mizuguchi M. [Diagnostic criteria of brain death for Japanese children]. Nippon Rinsho 2010;68(12):2317–21 [in Japanese].
164. Shemie SD, Pollack MM, Morioka M, et al. Diagnosis of brain death in children. Lancet Neurol 2007;6(1):87–92.
165. Joffe AR, Kolski H, Duff J, et al. A 10-month-old infant with reversible findings of brain death. Pediatr Neurol 2009;41(5):378–82.

Transient Global Amnesia

Gary Hunter, MD, FRCPC

KEYWORDS

• Transient global amnesia • Epileptic amnesia • DWI • CA1

The aptly named transient global amnesia (TGA) syndrome was initially described more than a century ago byRibot[1] and later in 2 independent case series.[2,3] It came to official recognition as a named syndrome after a large series described by Fisher and Adams.[4] Although the clinical syndrome is easily recognized and highly consistent in its characteristic features, the underlying pathophysiology has remained elusive. Proposed mechanisms include focal ischemic lesions, either related to arterial or venous dysfunction, paroxysmal neuronal discharges or epileptic phenomena, or local nonischemic energy failures of other causes. None of these, however, has been clearly demonstrated, although some evidence has been shown for all of these mechanisms. In the past, all investigations of these patients were normal, including brain imaging and electroencephalogram (EEG). With improvements and MRI technology, diffusion-weighted imaging (DWI) has been able to demonstrate focal areas of restricted diffusion, which seem entirely restricted to the CA1 sector of the hippocampus.[5] Nonetheless, the mechanism of this diffusion restriction is uncertain and does not necessarily indicate ischemia, leaving the exact nature of this seemingly benign disorder in doubt after many decades of study. The goal of this review is to summarize the pertinent clinical features, proposed pathophysiology, epidemiology, imaging, and future directions in understanding TGA.

CLINICAL FEATURES AND BASIC APPROACH

The definition of TGA includes an anterograde and retrograde amnesia lasting less than 24 hours, although significant variations from this time frame have been reported.[6] The clinical features are highly characteristic, but if this disorder is not considered, it can cause considerable diagnostic confusion. The usual presentation is a middle-aged patient brought in by family members concerned about stroke or other devastating brain disease. Most clinicians familiar with this syndrome agree that there is frequently a social or physical stress around the time of onset, but this has been difficult to prove in epidemiologic studies.[7–9] Proposed precipitating events

The author has no disclosures.
Division of Neurology, University of Saskatchewan, #112, 3502 Taylor Street East, Saskatoon, SK S7H 5H9, Canada
E-mail address: grwhunter@gmail.com

include social events such as family gatherings, travel, strenuous activity, pain, sexual intercourse, and even water contact or temperature change. The most characteristic feature is the tendency to repeat the same questions, and often forgetting conversations within just minutes. This can cause difficulty in explaining the diagnosis to patients, in that they often have insight into the fact that something is wrong and are frequently frightened. Reassuring these patients is a challenge because they readily forget that they have just had the condition explained.

The diagnosis of TGA requires that a patient is alert and otherwise seems well. Any encephalopathic patient should be presumed to have an underlying acute condition until proved otherwise. Language function is normal in TGA, as is the remainder of the neurologic examination, with the only deficit being isolated to anterograde memory, with lesser involvement of retrograde memory. Registration is generally preserved, but even brief delays before testing recall reveal dramatic impairment of anterograde memory. Associated symptoms may include headache, a vague sense of dizziness, nausea, fear of dying, and chills or flushes.[10] Many patients are anxious, because they quickly realize that something is wrong, at least partly because of the family's reaction to their behavior. Bizarre behavior out of character for a patient, loss of self-identity, forgetting names of family members, and dramatic retrograde memory impairment, however, are not characteristic of TGA and may be suggestive of a factitious memory disorder.

Basic investigations in an emergency department should include routine hematology and chemistry, glucose, screening for infection when indicated, and EEG and MRI when there is any doubt about the diagnosis. When the syndrome is clear, EEG and MRI need not be performed urgently, but MRI and EEG should be offered at least on a follow-up basis. In many cases, reassurance to the family and patient allows for discharge home in the care of family members with the patient can be observed until symptoms resolve. Hospital admission is always reasonable, however, to ensure resolution of symptoms and provide a safe environment for the patient, in general leading to the discharge of a healthy patient the following day. As symptoms clear, the period of time for which a patient is amnestic may decrease, but in general there is always some period of time that is never remembered. The prognosis is generally excellent, although some have suggested that long-term deficits in memory may persist in a subclinical fashion. Borroni and colleagues[11] subjected 55 patients who had suffered a TGA episode to standardized neuropsychological testing at least 1 year after the attack and found that they performed significantly worse on tests of memory compared with matched controls, whereas other cognitive domains were comparable.

Diagnostic criteria have been proposed[12], including: Witnessed anterograde amnesia, absence of encephalopathic symptoms or loss of personal identity, absence of cognitive deficits beyond amnesia, absence of focal neurologic deficits or symptoms of seizures, absence of recent head trauma, and resolution within 24 hours. These criteria can be further summarized to simply state that a patient must have isolated transient amnesia, with normal consciousness and other faculties intact, and rapid improvement. The duration criteria may be generous, because the mean duration of attacks is probably between 4 and 6 hours.[10,12]

Differential diagnostic possibilities are listed in **Box 1**. Consideration of seizures is important, especially in diabetic patients, because hypoglycemic seizures can produce an essentially identical transient amnestic syndrome in the postictal period.[13,14] This probably relates to selective metabolic stress to the CA1 region of the hippocampus in hypoglycaemia and seizures,[15] the same region thought to be affected in TGA. In young patients with apparent TGA, the history should always include questions of myalgias, tongue trauma, and nocturnal incontinence. Other

---

Box 1
Differential diagnosis of TGA

- Stroke involving mesial temporal area, thalamus, or fornix
- Delirium (often metabolic or infectious)
- Wernicke encephalopathy/Korsakoff syndrome (thiamine deficiency)
- Psychiatric disorder, dissociative fugue, conversion disorder
- Migraine
- Transient epileptic amnesia
- Nonconvulsive status epilepticus
- Hypoglycemic seizures
- Drug overdose or toxicity

---

temporal lobe seizures may also present with isolated postictal amnesia,[16] but this is less common in other disorders, such as mesial temporal sclerosis, compared with hypoglycemic seizures. A careful drug history is always advisable, specifically with respect to benzodiazepines, anticholinergics, and narcotics. Finally, factitious disorders should be considered when this classic description is not seen. Personal identity and recognition of family members are always intact in TGA.

In elderly patients, differential diagnosis should always include stroke, usually of the posterior cerebral artery, which supplies the medial temporal lobe and hippocampal regions. Isolated amnesia as a result of posterior cerebral artery stroke is uncommon, however, and careful assessment for hemianopia suggesting occipital lobe involvement is often revealing. Strategic infarcts of the medial or anterior thalamus or fornix can also produce isolated amnestic syndromes.[17–21] Thiamine deficiency should be considered in alcoholic patients, those with malabsorption syndromes, or those who have undergone abdominal surgeries that could affect nutritional status. Although this is generally considered a less acute problem, Wernicke encephalopathy certainly can present fulminantly, and consciousness may be relatively preserved. A variety of ocular motility disorders and gait impairment may be associated, but the safest approach is to administer thiamine intravenously if there is any doubt. MRI findings in Wernicke encephalopathy include abnormal signal or DWI changes in the medial thalami, mammillary bodies, periaqueductal region, and tectal plate[22,23] and less commonly in the cerebellar hemispheres.[24]

EPIDEMIOLOGY

The majority of TGA attacks occur in people between the ages of 50 and 70,[10] and it is rarely encountered in young patients; thus, more extensive investigations and hospital admission should be strongly considered in any patient younger than 40, even in otherwise classic cases. The reported incidence rate varies between 3 and 8 per 100,000 people per year.[25] There is no strong gender bias, with various investigators reporting higher prevalence in either gender.[10] Recurrences are relatively uncommon but may be as frequent as 6% to 10% per year.[10,25] Among 51 patients who were followed for 7 years, the recurrence rate was 8%.[26] Risk factors for a first attack or for recurrent TGA are not well defined, although there have been several valiant attempts. Factors that have been considered include hypertension, dyslipidemia, diabetes, seizures, and migraine, but none of these has consistent evidence of association, although migraine may be a risk factor in younger patients with TGA.[10] Personality traits may predispose patients to the development of TGA, with one study showing that 82% of 51 patients demonstrated pathologic avoidance behavior toward potentially fearful situations, such as crowded stores, seeing blood, or crossing a bridge.[8] A family history of psychiatric disorders may be a risk factor.[26]

PATHOPHYSIOLOGY

The localization of TGA has always been presumed to involve the mesial temporal structures or specifically the hippocampus. The physiologic mechanisms remain difficult to explain in full, however, because investigations (until recently) have been invariably negative, including EEG and neuroimaging. As discussed previously, there is no definite increased risk of transient ischemic attack (TIA) or stroke, seizures, or migraine among patients with TGA, although each of these has been weakly associated in some studies.[27] Abnormalities of venous flow have been investigated recently but without convincing evidence of a primary role for this mechanism in causing focal hippocampal dysfunction.[28,29] As with any studies using ultrasound, including those proposing venous abnormalities in multiple sclerosis,[30] operator dependence remains problematic in attaining objective results. In addition, the high variability of normal venous anatomy makes interpretation difficult.

The age of onset and sudden deficit are suggestive of ischemic mechanisms, but the prompt resolution of symptoms in all cases makes stroke less likely. Compared with patients with TIA, patients with TGA are less likely to suffer a stroke in the future.[31] Magnetic resonance angiography studies do not demonstrate abnormalities of the intracranial vessels, and perfusion-weighted imaging has also been normal, even during acute attacks.[32] Winbeck and coworkers[33] found that carotid atherosclerosis was more likely to be found among TGA patients with DWI changes compared with controls, using ultrasound examinations. They concluded that a subgroup of TGA patients may have symptoms resulting from ischemia, but this remains a loose association, and other vascular risk factors were not common in this group compared with TIA patients who served as controls. TGA patients did not show increased frequency of microvascular ischemic changes on MRI, again arguing against a primary arterial etiology.

The evidence for an association with migraine is complex. Without any definite causal association, migraine is associated with innumerable disorders, including epilepsy,[34] stroke,[35,36] patent foramen ovale,[37] high antiphospholipid antibody titers,[38] depression,[39] arterial dissection,[40] fibromyalgia,[41] and dementia,[42] to name a few. The ubiquity of the syndrome makes any association studies difficult to interpret. In the TGA population, some investigators have found a strong association with migraine,[43] whereas others have refuted this.[44] Nonetheless, a migrainous phenomenon is a reasonable candidate to explain TGA based on its well-described mechanisms of paroxysmal neuronal dysfunction with a comparable time course. Cortical spreading depression (CSD) of Leão[45,46] is generally accepted as the pathophysiologic correlate of migraine with aura and is characterized by transient neuronal depolarization and hyperperfusion, followed by hyperpolarization, hypoperfusion, and neuronal dysfunction, which spreads across the cortex at a rate of 3 to 5 mm per minute. This process can be seen in animal models, including in the hippocampal region, even leading to hypoxic states in the CA1 fields.[47] In 1986, Olesen and Jørgensen[48] proposed CSD as a mechanism for explaining TGA, because induction of CSD in animals produces comparable amnestic behavior that resolves spontaneously. They also proposed that the high hippocampal glutamate concentrations might explain the tendency of TGA to follow emotional events, which could trigger glutamate release. Since then, laboratory data have confirmed a selective vulnerability of the CA1 region to various metabolic stressors, resulting in glutamate excitotoxicity and calcium influx.[49] Experimentally, induction of hippocampal dysfunction is possible by initiating a stress response.[50] True abnormalities of DWI have not been described in migraines unless associated with stroke—however, abnormalities of apparent diffusion coefficient maps have been reported in patients with prolonged aura.[51] Although much of this experimental data does make CSD an attractive explanation, the epidemiology is not supportive because migraine aura is common in young individuals, but TGA is not. It might be hypothesized that in younger patients, compensatory mechanisms prevent the syndrome during CSD of the hippocampal regions. In addition, migraine headaches are generally not associated temporally with TGA attacks.[25] Ultimately, a potential but weak association with migraine is all that is possible in regards to explaining the physiology of TGA.

Epileptic phenomena have been suggested as a cause of transient amnesia since proposed by Hughlings-Jackson in 1889.[52] Quinette and colleagues[10] conducted EEG studies in 106 patients during or soon after an attack of TGA and found that 80% were unremarkable, with the remaining records showing minor, nonepileptiform abnormalities. In 52 patients recorded during the attack, 87% were normal. These findings, which have been consistent in the literature, in combination with the low likelihood of developing epilepsy in TGA patients, eventually led to a search for other mechanisms. There has been a resurgence of interest, however, in so-called transient epileptic amnesia[53] in recent years. Attacks of otherwise classic-appearing TGA associated with clear electrographic seizures have been reported[54] but with considerably shorter time courses of 1 to 3 hours as opposed to 24 hours for typical TGA. Similar clinical features may also be seen after otherwise typical complex partial seizures, with unresponsiveness, automatisms, or secondarily generalized seizures followed by an alert but amnestic state.[55] In a few cases recorded during an attack of apparent TGA, nonconvulsive status epilepticus has been found.[56–58] In one case, a temporal lobe tumor was presumed to have caused a 5-hour episode resembling TGA, with the EEG only showing wicket spikes (a benign variant).[59] The investigators proposed a possible underlying epileptic phenomenon. This syndrome should be considered when there is a history of epilepsy, when attacks are recurrent, or when the duration is atypical. Because up to 70% of patients with TEA may have normal interictal EEG,[54] continued surveillance may be necessary. Prolonged or ambulatory EEG studies in patients with TGA or TEA may be helpful in elucidating the nature of these attacks and better defining the frequency of TEA in a subgroup of patients.

NEUROIMAGING OF TGA

In the past, brain imaging was considered completely unrevealing for the vast majority of TGA cases. Over the last 2 decades, however, reports of DWI abnormalities suggesting ischemic injury have emerged.[60] Other investigators found no DWI changes during attacks of TGA[61] and recommended that if DWI changes are seen and thought to represent ischemic injury, a diagnosis of TGA should not be made. Since that time, there have been variable reports of DWI or apparent diffusion coefficient changes in TGA patients.[33,62,63] Ahn and colleagues[64] studied MRI scans of 203 cases of TGA over a 7-year period and found only 16 patients with DWI changes in the hippocampal region, among whom there were no apparent clinical differences. The overall mean time to MRI in this study was 6 hours, whereas those with DWI changes were studied at 9 hours ($P = .002$), suggesting that with careful timing of imaging, more abnormalities may be found. Supporting the importance of timing, Bartsch and coworkers[65] studied the evolution of MRI changes in 29 patients with TGA and found 34 DWI lesions localized to the CA1 sector of the hippocampus when studied between 24 and 72 hours. DWI normalization was seen at approximately day 10, which is similar to the time course for ischemic lesions,[66] leading the investigators to suggest a vascular origin for some TGA lesions. Optimal imaging protocols continue to be refined, but practical recommendations are available[25] and include a 3-T magnet, acquisition between 24 and 72 hours after onset, and a 3-mm DWI slice thickness.

Further evidence for local dysfunction of CA1 neurons comes from MR spectroscopy studies of hippocampal DWI lesions, which have demonstrated a lactate peak.[67] Positron emission tomography (PET) and single-photon emission CT (SPECT) studies have been conflicting but do generally support both hypoperfusion and hypometabolism of the hippocampal region.[68–70] In many cases, however, dysfunction has been seen elsewhere, including the thalamic, frontal, cerebellar, and striatal regions.[71–73] In most cases, resolution of these changes is expected, but in recurrent TGA, persistent hypoperfusion has been seen as late as 1 year after the initial attack.[74] In general, PET and SPECT studies are congruent with the findings from MRI studies, suggesting metabolic dysfunction in the mesial temporal lobes, although abnormalities in other anatomic regions are commonly seen as well. Unfortunately, this offers little additional insight into underlying mechanisms because altered perfusion and metabolism are also seen in migraine[75] and epilepsy.[76,77]

SUMMARY AND FUTURE DIRECTIONS

With the emergence of advanced imaging and laboratory techniques, the long-held belief that TGA is related to focal hippocampal dysfunction is no longer just a hypothesis. Clearly, there is metabolic stress, mainly localizing to the CA1 sector. Nonetheless, the precise etiology remains unclear, as are the exact triggers of attacks. Is it coincidental that stressors seem to precipitate episodes of TGA? Could this suggest a supply and demand phenomenon, wherein a threshold of metabolic stress is achieved causing energy failure in a metabolically fragile hippocampus? The frequency of DWI changes in TGA patients has not been clearly defined because the optimal imaging parameters have only recently been elucidated and are not available uniformly. The results of such studies may lead to uncertainty regarding treatment—should all patients with DWI lesions be treated as stroke or TIA patients, with initiation of secondary prevention measures? The epidemiology suggests otherwise, but imaging findings of presumed stroke make this less clear. Autopsy studies have not been performed and may be useful in clarifying whether the dysfunction relates to focal ischemia or energy failure of other causes. Prolonged or ambulatory EEG may be useful in identifying a subgroup of patients with epileptic syndromes, which should be considered in recurrent cases or those with unusually short duration. Fortunately, the prognosis for most cases of TGA remains excellent, and the mainstay of management remains recognition and reassurance.

REFERENCES

1. Ribot T. Diseases of memory. Appleton;1882.
2. Bender MB. Syndrome of isolated episode of confusion with amnesia. J Hillside Hosp 1956;5:212–4.
3. Guyotat M. Les ictus amnésiques. J Med Lyon 1956;37:697–9.
4. Fisher CM, Adams RD. Transient global amnesia. Acta Neurol Scand Suppl 1964; 40(Suppl 9):1–83.

5. Bartsch T, Alfke K, Stingele R, et al. Selective affection of hippocampal CA-1 neurons in patients with transient global amnesia without long-term sequelae. Brain 2006;129(Pt 11):2874–84.
6. Pai MC. Prolonged reversible amnesia: a case report. J Stroke Cerebrovasc Dis 2000;9(2):86–8.
7. Lewis SL. Aetiology of transient global amnesia. Lancet 1998;352(9125):397–9.
8. Inzitari D, Pantoni L, Lamassa M, et al. Emotional arousal and phobia in transient global amnesia. Arch Neurol 1997;54(7):866–73.
9. Rösler A, Mras GJ, Frese A, et al. Precipitating factors of transient global amnesia. J Neurol 1999;246(1):53–4.
10. Quinette P, Guillery-Girard B, Dayan J, et al. What does transient global amnesia really mean? Review of the literature and thorough study of 142 cases. Brain 2006;129(Pt 7):1640–58.
11. Borroni B, Agosti C, Brambilla C, et al. Is transient global amnesia a risk factor for amnestic mild cognitive impairment? J Neurol 2004;251(9):1125–7.
12. Hodges JR, Warlow CP. Syndromes of transient amnesia: towards a classification. A study of 153 cases. J Neurol Neurosurg Psychiatry 1990;53(10):834–43.
13. Holemans X, Dupuis M, Misson N, et al. Reversible amnesia in a Type 1 diabetic patient and bilateral hippocampal lesions on magnetic resonance imaging (MRI). Diabet Med 2001;18(9):761–3.
14. Chalmers J, Risk MT, Kean DM, et al. Severe amnesia after hypoglycemia. Clinical, psychometric, and magnetic resonance imaging correlations. Diabetes Care 1991;14(10):922–5.
15. Panickar KS, Purushotham K, King MA, et al. Hypoglycemia-induced seizures reduce cyclic AMP response element binding protein levels in the rat hippocampus. Neuroscience 1998;83(4):1155–60.
16. Maheu G, Adam C, Hazemann P, et al. A case of postictal transient anterograde and retrograde amnesia. Epilepsia 2004;45(11):1459–60.
17. Korematsu K, Hori T, Morioka M, et al. Memory impairment due to a small unilateral infarction of the fornix. Clin Neurol Neurosurg 2010;112(2):164–6.
18. Moudgil SS, Azzouz M, Al-Azzaz A, et al. Amnesia due to fornix infarction. Stroke 2000;31(6):1418–9.
19. Tomii Y, Kondo M, Hosomi A, et al. Two cases of hippocampal infarction with persistent memory impairment in which diffusion-weighted magnetic resonance imaging was useful. Rinsho Shinkeigaku 2008;48(10):742–5 [in Japanese].
20. Markowitsch HJ, von Cramon DY, Schuri U. Amnestic performance profile of a bilateral diencephalic infarct patient with preserved intelligence and severe amnesic disturbances. J ClinExpNeuropsychol 1993;15(5):627–52.
21. Miller LA, Caine D, Harding A, et al. Right medial thalamic lesion causes isolated retrograde amnesia. Neuropsychologia 2001;39(10):1037–46.
22. Cerase A, Rubenni E, Rufa A, et al. CT and MRI of Wernicke's encephalopathy. Radiol Med 2011;116(2):319–33.
23. Zuccoli G, Pipitone N. Neuroimaging findings in acute Wernicke's encephalopathy: review of the literature. AJR Am J Roentgenol 2009;192(2):501–8.
24. Kim HA, Lee H. Atypical Wernicke's encephalopathy with remarkable cerebellar lesions on diffusion-weighted MRI. EurNeurol 2007;58(1):51–3.
25. Bartsch T, Deuschl G. Transient global amnesia: functional anatomy and clinical implications. Lancet Neurol 2010;9(2):205–14.
26. Pantoni L, Bertini E, Lamassa M, et al. Clinical features, risk factors, and prognosis in transient global amnesia: a follow-up study. Eur J Neurol 2005;12(5):350–6.

27. Sander K, Sander D. New insights into transient global amnesia: recent imaging and clinical findings. Lancet Neurol 2005;4(7):437–44.

28. Cejas C, Cisneros LF, Lagos R, et al. Internal jugular vein valve incompetence is highly prevalent in transient global amnesia. Stroke 2010;41(1):67–71.

29. Sander D, Winbeck K, Etgen T, et al. Disturbance of venous flow patterns in patients with transient global amnesia. Lancet 2009;356(9246):1982–4.

30. Menegatti E, Genova V, Tessari M, et al. The reproducibility of colour Doppler in chronic cerebrospinal venous insufficiency associated with multiple sclerosis. IntAngiol 2010;29(2):121–6.

31. Hodges JR, Warlow CP. The aetiology of transient global amnesia. A case-control study of 114 cases with prospective follow-up. Brain 1990;113(Pt 3):639–57.

32. Toledo M, Pujadas F, Grivé E, et al. Lack of evidence for arterial ischemia in transient global amnesia. Stroke 2008;39(2):476–9.

33. Winbeck K, Etgen T, von Einsiedel HG, et al. DWI in transient global amnesia and TIA: proposal for an ischaemic origin of TGA. J NeurolNeurosurg Psychiatry 2005;76(3):438–41.

34. Davies PT, Panayiotopoulos CP. Migraine triggered seizures and epilepsy triggered headache and migraine attacks: a need for re-assessment. J Headache Pain 2011;12(3):287–8.

35. Caminero AB, Sánchez Del Río González M. Migraine as a cerebrovascular risk factor. Neurologia 2011. [Epub ahead of print].

36. Schürks M, Kurth T. Is migraine a predictor for identifying patients at risk of stroke? Expert Rev Neurother 2011;11(5):615–8.

37. Trabattoni D, Fabbiocchi F, Montorsi P, et al. Sustained long-term benefit of patent foramen ovale closure on migraine. Catheter Cardiovasc Interv 2011;77(4):570–4.

38. Cinzia C, Gianmatteo M, Filippo M, et al. Migraineurs show a high prevalence of antiphospholipid antibodies. J Thromb Haemost 2011. [Epub ahead of print].

39. Moschiano F, D'Amico D, Canavero I, et al. Migraine and depression: common pathogenetic and therapeutic ground? Neurol Sci 2011;32(Suppl 1):S85–8.

40. Demaerschalk BM. Migraine is associated with an increased risk of cervicocephalic arterial dissection. Cephalalgia 2011. [Epub ahead of print].

41. Evans RW. de Tommaso M.Migraine and fibromyalgia. Headache 2011;51(2):295–9.

42. Sas K, Párdutz A, Toldi J. Vécsei L.Dementia, stroke and migraine–some common pathological mechanisms. J Neurol Sci 2010;299(1/2):55–65.

43. Schmidtke K, Ehmsen L. Transient global amnesia and migraine. A case control study. Eur Neurol 1998;40(1):9–14.

44. Pantoni L, Lamassa M, Inzitari D. Transient global amnesia: a review emphasizing pathogenic aspects. Acta Neurol Scand 2000;102(5):275–83.

45. Leão AA. Spreading depression of activityin cerebral cortex. J Neurophysiol 1944;7:159–390.

46. Teive HA, Kowacs PA, MaranhãoFilho P, et al. Leao's cortical spreading depression: from experimental "artifact" to physiological principle. Neurology 2005;65(9):1455–9.

47. Pomper JK, Haack S, Petzold GC, et al. Repetitive spreading depression-like events result in cell damage in juvenile hippocampal slice cultures maintained in normoxia. J Neurophysiol 2006;95(1):355–68.

48. Olesen J, Jørgensen MB. Leao's spreading depression in the hippocampus explains transient global amnesia. A hypothesis. Acta Neurol Scand 1986;73(2):219–20.

49. Kosuge Y, Imai T, Kawaguchi M, et al. Subregion-specific vulnerability to endoplasmic reticulum stress-induced neurotoxicity in rat hippocampal neurons. Neurochem Int 2008;52(6):1204–11.

50. Zoladz PR, Park CR, Halonen JD, et al. Differential expression of molecular markers of synaptic plasticity in the hippocampus, prefrontal cortex, and amygdala in response to spatial learning, predator exposure, and stress-induced amnesia. Hippocampus 2011. [Epub ahead of print].
51. Belvís R, Ramos R, Villa C, et al. Brain apparent water diffusion coefficient magnetic resonance image during a prolonged visual aura. Headache 2010; 50(6):1045–9.
52. Hughlings-Jackson J. On a particular variety of epilepsy (intellectualaura), one case with symptoms of organic brain disease. Brain 1889;11:179–207.
53. Kapur N. Transient epileptic amnesia—a clinical update and areformulation. J Neurol Neurosurg Psychiat 1993;56:1184–90.
54. Bilo L, Meo R, Ruosi P, et al. Transient epileptic amnesia: an emerging late-onset epileptic syndrome. Epilepsia 2009;50(Suppl 5):58–61.
55. Pritchard PBI, Holmstrom VL, Roitzsch JC, et al. Epilepticamnesic attacks: benefit from antiepileptic drugs. Neurology 1985;35:1188–9.
56. Lee BI, Lee BC, Hwang YM, et al. Prolonged ictal amnesia with transient focal abnormalities on magnetic resonance imaging. Epilepsia 1992;33(6):1042–6.
57. Meo R, Bilo L, Striano S, et al. Transient global amnesia of epileptic origin accompanied by fever. Seizure 1995;4(4):311–7.
58. Vuilleumier P, Despland PA, Regli F. Failure to recall (but not toremember): pure transient amnesia during nonconvulsive statusepilepticus. Neurology 1996;46: 1036–9.
59. Huang CF, Pai MC. Transient amnesia in a patient with left temporal tumor: symptomatic transient global amnesia or an epileptic amnesia? Neurologist 2008; 14(3):196–200.
60. Ay H, Furie KL, Yamada K, et al. Diffusion-weighted MRI characterizes the ischemic lesion in transient global amnesia. Neurology 1998;51(3):901–3.
61. Budson AE, Schlaug G, Briemberg HR. Perfusion- and diffusion-weighted magnetic resonance imaging in transient global amnesia. Neurology 1999;53(1):239–40.
62. Huber R, Aschoff AJ, Ludolph AC, et al. Transient Global Amnesia. Evidence against vascular ischemic etiology from diffusion weighted imaging. J Neurol 2002;249(11):1520–4.
63. Matsui M, Imamura T, Sakamoto S, et al. Transient global amnesia: increased signal intensity in the right hippocampus on diffusion-weighted magnetic resonance imaging. Neuroradiology 2002;44(3):235–8.
64. Ahn S, Kim W, Lee YS, et al. Transient global amnesia: seven years of experience with diffusion-weighted imaging in an emergency department. Eur Neurol 2011; 65(3):123–8.
65. Bartsch T, Alfke K, Deuschl G, et al. Evolution of hippocampal CA-1 diffusion lesions in transient global amnesia. Ann Neurol 2007;62(5):475–80.
66. Fiebach J, Jansen O, Schellinger P, et al. Comparison of CT with diffusion-weighted MRI in patients with hyperacute stroke. Neuroradiology 2001;43(8): 628–32.
67. Bartsch T, Alfke K, Wolff S, et al. Focal MR spectroscopy of hippocampal CA-1 lesions in transient global amnesia. Neurology 2008;70(13):1030–5.
68. Stillhard G, Landis T, Schiess R, et al. Bitemporalhypoperfusion in transient global amnesia: 99m-Tc-HM-PAO SPECT and neuropsychological findings during and after an attack. J Neurol Neurosurg Psychiatry 1990;53(4):339–42.
69. Laloux P, Brichant C, Cauwe F, et al. Technetium-99m HM-PAO single photon emission computed tomography imaging in transient global amnesia. Arch Neurol 1992;49(5):543–6.

70. Jovin TG, Vitti RA, McCluskey LF. Evolution of temporal lobe hypoperfusion in transient global amnesia: a serial single photon emission computed tomography study. J Neuroimaging 2000;10(4):238–41.
71. Goldenberg G, Podreka I, Pfaffelmeyer N, et al. Thalamic ischemia in transient global amnesia: a SPECT study. Neurology 1991;41(11):1748–52.
72. Baron JC, Petit-Taboué MC, Le Doze F, et al. Right frontal cortex hypometabolism in transient global amnesia. A PET study. Brain 1994;117(Pt 3):545–52.
73. Eustache F, Desgranges B, Aupée AM, et al. Functional neuroanatomy of amnesia: positron emission tomography studies. Microsc Res Tech 2000;51(1): 94–100.
74. Lampl Y, Sadeh M, Lorberboym M. Transient global amnesia—not always a benign process. Acta Neurol Scand 2004;110(2):75–9.
75. Soriani S, Feggi L, Battistella PA, et al. Interictal and ictal phase study with Tc 99m HMPAO brain SPECT in juvenile migraine with aura. Headache 1997;37(1):31–6.
76. O'Brien TJ, Brinkmann BH, Mullan BP, et al. Comparative study of 99mTc-ECD and 99mTc-HMPAO for peri-ictal SPECT: qualitative and quantitative analysis. J NeurolNeurosurg Psychiatry 1999;66(3):331–9.
77. Newton MR, Berkovic SF, Austin MC, et al. SPECT in the localisation of extratemporal and temporal seizure foci. J Neurol Neurosurg Psychiatry 1995;59(1): 26–30.

Ethical Aspects of Disordered States of Consciousness

Emily B. Rubin, JD, MD[a,*], James L. Bernat, MD[b,c]

KEYWORDS

- Disordered consciousness • Coma • Minimally conscious state
- Vegetative state • Traumatic brain injury • Ethics
- Surrogate decision making • End-of-life care

STATES OF CONSCIOUSNESS

Consciousness has 2 clinical components: (1) wakefulness, which is mediated by the ascending reticular activating system of the brainstem and its thalamic and hemispheric projections, and (2) awareness of one's self and the environment, which is mediated by the cerebral cortex and its connections with itself, the thalami, and other subcortical structures.[1] A disordered state of consciousness results when one or both of these components are compromised. Disordered states of consciousness is a broad category that encompasses a spectrum of cognitive dysfunction, from mild confusional states, such as delirium, to dementia, coma, locked-in syndrome, vegetative state (VS), minimally conscious state (MCS), and brain death.

Coma is an eyes-closed pathologic state of unresponsiveness. Patients in a coma are neither awake nor aware and make no behavioral response to stimuli. Coma is caused by a structural or metabolic lesion that interferes with the reticular activating system. It is usually an unstable, transient state that leads within weeks to death, vegetative state, or recovery of awareness.[1]

Brain death is defined as the irreversible cessation of all functions of the entire brain, including the brainstem.[2] Patients who meet the criteria for brain death are legally dead in all jurisdictions. The locked-in syndrome, usually the result of a devastating vascular insult to the pons, is a state in which patients are awake and aware but profoundly paralyzed with only voluntary vertical eye movements. The locked-in syndrome is not a disorder of consciousness because both components of

The authors have nothing to disclose.
[a] Internal Medicine and Pediatrics, Massachusetts General Hospital, 55 Fruit Street, Boston, MA 02114, USA
[b] Dartmouth Medical School, 1 Rope Ferry Road, Hanover, NH 03755, USA
[c] Neurology Department, Dartmouth-Hitchcock Medical Center, One Medical Center Drive, Lebanon, NH 03756, USA
* Corresponding author. 29 Lawrence Street, Apartment B, Cambridge, MA 02139.
E-mail address: erubin3@partners.org

doi:10.1016/j.ncl.2011.07.007
neurologic.theclinics.com

consciousness are fully intact but is included because it can be confused diagnostically with VS or MCS by an unwary examiner.

As Jennett and Plum[3] first described in 1972, patients in a VS are awake but not aware. The Multi-Society Task Force on PVS defined VS as "a condition of complete unawareness of the self and the environment accompanied by sleep-wake cycles with either complete or partial preservation of brain stem and hypothalamic autonomic functions."[4] The most common causes of VS are traumatic brain injury and hypoxic-ischemic neuronal damage. Less common causes include stroke, degenerative disorders, and severe developmental malformations of the nervous system. A VS can result from 3 distinct neuropathologic patterns, all of which feature a disconnection of the cerebral cortex from the thalamus. These include (1) diffuse, widespread cortical damage, such as that resulting from hypoxic-ischemic encephalopathy suffered during cardiopulmonary arrest; (2) diffuse, widespread damage to the subcortical hemispheric white matter, such as that resulting from diffuse axonal injury in traumatic brain injury; and (3) profound damage to both thalami resulting from stroke, hypoxia-ischemia, or other injuries.[5] Although it was once thought that end-stage Alzheimer disease and other neurodegenerative disorders progressed over time to VS, it is now understood that few if any such patients ever reach a true VS.[6] The criteria for diagnosing the VS are listed in **Box 1** and the potential behavioral repertoire of patients in VS is listed in **Box 2**.

The MCS was first described in 2002 as "a condition of severely altered consciousness in which minimal but definite behavioral evidence of self or environmental awareness is demonstrated."[7] Patients in an MCS show evidence of cognitively mediated behavior, such as following simple commands; gesturing yes-or-no answers to questions; appropriate emotional responses, such as smiling or crying; and sustained gaze at moving targets. Such behaviors are typically intermittent and inconsistent but must be sustained or reproducible enough to allow distinction from reflex behavior. The criteria for diagnosing the MCS are listed in **Box 3**, and the potential behavioral repertoire of patients in an MCS is listed in **Box 4**.

Although defined as distinct diagnostic syndromes, VS and MCS are parts of the continuum of impaired consciousness seen in patients with diffuse brain injury.

Box 1
Criteria for diagnosing the vegetative state

- Unaware of self and the environment

- No interaction with others

- No sustained, reproducible, or purposeful voluntary behavioral response to visual, auditory, tactile, or noxious stimuli

- No language comprehension or expression

- No blink to visual threat

- Present sleep-wake cycles

- Preserved autonomic and hypothalamic function to survive for long intervals with medical/nursing care

- Preserved cranial nerve reflexes

- Bowel and bladder incontinence

Modified from Bernat JL. Chronic disorders of consciousness. Lancet 2006;367(9528):1181–92; with permission.

Box 2
Potential behavior repertoire of patients in a vegetative state

- Sleep-wake cycles with eyes closed, then open
- Spontaneous breathing
- Spontaneous blinking and roving eye movements
- Nystagmus
- Vocalization of sounds but no words
- Brief, unsustained visual pursuit
- Grimacing to pain, changing facial expressions
- Yawning; chewing jaw movements
- Swallowing of saliva
- Nonpurposeful limb movements; arching of back; decorticate limb posturing
- Flexion withdrawal from noxious stimuli
- Brief movements of head or eyes toward sound or movement
- Auditory startle
- Startle myoclonus
- Sleep-related erections

Modified from Bernat JL. Chronic disorders of consciousness. Lancet 2006;367(9528):1181–92; with permission.

Many patients who suffer traumatic brain injury, stroke, or hypoxic-ischemic injury as the result of cardiopulmonary arrest initially present in a coma. Then they either progress to brain death or transition to a vegetative state. Some VS patients transition to an MCS and some then recover to a state of higher consciousness in which they are able to reliably communicate and interact. VS and MCS can vary in severity and can be either chronic conditions or transient conditions that patients experience during the process of recovery from brain injury. It is also possible for patients in MCS at baseline to regress into VS, particularly in the context of superimposed metabolic or toxic illnesses.

Box 3
Criteria for diagnosing the minimally conscious state

- Globally impaired responsiveness
- Limited but discernable evidence of awareness of self and environment as demonstrated by the presence of one or more of the following behaviors:
  - Following simple commands
  - Gestural or verbal responses to yes-or-no questions
  - Intelligible verbalizations
  - Purposeful behavior: movements or affective behaviors that occur in contingent relation to relevant environmental stimuli and are not simply reflexive movements

Modified from Bernat JL. Chronic disorders of consciousness. Lancet 2006;367(9528):1181–92; with permission.

Box 4
Potential behavioral repertoire of patients in a minimally conscious state

- Follow simple commands
- Gesture yes-or-no answers
- Verbalize intelligently
- Vocalize or gesture in direct response to a question's linguistic content
- Reach for objects demonstrating a clear relationship between object location and direction of reach
- Touch and hold objects in a manner that accommodates the size and shape of the objection
- Sustain visual pursuit of moving stimuli
- Smile or cry appropriately to linguistic or visual content of emotional but not of affectively neutral topics or stimuli

Modified from Bernat JL. Chronic disorders of consciousness. Lancet 2006;367(9528):1181–92; with permission.

This article focuses on the MCS and VS because the care of patients in those states presents the most vexing and challenging ethical issues.

DETERMINING AND COMMUNICATING DIAGNOSIS

The foundation for rational medical decision making is accurate fact-finding and diagnosis. A primary professional and ethical obligation of physicians caring for patients with altered consciousness is to diagnosis a patient's condition accurately so that surrogates and other health care providers can make appropriate treatment choices on the patient's behalf.

Disordered states of consciousness present particular diagnostic challenges. It is impossible to fully appreciate the consciousness of another human being or to know with absolute certainty how aware another person is. The diagnosis of a patient's degree of awareness is, therefore, based by necessity on inference from the patient's demonstrated behavioral repertoire, which is thought to be a reasonable proxy for a patient's level of awareness and cognitive ability. Diagnostic studies, including MRI, functional MRI (fMRI), evoked potentials, electroencephalogram (and less frequently pathologic studies, such as biopsy), can aid in making a diagnosis but likewise are proxies for states of awareness and not absolute indicators.

Given that accurate diagnosis of patients with severe brain injury relies almost exclusively on the clinical examination, technical limitations and human error in the clinical examination can and do lead to inaccurate diagnosis. Several studies have, for example, convincingly demonstrated a high rate of misdiagnosis of the vegetative state. In one study by Andrews and colleagues[8] of 40 patients admitted to a long-term rehabilitation unit with a diagnosis of VS, 17 were considered as having been misdiagnosed. Many of the patients had been presumed vegetative for several years. After being rehabilitated and taught a method of communication that was compatible with their often profound visual and other physical impairments, nearly all of the 17 were aware enough to able to communicate their preference regarding quality-of-life issues.

Given the formidable diagnostic challenges presented by these patients, it is critical that examiners optimize the conditions of examination to give the patients every opportunity to demonstrate awareness. Examiners should use standardized examination techniques with standardized scoring scales for responses to stimuli,[9,10] discontinue medications that might confound the neurologic examination,[11] and address metabolic or other derangements that could contribute to altered mental status. All caretakers, including nurses and family members, should be engaged in the process and questioned thoroughly about any behaviors they have witnessed that could represent purposeful behavior by the patients. Examinations should be conducted by clinicians experienced in assessment of patients with severe brain injury and repeated over time. As Monti and colleagues[12] suggest, it is critical to "harness and nurture any available response, through intervention, into a form of reproducible communication, however rudimentary." Examiners should systematically apply the diagnostic criteria (described previously) to determine the most accurate diagnostic category for a patient.

A growing body of evidence generated by functional neuroimaging studies has highlighted the inherent limitations of the clinical examination in detecting the extent of patient cognition. This research ultimately may lead to changes in how patients with altered consciousness are understood and diagnosed. In 2006, Owen and colleagues[13] reported a 23-year-old woman with a diagnosis of VS 5 months after traumatic brain injury. She underwent fMRI while being walked by examiners through two mental imagery exercises. When asked to imagine playing tennis and think about the ball being hit back and forth across the net, her supplementary motor area was activated. When asked to imagine visiting each room in her house in sequence, there was activity in her parahippocampal gyrus, posterior parietal lobe, and lateral premotor cortex. These findings were consistent with cortical activations recorded in completely normal control subjects. Six months after these studies were done, she began to show evidence of awareness on clinical examination, suggesting that she might have been transitioning out of VS at the time the study was conducted.

In a larger series published in 2010, Monti and colleagues[12] studied 54 patients with disorders of consciousness, 23 of whom were diagnosed as vegetative and 31 of whom were diagnosed as being in an MCS. All patients underwent fMRI during which they were asked to perform 2 imagery tasks—1 motor and 1 spatial. The motor imagery exercise was to imagine standing on a tennis court swinging an arm to hit the ball back and forth to an instructor. The spatial imagery task was to imagine navigating the streets of a familiar city or to imaging walking from room to room in their home. The patients then were asked a yes-or-no question and asked to respond during an fMRI session by using one type of mental imagery for yes and the other for no. Six of these so-called communication scans were obtained for each patient to maximize statistical power. Five of the patients (4 diagnosed with VS and 1 with MCS, all of whom had traumatic brain injury as opposed to anoxic brain injury or cerebrovascular accident) were able to willfully modulate their brain activity during the imagery tasks. Additional clinical testing revealed some evidence of awareness in 3 of these patients. One patient was able to answer yes or no reliably during the communication scan, but no form of communication was possible at the bedside.

Di and colleagues[14] demonstrated activation of the perisylvian language cortex in patients previously diagnosed as in VS when hearing their names spoken in a familiar voice. These patients later developed clinical evidence of awareness, whereas the study subjects who did not demonstrate cortical activation on fMRI did not develop clinical evidence of awareness.

Some of the novel issues raised by the emerging use of these neuroimaging technologies to evaluate consciousness in patients with severe brain injury are discussed later.

DETERMINING AND COMMUNICATING PROGNOSIS

As difficult as it is to determine the proper diagnostic category for patients with severe brain injury, it can be even more challenging to accurately assess the prognosis of these patients. States of consciousness are clinical syndromes caused by different pathologies that can be fluid, with patients moving from coma to VS, VS to MCS, and sometimes from MCS back into VS, particularly in the context of infection or other cause of encephalopathy. The variability of these states can make it difficult to know when to establish prognosis and how definitive to be.

Under the guidelines established by the Multi-Society Task Force on PVS, VS is called persistent (PVS) if it lasts more than 1 month and permanent when irreversibility can be established with a high degree of certainty. In that regard, recovery from post-traumatic PVS after 12 months is considered extremely unlikely and recovery from nontraumatic PVS after 3 months exceedingly rare.[15] The degree to which patients in an MCS recover functioning over time is highly variable and is not well correlated with the duration of time in an MCS.[16]

Clinicians should be aware of several specific dangers in delivering prognosis for patients with severe brain injury, including the risk of making poorly informed summary judgments early in a patient's course, limitations on available data regarding prognosis, and the likelihood that personal bias will influence the framing of prognosis.[17]

Families are understandably eager to know the prospects for meaningful recovery when patients sustain severe brain injury and may exert pressure on physicians to state prognosis early in the course of brain injury. Some studies indicate that many decisions to withdraw life-sustaining treatment (LST) are made early in the course of treatment.[18] In the context of irreducible uncertainty, health care providers must strike a balance between early assessment of prognosis with the attendant risk of prematurely withdrawing support from a patient who might have experienced significant recovery over time, and waiting too long to deliver a prognosis, in which case suffering associated with living in a profoundly disordered state of consciousness might be prolonged. In addition, although withholding LST and withdrawing it have long been considered ethically equivalent, in practice there can be a greater reluctance on the part of surrogates and health care providers to withdraw LST once it has been initiated. The timing of delivering prognostic information can, therefore, affect the direction of a patient's care.

Clinicians should know and accurately portray to medical decision makers the objective data that are available about prognosis for a given condition and the limitations of any existing data in predicting prognosis of patients. Although it is appropriate to share available statistics, it is equally important to explain that statistics reflect only the mean outcomes for populations of people and do not provide specific information about what will happen in a particular patient's case. In addition, as Becker and colleagues[18] have articulated, it is important for physicians interpreting outcomes data for patients with severe brain injury to be aware that such data, which are typically based on retrospective studies, may be biased by the fact that LST is often withdrawn early in the course of severe brain injury, leading to a self-fulfilling prophecy of poor outcomes in such patients. Becker conducted a study of patients with intracerebral hemorrhage, 27 of whom had two features considered poor predictors of outcome under commonly used prognostic models—GCS less than or equal to 8 and hematomas greater than 60 cm^3. Six of these patients underwent surgery and 5 had unexpectedly positive results. In the study population as a whole, the most important overall prognostic variable in determining outcome after ICH was the level of medical support provided.

In addition to the inherent limitations of using statistical data to predict individual outcome, there are a few well-publicized cases of late recovery that can confuse the prognostic picture. Voss and colleagues,[19] for example, described the case of Terry Wallis, who sustained traumatic brain injury at age 19 and, after progressing from coma to VS to MCS, was in a stable MCS in which he was able only to nod and grunt. After 19 years in this state, he spontaneously began speaking in coherent full sentences. Diffusion tensor imaging suggested axonal regrowth in large regions of the posterior bilateral hemispheric white matter.

The presentation and framing of medical opinions about prognosis in cases of severe brain injury is inevitably subject to the bias of the medical professional offering the opinion. Framing of information in a medical context has a profound impact on the choices made by a decision maker.[20] Given evidence that a majority of physicians believe that living in a VS is a fate worse than death and that some physicians even believe that patients in VS should be considered dead,[21] the potential impact of physician bias on medical decision making by families of these patients is noteworthy.

In light of the many challenges inherent in delivering diagnostic and prognostic information in cases of severe brain injury, ethical care involves engaging in a fair and transparent process of shared decision making with surrogate decision makers. This process ideally involves striking a balance between undue pessimism regarding prognosis and provision of false hope, remaining vigilant about the possibility of personal bias, being aware of the influence that framing of information can have on surrogate decision makers, and consciously presenting the available information in as objective a manner as possible. Although it is understandably difficult for surrogates to make decisions in the face of prognostic uncertainty, ethical care involves being direct and honest about the limitations of available data regarding prognosis and appropriately humble about what can actually be known about a patient's true state of consciousness and the possibility of recovery over time.

DECIDING THE APPROPRIATE COURSE OF TREATMENT

Once a diagnosis and prognosis for a patient with severe brain injury are established as clearly as possible, decisions must be made about the direction of care for the patient, including the initiation and continuation of LST, tracheostomy, gastrostomy, artificial nutrition and hydration (ANH), and mechanical ventilation, although most patients in a stable VS or MCS do not require mechanical ventilation. These patients uniformly require surrogate decision makers for whom a host of ethical concerns can arise in the course of medical decision making, including issues regarding advance directives, surrogacy, and the appropriateness of certain medical interventions. The ultimate goal in each case is to provide the care that patients would want if they were able to make decisions for themselves.

Advance Directives

As in all medical situations involving difficult decisions about the direction of care, it is helpful if patients with severe brain injury had executed lawful advance directives before sustaining the brain injury. These directives ideally include both designation of a legal health care proxy (in some jurisdictions referred to as a health care agent or durable power of attorney for health care) and a living will or similar written directive that sets forth information about a patient's wishes regarding care in the event of serious illness or injury.

Unfortunately, only a minority of people execute advance directives. A 2005 Pew Research Center study revealed that only 29% of all Americans have living wills.[22]

Many patients with severe brain injury have suffered sudden, unexpected catastrophic events, such as trauma or cardiopulmonary arrest, and never have had occasion to specifically consider or discuss their wishes regarding LST in cases of impaired consciousness. In addition, living wills that set out patients' wishes regarding care often are too general to be of particular use and often cover only those situations in which a person has been determined to be terminally ill (the generally accepted definition of which is a life span not expected to exceed 6 more months). Many do not provide for situations in which a person's degree of consciousness is profoundly affected but whose life expectancy is not necessarily profoundly abbreviated.

Given the wide spectrum of potential disability and illness that an individual can face, it is impossible for any written directive to outline preferences in every possible scenario. In addition, there is a well-studied disconnect between the theoretic preferences that a person might express and a person's actual preferences once faced with the contemplated situation.[23] From a practical perspective, therefore, the most useful aspect of advance care planning is the designation of a legal health care proxy whom a patient trusts to make decisions consistent with the patient's goals, values, and wishes.

Principles of Surrogate Decision Making

Respect for patient autonomy and the related doctrine of informed consent are two ethical cornerstones of medical care. Because patients with severe brain injury are unable to communicate their wishes regarding their medical care, respect for patient autonomy in these cases involves adhering to the decisions made by surrogates on the patients' behalf. The concept of shared medical decision making, in which patients contribute their own goals and values and the health care team contributes knowledge and expertise about diagnosis and prognosis, should be applied in these situations via interaction with patients' surrogate decision makers.

The first issue that can arise in the context of an incapacitated patient is difficulty identifying the appropriate surrogate. Ideally a patient has specifically designated a legal health care decision maker. When a patient has no legally designated agent, state law governs who acts as a surrogate. The approach to this situation varies by jurisdiction, with some states setting out a statutory hierarchy of next of kin to act as surrogates[24] and others having no such hierarchy. In cases where there is no specified hierarchy of surrogacy and there are several interested family members, all interested next of kin should be treated as an informal surrogate group and invited to make decisions collectively. In cases without an available surrogate decision maker, a legal guardian should be sought and relevant hospital policies followed.

Surrogate is obligated, to the best of his ability, to make decisions for the patient that the patient would have made if he had the capacity to speak for himself. If the patient has specifically expressed wishes, in writing or otherwise, that apply directly to the situation at hand, the surrogate is obligated to follow those wishes regardless of whether they are consistent with the decision the surrogate would make for himself under the same circumstances.

If, as is usually the case, the patient has not specifically indicated what he would want for himself under the circumstances, the surrogate should apply the principle of substituted judgment, using his insight into the priorities and values of the patient and attempt to infer what the patient would decide if he were capable of speaking for himself. If there are no expressed or implied wishes to rely upon, the surrogate must then make the decision he believes is in the "best interest" of the patient, weighing the relative risks and benefits of the given treatment or intervention at issue.[25]

This procedure leaves a difficult decision for surrogates who lack prior knowledge of what patients would want done for themselves. Both the substituted judgment and the best interest standards have limitations. Shalowitz and colleagues[26] conducted a meta-analysis of 16 studies of surrogate decision making using a substituted judgment standard for end-of-life decision making. The pool of studies they analyzed involved 151 hypothetical scenarios with 2595 surrogate-patient pairs and 19,526 patient-surrogate paired responses. Surrogates predicted patients' treatment preferences with only 68% accuracy, and neither prior patient designation of a surrogate nor prior discussion of patient preferences with a surrogate improved the accuracy of surrogate prediction.

In patients with disorders of consciousness, it is difficult to exercise substituted judgment and perhaps even more difficult for a surrogate to determine the best interest of patients because prognostic information is usually ambiguous and optimum care for patients is heavily influenced by highly personal values and preferences. Acting in the best interest of patients in such a situation requires surrogates to balance the benefits and burdens of therapy. The ethical risk with a best interest determination is that a surrogate's balance of benefits and burdens might differ from the balance the patient would have struck.

Surrogate Refusal of Treatment

Where there is no clear, single surrogate decision maker (or even at times when the default surrogate is identified but there are other interested family members), disagreements among family members regarding the proper care of a patient can arise. In such cases, the health care team should first attempt to achieve consensus through family meetings, involving services such as social work, chaplaincy, and the patient's primary care physician, where appropriate. If disagreement among family members persists, assistance should be sought from the hospital ethics committee or a consent capacity board.

One question that arises repeatedly in different contexts is what limitations, if any, there should be on the ability of a lawful surrogate to make decisions to limit LST. Although ethical precepts are distinct from legal decisions, it is nevertheless instructive to explore some of the key legal cases that have addressed this issue.

In the landmark 1976 case of Karen Ann Quinlan, decided by the New Jersey Supreme Court, Quinlan was a 21-year-old woman in a PVS after an episode of cardiopulmonary arrest. Her father wanted to withdraw mechanical ventilation over the objection of medical personnel. The New Jersey Supreme Court held that Quinlan's right to privacy permitted her to decide to terminate her noncognitive, vegetative existence and that the only way to respect this right was by allowing her father to make a decision on her behalf to withdraw mechanical ventilation. Mechanical ventilation was withdrawn, but Quinlan survived another 9 years before dying of pneumonia.[27]

In the seminal 1991 case of Nancy Cruzan, a 30-year-old woman in a permanent vegetative state, Cruzan's parents wished to discontinue ANH once it was clear she would not recover. The U.S. Supreme Court held that it was lawful for the state of Missouri to require "clear and convincing evidence" that Cruzan would have wanted to die before physicians could discontinue LST.[28] The family ultimately provided such evidence and Cruzan died 12 days after discontinuation of ANH. The Supreme Court also found that every U.S. citizen has a constitutionally protected right to refuse all forms of LST, including ANH, and that right can be executed by a lawful surrogate.

In 1993, 42-year-old Robert Wendland was injured in an automobile accident leaving him in an MCS in which he could not be fed by mouth, was unable to control his bowels or bladder, and could not communicate consistently. He could follow certain 2-step commands with prompting and could answer some but not all yes-or-no questions. Prior to the accident, he had made several comments about not wanting to live if he were dependent on life support or unable to take care of himself and do the things he enjoyed. His feeding tube became repeatedly dislodged and most family members, including his wife, opposed replacing it based on what they believed Wendland would have wanted. His mother went to court to overrule this decision. Wendland died while the California Supreme Court was deliberating, but the court ultimately issued a unanimous ruling stating that the feeding tube could not have been discontinued. The court ruled that a health care agent may withhold or withdraw LST "for the purpose of causing [the patient's] death" only if there is "clear and convincing evidence" that the patient "wished to refuse life-sustaining treatment or that to withhold such treatment would have been in his best interest."[29]

The issue of when it is appropriate for a surrogate to decide to limit LST for a patient with severe brain injury was more recently and famously highlighted by the case of Theresa Schiavo, who had been in a VS for 15 years after a hypoxic-ischemic injury suffered during cardiac arrest at age 26. She had no written advance directives, but her husband (who was her lawful surrogate) refused further ANH for Schiavo, stating that discontinuation of ANH would be consistent with wishes she had expressed to him before her brain injury. Schiavo's parents objected to discontinuation of ANH, arguing that Schiavo would have wanted to continue living. After a protracted, highly publicized political and legal battle, in which several inappropriate attempts were made by the Florida state and national legislatures to intervene, nutrition and hydration were stopped and Schiavo was permitted to die.[30]

In the wake of the Wendland case, Lo and colleagues noted in an article critical of the legal deicison that "the court regarded an erroneous decision to withdraw treatment as more perilous than an erroneous decision to continue treatment, which is reversible and maintains the status quo." The intense political debate over the Schiavo case highlighted the apparently widely held perception that the default position should be continuation of all medical measures for vegetative patients in the absence of clearly expressed wishes to the contrary. Several states already have statutes requiring a specific prior directive from a patient in order for a proxy to withdraw ANH from patients in a VS and, in the wake of the Schiavo case, many more states have attempted to pass legislation that would make it impossible for surrogates to decide to withdraw ANH from vegetative patients in the absence of explicit expression by a patient that the patient would not have wanted ANH under such circumstances.[32] The logical implication of such statutes, which limit the ability of lawful surrogates to make decisions limiting ANH on behalf of patients in VS, is that surrogates have no authority to limit ANH on behalf of patients in less dire conditions, such as MCS.

The American Academy of Neurology has issued a position statement that opposes "all state and federal legislation that would presume to prescribe a patient's preferences for ANH or that gives legal standing to elected officials to intercede."[33] The authors agree that categorical limitations on the authority of lawful surrogates to make decisions on behalf of patients in VS or MCS are undesirable. This is especially true because, to the limited extent that patient preferences have been studied, the bulk of the evidence suggests that the vast majority of people would prefer not to continue living in the event they were to become profoundly cognitively impaired to the point of being unable to communicate with others, process information, or engage in any daily activities of living.[34–36] Although these population statistics do not indicate what any given individual might decide in such a situation, the authors believe they highlight the possibility that significant harm can be done and significant burdens caused to patients by continuing treatment that they might not have wanted.

The authors acknowledge that if surrogates are given unchecked authority to refuse LST on behalf of brain-injured patients, there is a risk that certain surrogates will seek to withdraw treatment from vulnerable patients out of self-interest or unwillingness to care for those patients. Given the extremely high stakes and the irreversibility of decisions to withhold or withdraw LST, utmost caution is required in evaluating patients with severe brain injury, ushering families through medical decision making, and guarding against the possibility of any conflicts of interest or hidden motives on the part of surrogates. The difficulty of drawing lines, however, should not lead to erring so far on the side of preserving life at all costs that these patients are effectively denied the right to refuse LST.

Although the focus in public discussion is frequently on the harm that can be done by withdrawing LST from vulnerable brain-injured patients, the continuation of LST of a severely brain-injured patient who might have found living in such a state intolerable has potential to cause significant harms: burdens on a patient's family that the patient would have wished to avoid, compromise of the dignity of a patient who would not have wished to live in such a dependent state, and imposition of medical procedures and treatment that a patient would not have wanted, ironically the very harm that the doctrine of informed consent originally was intended to avoid. Furthermore, it is impossible to know the extent of emotional suffering such patients might sustain on a daily basis living against their will in a severely compromised cognitive state.

Surrogate Insistence on Treatment

Just as difficult ethical dilemmas arise when a surrogate seeks to limit medical treatment without clear prior expression of a patient's wishes, equally problematic ethical questions arise when a surrogate seeks to initiate or continue medical interventions that a patient's health care providers believe are inappropriate. These types of disputes historically have been characterized in terms of medical futility. The notion that physicians are not required to provide aggressive medical treatments that are futile is iterated in multiple commission reports and codified in policies at major medical institutions.[37,38] Different observers over time have proposed different constructs for thinking about medical futility, including conflict between patient self-determination and physician autonomy, breakdown in patient-physician communication, and the assertion by physicians that it is their professional prerogative to decide what treatment they offer. Regardless of how medical futility is conceptualized, it has always proved impossible to define in a way that makes this concept easily applicable in practice.

Schneiderman and colleagues[39] stated that a medical act is futile if, based on empirical data, the desired outcome, although possible, is overwhelmingly improbable. There are two overarching notions of futility—quantitative and qualitative. A treatment may be considered quantitatively futile if it is extremely unlikely to accomplish its physiologic objective (eg, mechanical ventilation in brain death, which will not save a patient's life) and qualitatively futile if it is unlikely to improve a patient's life or condition in any meaningful way.

Qualitative benefit is inherently subjective and can be defined only in relation to highly personal, individual values regarding the quality of life. Clinicians, therefore, have no inherent advantage over lay people in determining what constitutes qualitative futility. Although many people regard as qualitatively futile the use of a ventilator to extend the life of a person who lacks the ability to communicate or think, some may see any extension of life as beneficial regardless of the circumstances. The issue then becomes which view of benefit should be permitted to prevail—that of a surrogate acting on behalf of a patient or that of the health care providers.

Aside from the question of whether a particular treatment is likely to benefit an individual patient in any meaningful way, the aggressive care of patients with limited or no awareness of self or the environment raises broader questions of distributive justice and the appropriate allocation of medical resources. Some observers have suggested just distribution of resources as a framework for thinking about medical futility.[40] This approach, however, seems to conflate two distinct considerations—first, whether a given treatment stands to benefit an individual patient in any meaningful way, and second, whether providing that treatment to that patient represents the most appropriate use of scarce medical resources. As Brock and Wartman describe,[41] what is a rational decision for an individual patient may not be rational for society as a whole.

It is generally understood that physicians are ethically obligated to serve the best interests of patients under their care. Physicians are also, however, charged with overseeing the use of finite medical resources (at least in the sense of triaging patients within their institution), although it remains controversial to what extent physicians should consider just allocation of resources in any given treatment decision. Encouraging physicians to make individual treatment decisions with a focus on just use of resources invites conflicts between the interests of individual patients and societal interests in optimizing use of limited resources. Moreover, if physicians emphasize allocation of resources in their treatment decisions, the treatment of individual patients might vary significantly depending on an individual physician's perspective on how to best allocate limited health care resources, creating an unacceptably arbitrary rationing of resources. Many argue that decisions about the rational distribution of health care resources should be made at the policy and societal level, separate from individual treatment decisions.[41,42]

As a practical matter, considerations of irresponsible resource allocation are bound to weigh into physician assessments of whether a particular treatment of a patient in VS or MCS is appropriate. It is essential, however, that physicians not summarily dismiss as futile any treatment that they believe irresponsible from a rationing perspective. In the interest of transparency, physicians must conceptually separate the determination that a given treatment is quantitatively or qualitatively futile for a particular patient from the determination that providing the treatment is an irresponsible use of finite resources.

The recent case in Canada of Samuel Golubchuck is instructive. Golubchuck was an 84-year-old orthodox Jew in Manitoba who suffered a severe brain injury after a fall and was in an MCS (his degree of consciousness remained in dispute, but all agreed that he was not in a vegetative state). He was mechanically ventilated and fed through a gastrostomy tube. His physicians wished to withdraw LST against the objections of his family members, who stated that Golubchuck himself would have opposed the removal of life support on religious grounds.

During the time the dispute over Mr Golubchuck's care was ongoing, the College of Physicians & Surgeons of Manitoba issued a guideline on the provision of LST stating that the minimum goal of LST is "the maintenance of or recovery to a level of cerebral function that enables the patient to achieve awareness of self; and achieve awareness of environment; and experience his/her own existence." The guideline provides that where a determination has been made that the minimum goal is not achievable, physicians can withdraw LST over objection of family members after an implementation procedure involving consultation with other physicians.[43] The Golubchuck family sought and received an emergency order to prevent the hospital from withdrawing ANH, which was upheld by a higher court. Golubchuck ultimately died from natural causes.

The Golubchuck case stimulated vigorous debate, with some observers arguing strenuously that respect for patient autonomy should be the prevailing ethical principle and that physicians should not have the right to override a lawful surrogate's wishes for continuing LST, regardless of the prospect for return of awareness.[42] Others defended the regulation, arguing that the emphasis on patient autonomy has become excessive, that respect for patient autonomy should not be interpreted as an absolute right to demand treatment of any kind under any circumstances, and that health care providers should be able to exercise their own professional autonomy by refusing to provide treatment that may be physiologically effective in extending life but that they believe will provide no meaningful benefit to a patient.[44,45]

The authors agree with Lo and colleagues,[31] who commented on the Wendland case: "[f]ear of legal liability should not drive physicians to provide interventions that contradict widely accepted standards of practice and sound clinical judgment." Nevertheless, in the vast majority of cases in which a patient's right to demand treatment over physician objection has been adjudicated, courts have found in favor of the patient.[46–49] Judges, however, have typically decided these cases on procedural grounds and have avoided making definitive decisions regarding whether the medical treatment at issue is futile. In the 1991 case of Helga Wanglie, for example, the physicians caring for an 86-year-old woman who had been in VS for over a year after anoxic injury wanted to discontinue mechanical ventilation over the objection of her husband. The court ultimately decided the case without commenting on the futility question, determining only that her husband was her lawful surrogate.[47]

With the impossibility of objectively defining medical futility, in the presence of a dispute about the appropriateness of a particular course of treatment, the focus should be on the process of airing the dispute and providing due process to a patient whose surrogate is requesting treatment that a clinician is reluctant or unwilling to provide. To this end, clinicians should make every effort to fully hear and understand the perspectives of a patient's surrogate and to transparently explain their perspective and why they believe such a treatment would not be beneficial to the patient, engaging services such as palliative care consultation, social work, and chaplaincy, when useful. When disputes remain intractable, the assistance of a hospital ethics committee should be sought. Families should be offered an opportunity to seek transfer of the patient to another clinician or hospital willing to provide the services they are seeking (although given the time-sensitive nature of many of these decisions, this often is impractical). Finally, futility policies should emphasize the principles of palliative care at the end of life, as elucidated by the Society of Critical Care Medicine.[50] The American Medical Association Council on Ethical and Judicial Affairs has recommended an algorithm for physicians facing disputes about treatment in end-of-life care, which is reproduced in **Box 5**.[51]

ETHICAL CHALLENGES POSED BY NEW TECHNOLOGIES

Functional neuroimaging technologies, such as fMRI, raise the possibility of refining understanding of human cognition and awareness in severely brain-injured patients.[52] This is a promising development in terms of enhancing the ability to provide accurate prognostic information and possibly treatment options to patients with severe brain injury. The increasing use of these technologies will, however, inevitable present a new set of ethical challenges as we move towards a new understanding of complex states of consciousness. As Fins observed, "confusion will be the price of incremental progress."[53]

The few reports from small-scale studies are provocative and have received intense media attention. Given the uncertainty of clinical diagnosis of patients with severe brain injury, there undoubtedly will be pressure from families to use such technologies clinically before they are appropriately refined or understood. Research on a larger

---

Box 5
An algorithm for physicians faced with futility disputes in the ICU

1. Deliberate values with surrogates, and transfer patients to the care of another physician if the values conflict.

2. Conduct joint shared decision making using outcome data and value judgments.

3. Involve consultants if disagreements about data arise.

4. Involve the hospital ethics committee if disagreement continues.

5. Attempt to transfer the patient to another physician within the institution if disagreement continues.

6. Consider transfer to another hospital, if possible.

7. Only if all these measures fail and disagreement continues can physicians unilaterally cease the futile intervention.

Modified from American Medical Association Council on Ethical and Judicial Affairs. Medical futility in end-of-life care: report of the Council on Ethical and Judicial Affairs. JAMA 1999; 281(10):937–41; with permission.

---

scale is necessary, however, before functional neuroimaging can ethically be integrated into clinical practice.[54]

Until the various testing modalities are validated and their sensitivity and specificity are known, the communication of the results of such studies will be subject to ad hoc variability depending on who is interpreting them and discussing them with families. In the short term, it will be difficult to know how to integrate the results of any such testing with the behavioral repertoires exhibited by patients that are currently used as the foundation for diagnosis. Such uncertainties raise the question of whether it is ethical to perform testing on patients in a clinical setting when such testing has no clear implication for either treatment or prognosis.

The use of functional neuroimaging technologies ultimately has the capacity to exacerbate some of the issues of surrogate decision making (discussed previously).[55] For example, will those who seek to limit the right of surrogates to make decisions to withdraw LST from severely brain-injured patients use the results of functional neuroimaging tests that show some evidence of intact cognition to support their cause? Might evidence of cognition detected by functional neuroimaging lead to prolongation of life in more patients who might not want to live under such circumstances? Before physicians uncritically strive to achieve more tailored diagnosis and prognosis based on individual imaging findings in a patient with severe brain injury, serious consideration must be given to the benefits and risks this approach might provide to patients and their families.

REFERENCES

1. Posner J, Saper CB, Schiff ND, et al. Plum and posner's diagnosis of stupor and coma. 4th edition. New York: Oxford University Press; 2007.

2. Wijdicks EF, Varelas PN, Gronseth GS, et al. Evidence-based guideline update: determining brain death in adults: report of the Quality Standards Subcommittee of the American Academy of Neurology. Neurology 2010;74(23):1911–8.

3. Jennett B, Plum F. Persistent vegetative state after brain damage. A syndrome in search of a name. Lancet 1972;1(7753):734–7.

4. The Multi-Society Task Force on PVS. Medical aspects of the persistent vegetative state (2). N Engl J Med 1994;330(22):1572–9.
5. Kinney HC, Samuels MA. Neuropathology of the persistent vegetative state. A review. J Neuropathol Exp Neurol 1994;53(6):548–58.
6. Volicer L, Berman SA, Cipolloni PB, et al. Persistent vegetative state in Alzheimer disease. Does it exist? Arch Neurol 1997;54(11):1382–4.
7. Giacino JT, Ashwal S, Childs N, et al. The minimally conscious state: definition and diagnostic criteria. Neurology 2002;58(3):349–53.
8. Andrews K, Murphy L, Munday R, et al. Misdiagnosis of the vegetative state: retrospective study in a rehabilitation unit. BMJ 1996;313(7048):13–6.
9. Pape TL, Heinemann AW, Kelly JP, et al. A measure of neurobehavioral functioning after coma. Part I: theory, reliability, and validity of disorders of consciousness scale. J Rehabil Res Dev 2005;42(1):1–17.
10. Pape TL, Senno RG, Guernon A, et al. A measure of neurobehavioral functioning after coma. Part II: clinical and scientific implementation. J Rehabil Res Dev 2005; 42(1):19–27.
11. Strens LH, Mazibrada G, Duncan JS, et al. Misdiagnosing the vegetative state after severe brain injury: the influence of medication. Brain Inj 2004;18(2):213–8.
12. Monti MM, Vanhaudenhuyse A, Coleman MR, et al. Willful modulation of brain activity in disorders of consciousness. N Engl J Med 2010;362(7):579–89.
13. Owen AM, Coleman MR, Boly M, et al. Detecting awareness in the vegetative state. Science 2006;313(5792):1402.
14. Di HB, Yu SM, Weng XC, et al. Cerebral response to patient's own name in the vegetative and minimally conscious states. Neurology 2007;68(12):895–9.
15. The Quality Standards Subcommittee of the American Academy of Neurology. Practice parameters: assessment and management of patients in the persistent vegetative state (summary statement). Neurology 1995;45(5):1015–8.
16. Lammi MH, Smith VH, Tate RL, et al. The minimally conscious state and recovery potential: a follow-up study 2 to 5 years after traumatic brain injury. Arch Phys Med Rehabil 2005;86(4):746–54.
17. Bernat JL. Ethical aspects of determining and communicating prognosis in critical care. Neurocrit Care 2004;1(1):107–17.
18. Becker KJ, Baxter AB, Cohen WA, et al. Withdrawal of support in intracerebral hemorrhage may lead to self-fulfilling prophecies. Neurology 2001;56(6): 766–72.
19. Voss HU, Uluc AM, Dyke JP, et al. Possible axonal regrowth in late recovery from the minimally conscious state. J Clin Invest 2006;116(7):2005–11.
20. Tversky A, Kahneman D. The framing of decisions and the psychology of choice. Science 1981;211(4481):453–8.
21. Payne K, Taylor RM, Stocking C, et al. Physicians' attitudes about the care of patients in the persistent vegetative state: a national survey. Ann Intern Med 1996;125(2):104–10.
22. Pew Center report. More Americans discussing and planning end-of-life treatment. 2006.
23. Ubel PA, Loewenstein G, Schwarz N, et al. Misimagining the unimaginable: the disability paradox and health care decision making. Health Psychol 2005; 24(Suppl 4):S57–62.
24. Menikoff JA, Sachs GA, Siegler M. Beyond advance directives—health care surrogate laws. N Engl J Med 1992;327(16):1165–9.
25. Bernat JL. Plan ahead: how neurologists can enhance patient-centered medicine. Neurology 2001;56(2):144–5.

26. Shalowitz DI, Garrett-Mayer E, Wendler D. The accuracy of surrogate decision makers: a systematic review. Arch Intern Med 2006;166(5):493–7.
27. In re Quinlan, 70 NJ 10; 355 A2d 647 (1976).
28. Cruzan v Missouri Department of Health, 497 US 261, 110 S Ct 2841 (1990).
29. Wendland v Wendland, 26 Cal 4th 519, 28 P3d 151 (2001).
30. Quill TE. Terri Schiavo–a tragedy compounded. N Engl J Med 2005;352(16): 1630–3.
31. Lo B, Dornbrand L, Wolf LE, et al. The Wendland case—withdrawing life support from incompetent patients who are not terminally ill. N Engl J Med 2002;346(19): 1489–93.
32. Larriviere D, Bonnie RJ. Terminating artificial nutrition and hydration in persistent vegetative state patients: current and proposed state laws. Neurology 2006; 66(11):1624–8.
33. Bacon D, Williams MA, Gordon J. Position statement on laws and regulations concerning life-sustaining treatment, including artificial nutrition and hydration, for patients lacking decision-making capacity. Neurology 2007;68(14): 1097–100.
34. Frankl D, Oye RK, Bellamy PE. Attitudes of hospitalized patients toward life support: a survey of 200 medical inpatients. Am J Med 1989;86(6):645–8.
35. Pearlman RA, Cain KC, Patrick DL, et al. Insights pertaining to patient assessments of states worse than death. J Clin Ethics 1993;4(1):33–41.
36. Fried TR, Bradley EH, Towle VR, et al. Understanding the treatment preferences of seriously ill patients. N Engl J Med 2002;346(14):1061–6.
37. Council on Ethical and Judicial Affairs, American Medical Association. Guidelines for the appropriate use of do-not-resuscitate orders. JAMA 1991;265(14): 1868–71.
38. President's Commission for the Study of Ethical Problems in Medicine and Biomedical and Behavioral Research. Deciding to Forego Life-Sustaining Treatment: Ethical MaLIiTD.
39. Schneiderman LJ, Jecker NS, Jonsen AR. Medical futility: its meaning and ethical implications. Ann Intern Med 1990;112(12):949–54.
40. Jecker NS, Schneiderman LJ. Futility and rationing. Am J Med 1992;92(2): 189–96.
41. Brock DW, Wartman SA. When competent patients make irrational choices. N Engl J Med 1990;322(22):1595–9.
42. Jotkowitz A, Glick S, Zivotofsky AZ. The case of Samuel Golubchuk and the right to live. Am J Bioeth 2010;10(3):50–3.
43. Statement by the College of Physicians and Surgeons of Manitoba. 2007. Available at: http://www.cpsm.mb.ca/1_3_3_1_ethics.php. Accessed July 6, 2011.
44. Cantor NL. No ethical or legal imperative to provide life support to a permanently unaware patient. Am J Bioeth 2010;10(3):58–9.
45. Paris JJ. Autonomy does not confer sovereignty on the patient: a commentary on the Golubchuk case. Am J Bioeth 2010;10(3):54–6.
46. In re Baby K, 16 F3d 590 (4th Cir), cert denied, 115 S Ct 91 (1994).
47. In re Conservatorship of Wanglie, No PX-91–283 (D Minn P Div July 1, 1991).
48. In re Jane Doe, 418 SE2d 3 (Ga 1992).
49. Paris JJ, Crone RK, Reardon F. Physicians' refusal of requested treatment. The case of Baby L. N Engl J Med 1990;322(14):1012–5.
50. Truog RD, Cist AF, Brackett SE, et al. Recommendations for end-of-life care in the intensive care unit: the Ethics Committee of the Society of Critical Care Medicine. Crit Care Med 2001;29(12):2332–48.

51. Medical futility in end-of-life care: report of the Council on Ethical and Judicial Affairs. JAMA 1999;281(10):937–41.
52. Coleman MR, Davis MH, Rodd JM, et al. Towards the routine use of brain imaging to aid the clinical diagnosis of disorders of consciousness. Brain 2009;132(Pt 9): 2541–52.
53. Fins JJ. Neuroethics and neuroimaging: moving toward transparency. Am J Bioeth 2008;8(9):46–52.
54. Fins JJ, Illes J, Bernat JL, et al. Neuroimaging and disorders of consciousness: envisioning an ethical research agenda. Am J Bioeth 2008;8(9):3–12.
55. Wilkinson DJ, Kahane G, Horne M, et al. Functional neuroimaging and withdrawal of life-sustaining treatment from vegetative patients. J Med Ethics 2009;35(8): 508–11.

Index

Note: Page numbers of article titles are in **boldface** type.

Neurol Clin 29 (2011) 1073–1093
doi:10.1016/S0733-8619(11)00099-5
0733-8619/11/$ – see front matter © 2011 Elsevier Inc. All rights reserved.

neurologic.theclinics.com

Moving?

Make sure your subscription moves with you!

To notify us of your new address, find your **Clinics Account Number** (located on your mailing label above your name), and contact customer service at:

Email: **journalscustomerservice-usa@elsevier.com**

800-654-2452 (subscribers in the U.S. & Canada)
314-447-8871 (subscribers outside of the U.S. & Canada)

Fax number: **314-447-8029**

Elsevier Health Sciences Division
Subscription Customer Service
3251 Riverport Lane
Maryland Heights, MO 63043

Printed and bound by CPI Group (UK) Ltd, Croydon, CR0 4YY

03/10/2024

01040457-0014